SO-BMT-526

www.harcourt-international.com

Bringing you products from all Harcourt Health Sciences companies including Baillière Tindall, Churchill Livingstone, Mosby and W.B. Saunders

▶ **Browse** for latest information on new books, journals and electronic products

▶ **Search** for information on over 20 000 published titles with full product information including tables of contents and sample chapters

▶ **Keep up to date** with our extensive publishing programme in your field by registering with eAlert or requesting postal updates

▶ **Secure online ordering** with prompt delivery, as well as full contact details to order by phone, fax or post

▶ **News** of special features and promotions

If you are based in the following countries, please visit the country-specific site to receive full details of product availability and local ordering information

USA: www.harcourthealth.com

Canada: www.harcourtcanada.com

Australia: www.harcourt.com.au

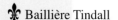 Baillière Tindall   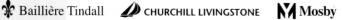 CHURCHILL LIVINGSTONE   Mosby   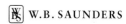 W.B. SAUNDERS

Tropical Medicine and Parasitology

FIFTH EDITION

Commissioning Editor: Deborah Russell
Project Manager: Cheryl Brant
Design Manager: Jayne Jones
Illustration Manager: Mick Ruddy

Tropical Medicine and Parasitology

FIFTH EDITION

Wallace Peters

MD (London), DSc (London), Docteur Honoris Causa (Université René Descartes, Paris)
FRCP, DTM&H
Emeritus Professor of Medical Protozoology, London School of Hygiene and Tropical Medicine
Director, Tropical Parasitic Diseases Unit, Northwick Park Institute for Medical Research
Harrow, London, England

Geoffrey Pasvol

MA (Oxon), MB ChB, DPhil (Oxon), FRCP, FRCPE
Professor of Infection and Tropical Medicine, Imperial College School of Medicine, Northwick Park
and St. Mary's Hospitals, London, England

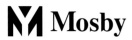 Mosby

London   Edinburgh   New York   Philadelphia   St Louis   Sydney   Toronto   2002

MOSBY
An imprint of Harcourt Publishers Limited

© Mosby International Limited 2002

 is a registered trademark of Harcourt Publishers Limited

The rights of Wallace Peters and Geoffrey Pasvol to be identified as authors of this work has been asserted by them in accordance with the Copyright, Designs and Patents Act 1988

All rights reserved. No part of this publication may be reproduced, stored in a retrieval system, or transmitted in any form or by any means, electronic, mechanical, photocopying, recording or otherwise, without either the prior permission of the publishers (Harcourt Publishers Limited, Harcourt Place, 32 Jamestown Road, London NW1 7BY), or a licence permitting restricted copying in the United Kingdom issued by the Copyright Licensing Agency, 90 Tottenham Court Road, London W1P 0LP.

First published in 1995 by Mosby-Wolfe, Times Mirror International Publishers Ltd

ISBN 0 7234 3191 4

British Library Cataloguing in Publication Data
A catalogue record for this book is available from the British Library

Library of Congress Cataloging in Publication Data
A catalog record for this book is available from the Library of Congress

Note
Medical knowledge is constantly changing. As new information becomes available, changes in treatment, procedures, equipment and the use of drugs become necessary. The editors/authors/contributors and the publishers have taken care to ensure that the information given in this text is accurate and up to date. However, readers are strongly advised to confirm that the information, especially with regard to drug usage, complies with the latest legislation and standards of practice.

Existing UK nomenclature is changing to the system of Recommended International Nonproprietary Names (rINNs). Until the UK names are no longer in use, these more familiar names are used in this book in preference to rINNs, details of which may be obtained from the British National Formulary.

The publisher's policy is to use **paper manufactured from sustainable forests**

Printed in China

Contents

Acknowledgements

In 1977 the first edition of this atlas was published from a manuscript prepared jointly by Professor Herbert M Gilles and the present senior author. The success of that work led to the production by the same authors of three further editions, in 1981, 1989 and 1995, respectively. The authors of this, the fifth edition, would like to express their gratitude to Professor Gilles for his clinical contributions to the earlier editions, all of which have served as valuable teaching aids to a multitude of students and graduates in the fields of tropical medicine and parasitology in many countries for over 20 years.

Unless otherwise stated, the copyrights of individual figures belong to those colleagues or organisations against whose names they are listed here:

Dr D T D J Abeysekara, 30; Dr G Adhia, **979**; Professor M Aikawa, **122**; Professor J F Alderete, **989**; Professor A D'Alessandro and the *American Journal of Tropical Medicine and Hygiene*, **762**; Dr J O'D Alexander, **920–922, 929, 939**; Professor H de Oliveira Almeida, **200**; Drs J Anderson and H Fuglsang, **320, 332, 343, 346, 348, 349**; Dr M A Ansari, **945**; Professor P Anthony, **676**; Dr Kemal Arab, **667**; The Director, Armed Forces Institute of Pathology, Washington, DC, **20, 65, 353, 396, 434, 562, 580, 772, 862, 1027**; Professor V S Arean, **430**; Dr O P Arya, **344, 815, 1000**; Professor L R Ash, **432, 632**; Professor R W Ashford, **212, 213, 412, 636, 647**; Professor N Ashton, **961**; Dr D A T Baldry, **162, 167, 168, 176, 328, 345**; Dr G L Barbosa, **908**; Dr D Baxby, **823**; Becton Dickinson Tropical Disease Diagnostics, **102**; Dr F Beltran, **436**; Professor E Bengtsson★, **751**; Dr R Ben-Ismail, **239**; Professor J K A Beverley★ and Royal Sheffield Hospitals, **654**; Professor A E Bianco, **295**; Drs A Biglino and A Casabianca, **366**; Dr R G Bird★, **34, 46**; Dr A Björkman, **783**; Dr S Bowman and The Sanger Centre, Cambridge, **Frontispiece (Background)**; Dr J G Breman, **826, 827**; Dr S G Browne★, **849, 853, 864**; Professor A Bryceson, **43, 169, 171, 204, 270, 347, 569, 578, 749, 832, 834, 817–819, 942, 951, 987, 998**; Dr A Buck, **880**; Professor D Bunnag, **529, 530**; Dr D A Burns, **936**; Dr T Butler, **62, 63, 66**; Dr P Caramello, **753, 756**; Dr J L Champalimaud, **177**;

Dr M L Chance, **10**; Mr A R Chandler and Smith Kline & French Laboratories, **182**; Professor Shiu-Nan Chen, **507, 518, 536, 677, 679**; Dr R Chojniak and *Revista da Sociedade Brasiliera de Medicina Tropical*, **907**; Dr I L Chrystie, **566**; Dr A C Chu, **934**; Dr J D Chulay, **232**; Professor M J Clarkson, **427**; Dr R Cooke, **123, 589, 649, 733, 813, 900, 912, 968, 1033**; Cooper, McDougall & Roberston Ltd, **78**; Professor G O Cowan OBE, **41, 980**; Dr J Croese and Dr P Prociv, **402**; Dr J C Crook, Royal Army Medical College, **672, 682**; Dr J H Cross **311**; Dr A Crump, **26, 178, 205**; Dr N Cumberlidge, **546**; Professor C Curtis, **276**; Dr I Davidson, **249**; Dr R N Davidson, **486**; Dr J E Dawson, **49**; Professor J-P Dedet, **263**; Dr D T Dennis, **64, 311**; Professor S P Deshpande, **933**; DiaMed, **103**; Professor A S Dissanaike, **368**; Dr P Dobson, **428**; Dr N Dorrell, **586**; Dr W S Douglas, **944**; Dr C C Draper, **467, 556**; Dr B Duke, **333, 337**; Dr M Dynski-Klein, **652**; Professor J Eckert, **759**; Professor G Edington★, **1025**; Dr D S Ellis, **278, 279, 658, 659, 779, 798, 917, 1016**; Dr D W Ellis-Jones, **775**; Professor A El-Rooby, **465**; Professor R T D Emond and Dr H A K Rowland, **820**; Drs A Evangelopoulos, G Spanakos, E Patsoula, N Vakalis and N Legakis, **611**; Dr D A Evans, **231, 236**; Professor Z Even-Paz, **246**; Professor L A F Eyckmans, **172**; Mr M G Falcon, **886**; Professor A M Fallis, **397**; Professor W E Farrar, **27, 35, 45, 69, 428, 563, 565, 575, 576, 587, 668, 785, 829, 839, 966, 970, 1026, 1099**; Dr C F Farthing, **56, 218, 220**; Professor F Fenech, **591, 592**; Mr J Ferguson, **308**; Drs S Ferrero, I Arnaudo, M B Sessa and A Pisacane, **410, 411**; Professor C D Forbes and Dr W F Jackson, **650, 652, 806, 875, 967, 983, 999, 1001**; Dr H Fraiha Neto, **1074–1076**; Dr N Francis, **125**; Dr P J Gardener, **211**; Dr P Garen, **829**; Dr A M Geddes, **582**; Dr L Gern, **80**; Professor J D Gillett★, **87**; Drs R Gilman and F Koster, **587**; Dr J M Goldsmid, **414, 424, 739**; Dr J D Goldstein, **367**; Dr L Gomulski, **12**; Professor B M Greenwood, **181, 974**; Professor D Greenwood, **415, 416, 456, 526, 664, 742, 743**; Dr med C Grewe, **777, 778**; Dr W A D Griffiths, **240, 1036**; Professor E M Grosshans, **930**; Professor Y Gutierrez, **362**; Dr B W Halstead, **1042–1044, 1046, 1047, 1049, 1050**;

Professor P Hamilton★ 153, 1038; Professor T Harinasuta, 515, 531, 629; Dr C Hatz, 477, 481; Professor R Hay, 910; Professor R Hendrickse, 572, 833, 965, 985, 991, 995, 1007, 1022, 1039, 1040; Dr R H Heptinstall and Department of Pathology, Johns Hopkins University, 671; Dr B Heyworth, 571, 688, 689; Dr H Higo, 549; Dr S L Hinrichsen, 81; Dr P R Hira, 750, 757; Dr H Hoogstraal★, 468; Dr J Horton and Professor Kraivichian, 696–699; Professor R E Howells, 385, 445–452, 503, 763, 769; Professor Hung Tao, 1019, 1020; Dr M P Hutchinson★, 175; Professor W M Hutchinson★, 646; Professor M S R Hutt★, 123, 154, 155, 621, 835, 1030–1032, 1096; Professor K P Hwang, 683; Professor H L Ioachim, 786, 796; Professor A Ishii and Dr N Suzuki, 453, 558; Dr J M Jewsbury, 495–502; Mr Ken Jones, 160; Dr G J Kane, Wellcome Reagents Ltd, 655, 670; Dr J F Kassel★, 292, 293; Professor D Katamine, 297; Dr G Khalil and Professor J F Schacher, 765, 766; Dr S Knutton, 575, 576; Professor F Köberle★, 198, 199, 203; Dr J A Kovacs, 795; Ms E Kritzinger, 650; Dr W A Krotoski and the *American Journal of Tropical Medicine and Hygiene*, 94; Professor R E Kuntz, 228; Professor R Lainson FRS, 215, 261, 266, 1077; Dr R Lane, 960; Professor Y Larsson, 870; Dr C Lavaissière, 185; Dr C Lemaire, 1071; Dr med H Lieske, 19, 33, 51, 911, 935, 941; Dr R Lindner, 342; Dr S Lindsay, 928; Liverpool School of Tropical Medicine, 160, 611, 882; Dr L E Llewellyn, 1048; Professor S Looareesuwan, 593, 594; Dr J R Lucas, 158, 574, 949, 1084; Professor S Lucas, 124, 126, 179, 196, 365, 407, 429, 457, 458, 466, 470, 482, 521, 555, 615, 622, 630, 631, 643, 651, 660, 661, 711, 712, 736, 754, 760, 781, 788, 797, 802, 803, 1014, 1034; Dr Lily Ma, 522; Drs A Macor, R Ruffatto, A M Pisicane and M L Soranzo, 801; Sir Ian McAdam★, 676; Mr S N McDermott 230; Professor W W Macdonald, 15, 16, 282; Professor C D Mackenzie, 336, 339, 340, 730, (and University of Chicago Press) 335; Dr D McClaren, 967, 999; Dr A W R McCrae, 1068, 1069, 1083; Dr I Maddocks and the Medical Learning Resources Unit, University of Papua New Guinea, 588, 625; Professor B G Maegraith★, 508; Dr D Magnaval, 431; Professor El Sheikh Mahgoub, 896–899; Professor Osman Malik, 1028; Dr K Markwalder, 734; Professor P Marsden★, 1085; Dr C Marty, 1065, 1072, 1078; Professor E Mathai and Dr S David, 300; Dr T M Mather, Harvard School of Public Health 79; Dr B E Matthews (reprinted with permission from the *Journal of Nematology*), 386–390, 421; Dr U G Meneghelli, 761; Professor M Miles, 195; Professor L E Millikan, 932, 1063, 1079; Professor C D Mimms, 582; Dr A Mindel, 804, 805, 916; Dr D Minter, 67; Dr J J Misiewicz, 1099; Professor I Miyazaki★, 357, 487, 511, 520, 529, 530, 549–551, 554, 557, 694; Professor D H Molyneux, 186, 221, 351; Professor M Molyneux, 114; Mr P Montague, 578; Professor P Morera, 684; Professor H Morgan, 927; Professor D Morley and TALC, 476; Professor S A Morse, 780, 811, 814, 816, 838; Dr R Muller, 350, 363, 491, 492, 538, 681, 730, 752; Dr phil K Y Mumcuoglu, 954; Dr L E Munstermann, 4; Dr F A Murphy, 1012; Dr M Murray, 539, 542; Dr P Myak, 599, 600;

Professor G S Nelson, 740; Dr J Newman, 563, 1026; Dr F Noireau, 318; Dr T B Nutman, 319, 337; Professor B Ochoa, 425, 426; Dr T O Ogunlesi, 471; Ms Lisa Oke, 8, 276; Dr G F Otto, 671; Dr R Owen, 741; Professor H E Parry, 567; Professor F M Paul, 30; Dr P L Perine, 36, 809; Dr W Petana, 202; Dr H-W Pfister, 77; Dr E H Pike, 726; Dr A M Polderman, 675; Dr M A Prentice, 327; Dr E Price★, 1101; Professor P Pruaphadit, 31; Dr R Quick, 584; Professor A J Radford, 865, 866, 878, 976, 985, 997; Dr M Radmanesh, 963, 1052, 1054–1056; Dr G Rapeport, 629; Dr S R Rathinam, 598; Dr J Raven, 1057; Dr P Ready, 256; Dr H A Reid★, 1087, 1093; Dr S Reuter and Professor P Kern, 758; Dr G L Ridgway, 839; Professor J A Rioux, 250; Dr W M S Romosser, 32; Ms S Ryall, 609; Dr P Sarathchandra, 639; Dr P Sargeaunt, 608, 610, 616; Dr I Sato, 690–692; Dr G D Scarrow, 994, 996, 1041; Professor Dr K F Schaller, 338, 1004, 1035; Dr P M Schantz, 761; Professor H Schenone, 190, 1059, 1060; Drs Y Schlein and R Seltser and the *International Journal of Oral and Maxillofacial Surgery*, 953; Dr C W Schraft Jr, 623; Dr A Schrank, 812; Dr D Scott, 175; Professor J T Self, 770, 771; Dr T F Sellers Jr, 668; Professor V Šěry, 238; Professor J J Shaw, 266; Shell International Chemical Co. Ltd, 454, 473, 484; Dr A J Shelley, 943, 959; Colonel H E Shortt★, 216 (for preparation of the specimen); Professor D I H Simpson, 1016, 1017; Professor R Sinden, 91; Dr David Smith★, 184; Dr J A Smith and Ibadan University, 773; Dr M Smith, 78; Dr S R Smith, 1034; Dr J W Snow, 947; Dr R V Southcott and the Adelaide Children's Hospital, 1070; Professor A Spielman, 77; Air Vice Marshall W Stamm★, 626; Dr M V Steniowski, 826, 827; Professor G T Strickland, 75; Dr H Striebel, 444; Dr R Sturrock, 443; Professor S Sucharit, 1080; Mr R Suswillo, 299, 334; Drs I M Sulaiman, L Xiao, C Yang, L Escalante, A Moore, C B Beard, M J Arrowood and A A Lal, 644; Professor M Suzuki, 517, 519; Dr P Syrdalen, 962; Dr J S Tatz, 634; Dr R Tauxe, 584; Dr Ahmed Tayeh, 704; Dr A C Templeton, 764; Dr D Theakston, 150; Dr B Thylfors, 359; Dr Tin Chua Kian, 25; Mr G Tovey, 658, 659; Professor H Townson, 280, 281; UNDP/World Bank/WHO Special Programme for Research and Training in Tropical Diseases, 26, 178, 295; US Department of Agriculture, 946; Dr S Vajasthira, 506, 512, 516, 523, 524, 527, 547; Dr G S Visvesvara, 657, 799, 884, 885, 887; Dr F L Vichii, 197; Dr Anthony du Vivier and St. John's Hospital for Skins, 846, 891; Dr A Voller, 206; Dr J Walters, 356, 408, 653, 895, 1097, 1098; Dr A Warburg, 237; Professor D C Warhurst, 612, 883; Professor D Warrell, 30, 40, 73, 97, 113, 115–117, 120, 595, 789, 830, 831, 888, 909, 972, 1014, 1045, 1061, 1062, 1066, 1073, 1081, 1086, 1088–1092, 1094; Professor J Waterlow FRS, 990, 991, 1005; Wellcome Museum of Medical Science and Dr A J Duggan, 701, 1028; Professor G Wernsdorfer, 83; Mr J Williams, 183, 640–642, 923; Dr M L Wilson, 1009; Dr S Wilson, 231; Dr A Wisdom, 821; Professor M Wittner, 309, 490, 548; Professor A Woodruff★, 358; Professor T Woodward, 44; WHO, 350, 405, 417, 505, 826, 827, 837, 840, 841; WHO/ODA 257; Dr T Yamamoto, 579; Professor Y Yoshida, 553; Professor K

Yoshimura, **690–692**; Dr M Young, **919**; Dr H Zaiman, **747**; Professor V Zaman, **287, 959, 1067**; Professor A J Zuckerman, **559, 561, 1021**.

*[*Now deceased.]*

In addition to those whose assistance we acknowledged in the earlier editions of this work, we wish to thank especially Dr David Ellis, Professor R Killick Kendrick, Professor Sebastian Lucas, Professor P Marsden*, Professor Ishiro Miyazaki* and Professor David Warrell for valuable comments and advice. Several staff members of the US Centers for Disease Control and Prevention generously gave us their time as well as freely contributing the illustrations that are attributed to them above. Mr Richard Tranfield of the International Institute of Parasitology kindly helped with the production of several photographs as did various members of the staffs of the Departments of Medical Illustration of the Liverpool School of Tropical Medicine, the London School of Hygiene and Tropical Medicine and the Northwick Park Institute for Medical Research. We wish to acknowledge especially the work of Ms Andrea Darlow who produced with great skill all the maps and diagrams of life cycles in this book.

Figure **24** is from Burgess NHR and Cowan GO (**1993**) *A Colour Atlas of Medical Entomology* (Figure **15.16**) and is reproduced by permission of Chapman and Hall. Figures **338** and **1004** are from Schaller K F (ed.) (**1994**) *Colour Atlas of Tropical Dermatology and Venerology* (Figures **9.34** and **12.7**) and are reproduced by permission of Springer-Verlag. Figure **266** is modified from Lainson R and Shaw J J **In:** Cox F E G, Kreier J P and Wakelin D (eds) (**1998**) *Topley and Wilson's Microbiology and Microbial Infections, 9th edn. Vol 5 Parasitology* (Figure **13.4**) and is reproduced by permission of Arnold Publishers. Figures **366, 410, 411, 753, 756** and **801** are reproduced by kind permission of Dr P Caramello from the *Atlas of Medical Parasitology* and the individual colleagues listed above. Figure **611** is reproduced with permission of the Liverpool School of Tropical Medicine. Figure **64** is reproduced by kind permission of Dr D T Dennis. Figures **674** (by Professor van Marck, Antwerp) and **675** (by Professor A M Polderman, Leiden) are published here by courtesy of the 'Oesophagostomum project Leiden-Togo-Ghana.'

Our sincere thanks go again to the editorial staff of the publishers for their continuous help and guidance in the preparation of this new edition. Finally, we would like to express our gratitude to the reviewers of the first four editions of this atlas for their constructive comments, all of which we have taken into account while preparing the present work.

A century of progress in parasitology

Foreground—**Original figure of *Plasmodium falciparum* in a fresh, unstained, thin blood film**
A French military surgeon, Charles Louis Alfonse Laveran, discovered pigmented bodies and motile
flagellates in the erythrocytes of a patient with malignant tertian malaria in 1880. In this figure from
his book entitled *Paludism*, published in 1893, the following stages can be recognised: *a*, young
intraerythrocytic trophozoite; *b*, free trophozoites in plasma; *c*, intraerythrocytic schizont; *d*, probably a
macrogamete in plasma; *e*, exflagellating microgamete; *f*, free microgamete; *g*, microgametocytes;
h, haemozoin-containing phagocyte; and *l*, normal polymorphonuclear leucocyte (× *500*). (The figure
has been modified slightly from the original.)

Background—**Part of the genome of *Plasmodium falciparum***
The revelation of the genomic structure of this malaria parasite by molecular biological techniques
opens new roads to the rational design of drugs and vaccines to combat this parasite. A fraction of the
genome of chromosome 4 as revealed by nucleotide sequencing in the year 2000 forms the basis of
the pattern used in the background.
(Courtesy of Dr Sharen Bowman, The Sanger Centre, Cambridge, © The Sanger Centre.)

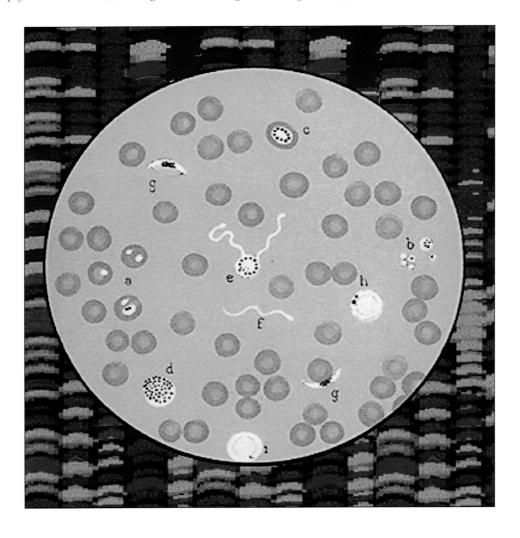

List of Tables

Introduction

The creation of a new edition of this book after only five years initially gave us some concern as to whether there was sufficiently new material to justify the task. However, in the course of our revision it soon became apparent not only that there were new diseases to present but, more importantly, that the causes of morbidity and mortality had changed significantly throughout the world and were continuing to change. The impact of such change is especially evident in the tropics.

Dominating the scene more than ever is the spectrum of disease and death caused by pandemic infection with the human immunodeficiency virus (HIV1) and its close retroviral relatives. Of all the opportunistic infections associated with HIV, tuberculosis has emerged as a leading problem and one that is compounded by the rapid spread of multidrug resistance. To date, no sure way has been found to limit the spread of HIV beyond attempting to spread the gospel of 'safe sex' through health education. Moreover, multidrug resistance both in HIV and a broad range of bacterial pathogens is of serious concern.

Rapid advances in knowledge of the molecular basis of several major pathogens hold out hope for the future, but that future is by no means just around the corner. Nevertheless some major advances in the reduction of tropical diseases have been achieved and these are considered in the following, brief summary. In general terms, certain negative factors in the balance sheet demand attention. Global warming which, by now, even the most critical authorities have to accept as a reality, is already resulting in a creeping extension of the geographical limits of several infections, the spread of which depends in part on the environmental temperature and humidity. Malaria, for example, is spreading to higher altitudes in certain tropical countries and beyond its normal northern and southern confines in others. Increasing drug resistance is of major concern in its control. Some arboviruses, along with their vectors, are extending their geographical horizons. The current enzootic of West Nile fever in North America is an example. Other negative factors appear unavoidable. These are the natural disasters that such events as major drought, famine, floods and earthquakes bring in their wake. Of the man-made catastrophes (in addition to global warming), war and genocide go hand in hand with disease and starvation. Now a new threat hangs over human kind, that of biological warfare.

There are, however, some remarkable factors on the positive side of the balance sheet that are considered here in relation to the individual chapters of this atlas. The **frontispiece** draws attention to the spectacular progress that has been made in exploring the genome of the malignant malaria parasite, *Plasmodium falciparum*. This knowledge will, it is foreseen, lead to the development of new drugs and vaccines to combat a parasite that, in the face of all efforts to conquer it, remains so far the most lethal parasitic disease of the tropics—one that afflicts between 300 and 500 million people every year and kills about one million African children under five years of age. New techniques in medicinal chemistry promise to yield radically new drugs in addition to novel developments based on artemisinin (the active constituent of Chinese wormwood). Immunological research seems to be approaching the holy grail of a range of malaria vaccines. Effective intercountry collaboration fostered by the WHO has made considerable progress in reducing the burden of Chagas' disease in Latin America. Leishmaniasis, however, remains a problem, although new drugs hold out some hope of reducing the morbidity from this condition. New therapeutic developments also offer strong hopes that the burden of lymphatic filariasis will be greatly diminished during the next decade, whereas the international programme to control river blindness caused by *Onchocerca volvulus* has already succeeded in arresting transmission in much of its former distribution, especially in Africa.

As regards the reduction of the soil-mediated helminthiases, progress has been made but only on a limited scale, and these infections continue to contribute to morbidity in the poorer populations of the developing world. Similarly, relatively little progress has been made in most countries in the prevalence of snail-mediated helminthiases, with the exception of certain countries in Southeast Asia and the Far East. The schistosomiases continue to afflict some 200 million people worldwide, but health education and other measures have succeeded in reducing the number of people infected with *Fasciolopsis buskii* from 15 to about 0.2 million in the past few years.

Of the infections acquired through the gastrointestinal tract, only poliomyelitis is nearing total eradication. Effective vaccines are now available to protect against some of the viruses causing hepatitis. Moreover, there is now a strong likelihood that the genetic manipulation of certain plant genes will lead to the production of extremely cheap vaccines to protect against such pathogens as the hepatitis B virus (HBV), which would bring in its train a significant reduction of hepatic carcinoma. On the other hand, hepatitis C virus (HCV) seems to be increasingly prevalent in many countries. The threatened pandemic of cholera caused by serovar O: 139 has, fortunately, not materialised, whereas the widescale administration of simple rehydration fluids has greatly reduced the mortality of those affected by the less virulent forms such as El Tor. Banal infectious diarrhoeas caused by viruses or bacteria other than *Vibrio cholerae*, however, continue to impose a heavy loss of life in newborns and infants in developing countries. With the recent recognition that carriers of large gut amoebae are mainly infected with the harmless *Entamoeba dispar* and not the pathogenic *E. histolytica*, amoebiasis is no longer considered to be the common pathogen that it was formerly believed to be although, when the latter parasite is present, radical chemotherapy is still essential. Among the many helminth infections acquired through the gastrointestinal tract, *Dracunculus medinensis*, the Guinea worm, has been almost totally eradicated over the past five years, mainly through health education and the deployment of extremely simple, cheap methods of control such as the filtering of drinking water through a fine plastic mesh sieve! There

was no need for sophisticated technology in this exceptional case.

When the first edition of this book was published in 1977, HIV was unknown. The exponential spread of this virus and its associated mortality has exceeded all expectations, while current progress in preventing or treating AIDS offers little hope of slowing down its advance, especially in the African continent and Southeast Asia. HIV/AIDS and other sexually transmitted diseases have become of such importance that they are now dealt with in this edition in a new and separate chapter.

Of the other infections acquired through the skin and mucous membranes, considerable progress has been made in the reduction of leprosy as a public health problem. This has been achieved mainly by a concerted, international effort to identify cases, to administer multiple drug therapy and to reduce the physical damage caused by the disease. From a global prevalence rate of 21.1 per 10 000 population in 1985, the rate was reduced to 5.7 in 1992 and, at the beginning of 2000, still lower to 1.25 per 10 000. Although the aim of eliminating leprosy by the end of the year 2000 could not be attained, it is very probable that this will be achieved in the near future. Deaths from neonatal tetanus have been reduced by over 40% since the introduction, in 1989, of a mass campaign to vaccinate pregnant women and improve delivery care.

Although the most important airborne infections continue to afflict the inhabitants of the tropics and subtropics, the increasing deployment of such weapons as vaccines against measles and the meningococcus are making an impact. However, the spread of multidrug-resistant tuberculosis, especially in association with HIV/AIDS, poses a further burden on some of the world's most disadvantaged people.

Malnutrition remains a killer of major proportions against which medical science can do little. Both natural and man-made disasters contribute and will continue to contribute to the shortage of essential foodstuffs in many countries, and even the best-intended international efforts to supplement locally available food are but of temporary help. Sustainable aid designed to increase local food production may, however, follow the provision, for example, of genetically modified crops such as rice or maize, that represent the staple diet in many areas. When it is realised that the global population of 5.35 billion in 1991 is estimated to rise to 8.66 billion by the year 2030, it will be appreciated that it will be possible to avoid mass starvation in many parts of the world only if drastic steps are taken without delay to improve radically both the production and distribution of the available food resources, as well as to limit population growth.

Among the miscellaneous disorders with which this book concludes are a number of potentially lethal, zoonotic virus infections, mainly spread from rodents, for example those caused by different species of *Hantavirus* and *Arenavirus* (*see* **Table 25**). Up to now they have affected relatively small numbers of people, but some of them possess the potential for rapid spread in human communities and demand constant vigilance to contain them. Ebola haemorrhagic fever, a *Filovirus* with an unknown wild reservoir and a mortality up to 88%, has caused several epidemics in tropical Africa. No vaccine is available nor any specific drug with which to treat established infections. The reduction through large-scale vaccination of infection with HBV should,

as mentioned above, in time reduce the prevalence of hepatic carcinoma.

Throughout this edition attention is drawn to newer diagnostic procedures, including ones based on immunological or molecular biological principles, as well as current types of medical imaging. We have attempted to lay emphasis on procedures that are likely to be of value not only for those engaged in medicine in the Western World, but also for practitioners in less well resourced environments. As vast numbers of travellers from the west now devote time to exploring what are for them exotic places, they are likely to encounter virtually any of the exotic pathogens and parasites that exist there. For this reason we have included a number of less common conditions so that their presence is less likely to be overlooked in differential diagnosis. The bibliography has also been expanded to provide more detailed source material than can be included in the text of this book.

CHAPTER 1

Arthropod-borne Infections

Numerically speaking, mosquitoes are probably responsible for more disease than any other group of arthropods, but other insects too are of great importance. Whereas *Anopheles* mosquitoes carry malaria, various viral infections and some types of filariasis, other viruses and filarias are transmitted by culicines. Different types of biting flies transmit African trypanosomiasis, leishmaniasis, bartonellosis and several kinds of filariasis. Fleas carry plague and one species of typhus, lice carry epidemic typhus, and mites and ticks carry other varieties of typhus. Ticks are also responsible for transmission of some of the haemorrhagic and relapsing fevers as well as Lyme disease and the human Ehrlichioses. The arthropod vectors of disease are classified in **Table 1**.

The important arthropod-borne (arbo) viruses considered here are yellow fever, dengue, Rift Valley fever and Japanese encephalitis. These are representative of the arbovirus diseases, which include many other infections of humans in the tropics (**Table 2**). In spite of the availability of protective vaccination, yellow fever remains a serious public health problem, particularly in Sub-Saharan Africa. The incidence and geographical spread of dengue has increased dramatically over the past 30 years. It is estimated that 2.5 billion of the world's population are at risk and that 100 million cases arise annually, including 500 000 cases of dengue haemorrhagic fever. Rift Valley fever made its first appearance beyond the African mainland in September 2000 as

an enzootic/epidemic outbreak in the southwest of Saudi Arabia and adjoining areas of Yeman. In spite of an intensive, international programme of insecticiding to destroy potential mosquito vectors, by mid-January 2001 the virus had killed at least 230 people (a mortality rate of 11.5% in about 2000 known to be infected and more than 3000 sheep, cattle and goats.

The geographical distribution of West Nile virus is also increasing significantly. Late in 1999 this pathogen was identified as the cause of an extensive epidemic and enzootic in several of the northeastern states of the USA. A serological survey in the Queens district of New York city indicated that as many as 2.6% of the population had been infected. Most cases were mild, but seven people died. Local transmission was by peridomestic *Culex pipiens* mosquitoes. A third of a large sample of birds found dead in the affected areas were positive for the virus. The virus, which spread further during 2000 and was isolated from other species of culicines and birds in a widening geographical area, is now likely to have become permanently established in the New World.

The worldwide dissemination of a dangerous arbovirus vector, *Aedes (Stegomyia) albopictus*, poses a very serious new threat for the coming years in relation to a number of diseases, including dengue. Of the rickettsioses, louse-borne typhus due to *Rickettsia prowazeki* is potentially the most important, but tick typhus is fairly common in some

Class	Order	Vectors	Diseases transmitted
ARACHNIDA	Acarina	hard ticks	spotted and Q fevers, virus encephalitides, Lyme disease
		Ornithodorus spp. (soft ticks)	endemic relapsing fever
		mites	scrub typhus, Rickettsial pox, scabies
CRUSTACEA	Cyclopoida	*Cyclops* spp. (water fleas)	guinea worm, fish tapeworm
	Decapoda	crayfish, freshwater crabs	paragonimiasis
INSECTA	Dictyoptera	cockroaches	*Hymenolepis diminuta* (rat tapeworm)
	Hemiptera	Reduviidae (assassin bugs)	Chagas' disease
	Phithiraptera		
	Anoplura	*Pediculus humanus* (body louse)	epidemic typhus, epidemic relapsing fever
	Mallophaga	chewing lice	*Dipylidium caninum* (dog tapeworm)
	Coleoptera	beetles	rat tapeworms
	Lepidoptera	grain moths	rat tapeworms
	Diptera	*Anopheles*	malaria, filariasis (*Wuchereria bancrofti, Brugia malayi*)
		culicines	filariasis (*W. bancrofti, B. malayi*), arboviruses (including yellow fever, dengue)
		Culicoides	filariasis (*Mansonella ozzardi, M. perstans, M. streptocerca*)
		Simulium	onchocerciasis (*Onchocerca volvulus*)
		Chrysops	filanasis (*Loa loa*)
		Phlebotomus	sandfly fever, bartonellosis, leishmaniases
		Lutzomyia	New World leishmaniases
		Glossina	African trypanosomiases
	Siphonaptera	fleas	plague, murine typhus, rat and dog tapeworms

Table 1 Arthropod vectors of disease

(see *also* **Chapter 6**, Ectoparasitic arthropods and **Table 23**)

areas (e.g. East Africa) and mite-borne scrub typhus (tsutsugamushi disease) in Southeast Asia and the Southwest Pacific. The sandfly-transmitted organisms (*Bartonella bacilliformis*) that cause bartonellosis (Carrión's disease—a disease limited to mountainous areas of western South America) have recently been shown to have some genetic relationship to the rickettsias.

Plague due to *Yersinia pestis* is still endemic in certain tropical and subtropical areas, and localised outbreaks are not uncommon, especially in the disrupted social and ecological situations brought about by wars. Relapsing fever in Africa is also geographically limited but may occur in epidemics under wartime conditions, as witnessed in 1991 in Ethiopia.

Among the protozoal infections, African trypanosomiasis is increasing in both West and East Africa but, in numerical terms, is still mainly of importance for its effect on domestic animals. Fifty million Africans are still at risk, and about 25 000 new cases occur each year. South American trypanosomiasis (Chagas' disease) spread by reduviid bugs extends through much of the subcontinent and is responsible for considerable ill health in parts of its distribution. Of the 90 million people at risk, between 16 and 18 million are believed to be infected. Two major, multinational, vector-control programmes, one in the 'Southern Cone' countries (Argentina, Brazil, Bolivia, Chile, Paraguay and Uruguay) and the other in the Andean and Central American countries (*see* **187**), are now making a major impact on transmission. These programmes are based on the use of fumigant canisters and insecticidal paints, together with screening of blood donors, although transfusion infection remains a

Table 2 Arboviruses that infect humans[1]

Family	Genus	Virus or Disease	Vectors	Reservoir hosts	Amplifier hosts
Togaviridae	*Alphavirus*	Chikungunya	*Aedes*	monkeys, ? rodents	
		Eastern equine encephalitis	*Culiseta*	birds	horses
		Mayaro	*Aedes, Anopheles*	wild vertebrates	
		Mucambo	culicines	?	
		O'Nyong-Nyong	*Anopheles*	humans	
		Semliki Forest	mosquitoes	?	
		Ross River	*Aedes*	? wallabies	
		Sindbis	culicines	birds	
		Venezuelan equine encephalitis	*Aedes, Culex* spp.	rodents	horses
		Western equine encephalitis	*Culex*	birds	horses
	Flavivirus (mainly mosquito-borne)	Banzi	culicines	?	
		Bussuquara	culicines	rodents	
		Dengue 1,2,3,4	*Aedes*	mosquitoes[2]	? monkeys
		Ilheus	culicines	birds	
		Japanese encephalitis	*Culex, Anopheles*	birds	pigs, equines
		Kunjin	culicines	birds	
		Murray Valley encephalitis	culicines	birds	
		Rocio	*Psorophora* spp.	birds	
		St. Louis encephalitis	culicines	mosquitoes[2], birds	
		Spondweni	culicines	?	
		Wesselbron	culicines	rodents	
		West Nile	*Culex*, ixodids, argasids	birds, bats, rodents	
		Yellow fever	*Aedes (Stegomyia)*	mosquitoes[2]	monkeys
			Haemagogus spp.	mosquitoes[2], rodents	monkeys
		Zika	culicines	?	
	Flavivirus (mainly tick-borne)	Absettarov	ixodids	?	
		Hanzalova	ixodids	?	
		Hypr	ixodids	rodents	
		Kumlinge	ixodids	rodents, birds	
		Kyasanur Forest disease	ixodids, argasids	forest rodents	monkeys
		Louping ill	ixodids	rodents, birds	
		Negishi	ixodids	?	
		Omsk haemorrhagic fever	ixodids	ticks[2,3], rodents	
		Powassan	ixodids	rodents	
		Russian spring-summer encephalitis	ixodids	rodents, birds	
		Dakar bat virus	?	bats	
Reoviridae	*Orbivirus*	Colorado tick fever	ixodids, argasids	rodents	
Bunyaviridae	*Nairovirus*	Crimea–Congo haemorrhagic fever	ixodids	ticks[2], birds, leporids, rodents	sheep
	Hantavirus	Hantaan virus[4]	? ticks	murine rodents	
	Bunyavirus	California encephalitis group	mosquitoes	*Aedes*[2], rabbits	
		Oropuche	mosquitoes	monkeys, sloths	
		Brazilian group	mosquitoes	?	
		Bunyamwere group	culicines	?	
	Phlebovirus	Rift Valley fever	mosquitoes	? rodents	cattle, sheep
		sandfly fever	*Phlebotomus*	sandflies[2]	? sandfly, mites

? Not yet known.
[1] *See also* **Table 25**
[2] Vertical transmission occurs in vectors.
[3] Infection may occur from handling carcasses or pelts of infected rodents, e.g. muskrats.
[4] One species is the cause of Korean haemorrhagic fever; other viruses in this group, which are spread by murine rodent excreta, cause haemorrhagic fever with renal syndrome (HFRS) and nephropathia epidemica.

serious problem. The aim is to eliminate the transmission of Chagas' disease by 2005.

Malaria and the leishmaniases are both widespread and increasing—sometimes in epidemic fashion—despite measures to control them. Malaria, to which over half of the world's population is exposed, continues to cause severe morbidity and mortality in many countries, with the problem being aggravated by the existence, on an increasing scale, of the vectors' resistance to insecticides and the parasites' resistance to antimalarial drugs. About 270 million people are believed to be chronically infected, with over 100 million new cases arising each year and between one and two million deaths. Fortunately, a new class of drugs based on artemisinin (the active constituent of Chinese wormwood—*Artemisia annua* Linn.) is being developed, and these are proving, for the time being at least, very effective in reducing morbidity and mortality from severe malaria. It is to be hoped that the current, intensive effort to develop a vaccine against malaria will, in time, provide a new and powerful weapon with which to combat this persistent and deadly disease. A malarial parasite resembling a simian species, *Plasmodium simiovale*, that was originally described in *Macaca sinica* in Sri Lanka, has recently been identified by immunological detection of a species-specific peptide sequence in a small number of human patients in Papua New Guinea, Indonesia, Madagascar, Brazil and Guyana. It is reported to produce an infection resembling that normally associated with *P. vivax* but more severe.

Of over 750 million people exposed to lymphatic filariasis, about 79 million are infected in 76 countries. Of the tissue filariases, those due to *Wuchereria bancrofti* and *Brugia malayi* may produce serious deformity, whereas infection with the skin-dwelling parasite *Onchocerca volvulus* remains a problem in parts of tropical Africa and Central America. However, thanks to an extensive control campaign to destroy the aquatic stages of the vectors of onchocerciasis (species of *Simulium*) and to the introduction of ivermectin, the most serious complication, blindness, is being conquered and should become a thing of the past.

Whereas the diagnosis of the viral and bacterial infections must be confirmed by appropriate serological and cultural techniques, most protozoal and helminthic infections are readily recognised, if not on clinical grounds alone, then by fairly simple techniques designed to demonstrate the presence of the causative parasites. Powerful and sophisticated diagnostic agents in the form of highly sensitive and specific, simple monoclonal antibody tests are being developed. However, molecular biological tests using DNA probes and polymerase chain reaction primers are likely to be of limited practical application for the foreseeable future in many developing countries.

THE ARBOVIRUSES

(See **Table 2.**)

YELLOW FEVER

1 Distribution map of yellow fever virus
Focal outbreaks of mosquito-borne yellow fever still occur in South America but are especially a problem in tropical Africa where the disease is endemic in 34 countries with a total population of 468 million. It has been estimated that more than 200 000 cases with up to 30 000 deaths occur annually, the great majority in Africa. Vaccination provides a high level of protection for 10 years and is a legal requirement for travellers entering endemic countries. The virus is transmitted by mosquitoes of the

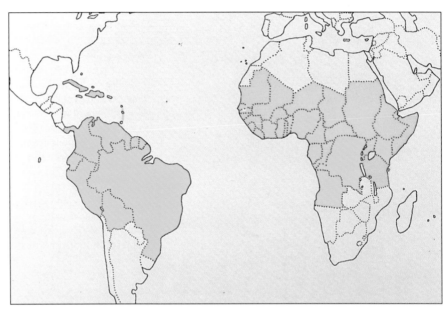

genus *Aedes*. It is now accepted that the main reservoirs are the susceptible mosquitoes, in which the virus is transmitted from generation to generation by transovarial infection. The map indicates the countries at risk (light and dark yellow) and those in which at least one outbreak was reported between 1985 and 1998 (dark yellow). Nine epidemics occurred in Nigeria between 1986 and 1994. The main differential characters of the principal families of mosquito vectors of disease are shown in the next figures. (See *also* **87, 273–282** *and* **284.**)

2 Newly emerged female *Aedes (Stegomyia) aegypti*
The main vector of yellow fever within village and urban settlements in both the Old and New Worlds is *Ae. (Stegomyia) aegypti.* Over the centuries, its eggs have been transported in man-made containers from Africa so that this species is now found in most parts of the tropics and subtropics. It breeds readily in all types of domestic and peridomestic collections of fresh water, including flower vases, water drums, tin cans, broken coconut shells etc. (× *12.*)

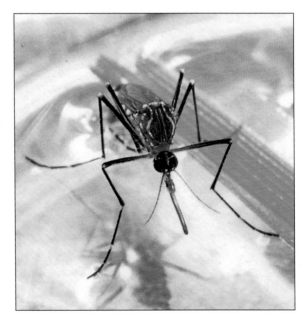

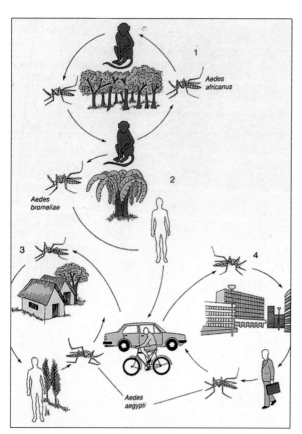

Aedes africanus

Aedes bromeliae

Aedes aegypti

3 Transmission cycles of yellow fever

'Jungle' yellow fever is enzootic among monkeys in the tropical forests of Africa and South America. Although the main reservoirs are now generally believed to be the mosquito vectors, the virus is enzootic in Africa in species of *Cercopithecus* (vervets), *Cercocebus* (mangabeys), *Colobus* and *Papio* (baboons) in which the infections are usually inapparent. Epidemics of yellow fever occur in Africa when the virus is passed by a succession of *Aedes (Stegomyia)* species between the monkey reservoirs and humans. The infection is maintained in the forest (1) by several species of mosquito, including *Aedes (Stegomyia) africanus* and *Ae. (Stegomyia) bromeliae*. The latter may leave the forest to breed in plantations (2) where farmers can become infected. The virus that causes sylvatic yellow fever in East Africa differs from that which is responsible for urban epidemics in the west of the continent. There, villagers (3) who acquire viraemia serve as a source of infection, which is readily transmitted in more urban areas (3) by *Ae. (Stegomyia) aegypti* that breeds in domestic and peridomestic sites, thus starting the urban cycle of transmission (4). In South America, epidemics are usually preceded by severe enzootics in which large numbers of forest monkeys may die. (Adapted from *Service*, 1986.)

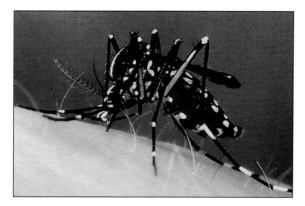

4 Female *Aedes (Stegomyia) albopictus*

Imported in tyres sent from Japan to Houston in the USA in 1985, *Ae. (Stegomyia) albopictus* (the 'Asian tiger mosquito') has now colonised most states of the USA. *Ae. (Stegomyia) albopictus* has been shown to be capable of supporting the development of over 24 arboviruses, including those causing yellow fever, dengue 1–4 (with which it has been found naturally infected), eastern, western and Venezuelan encephalitides, chikungunya and La Crosse encephalitis. It can truly be considered as the '*Aedes aegypti* of the 1990s,' and could readily cause epidemic yellow fever if the virus is reintroduced into the southern parts of the USA. Moreover, this mosquito has genetically adapted to higher temperatures and has already invaded Latin America and parts of West Africa. *Ae. (Stegomyia) albopictus* may prove to be a far more dangerous vector of arboviruses than *Ae. (Stegomyia) aegypti* because of its ability to thrive in both cold and hot climates. (× 7.5.)

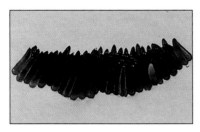 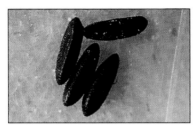 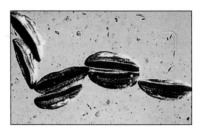

5–7 Mosquito eggs
Culex eggs (**5**, left) are deposited on the water surface in 'rafts'; *Aedes* eggs (**6**, centre) are laid singly and often have a conspicuously sculptured surface; *Anopheles* eggs (**7**, right) have lateral floats and tend to aggregate on the water surface, forming 'Chinese figure' patterns. (**5** × 25; **6,7** × 27.)

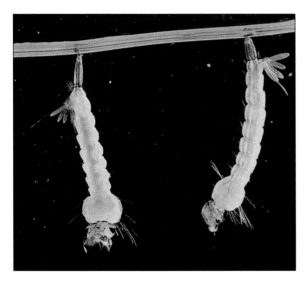

8 Third stage larvae of *Culex (Culex) quinquefasciatus* and *Aedes (Stegomyia) aegypti*
The larvae of *Culex* and *Aedes* are suspended under the air–water interface by their siphons. This figure illustrates the differences between the larvae of the two genera—*Culex* (left) with a long siphon and several tufts of lateral siphon hairs, *Aedes* (right) with a short siphon and single hair tuft. (× 9.)

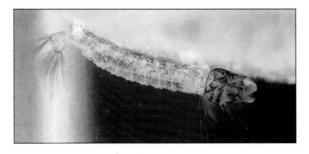

9 Third stage larva of *Anopheles*
The larvae of *Anopheles* lie parallel to the water surface. (× 9.)

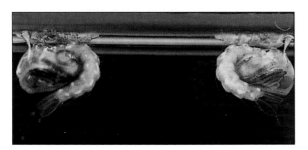

10 Pupae of *Culex*
Pupae of *Culex*, *Aedes* and *Anopheles* are very similar. They obtain air through siphons on the cephalothorax. (× 9.)

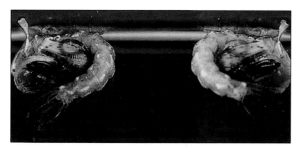

11 Pupae of *Anopheles*
Compare the shorter siphon of this pupa with that of *Culex* (**10**). (× 9.)

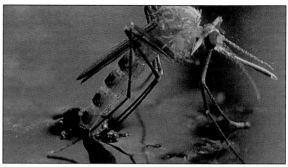

12 Adult *Culex (Culex) quinquefasciatus* hatching from pupa
The mature pupa, with the siphons penetrating the surface film, splits open and the adult mosquito, in this case a female, emerges, allowing its wings to expand and harden. (× 8.)

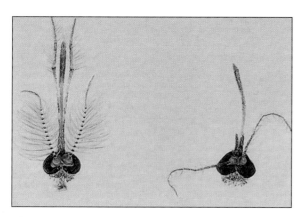

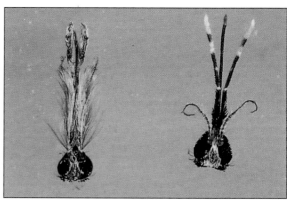

13 & 14 Heads of adult culicine and anopheline mosquitoes
The adults are distinguished by the form of the antennae and palps. *Culex* ♂ (left) ♀ (right) (**13**, left); *Anopheles* ♂ (left) ♀ (right) (**14**, right). (× 16.) *Aedes* males and females are similar to those of *Culex*. Compare the short palps of the female *Culex* with the long ones of the female *Anopheles*.

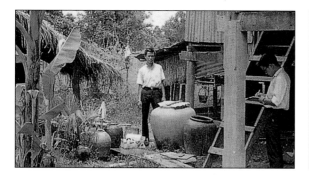

15 Larval breeding in water storage jars
Such containers attract *Aedes (Stegomyia) aegypti* and *Ae. (Stegomyia) albopictus*, which readily colonise them even when the jars are covered. Generally, the lids are ill fitting and do not keep the female mosquitoes out (as seen in this Thai village).

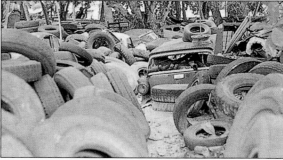

16 Larval breeding in discarded motor tyres
In recent years, the eggs of *Aedes (Stegomyia) aegypti* and *Ae. (Stegomyia) albopictus* have been carried from continent to continent in motor tyres, which are often sent to central collection areas for recycling. While awaiting transport, the tyres are usually left in dumps exposed to the rain, and such dumps provide ideal sites for egg laying.

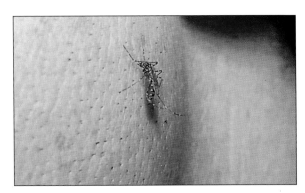

17 *Aedes* biting
Photograph taken at midday in a rain forest near Belém, Brazil, at the mouth of the River Amazon. Mosquitoes of the genera *Aedes (Stegomyia)* and *Haemagogus* transmit yellow fever virus to forest monkeys in which there is a sylvatic reservoir, from monkeys to humans, and subsequently from humans to humans. Viraemia in monkeys, as in humans, is short lived. (× 2.)

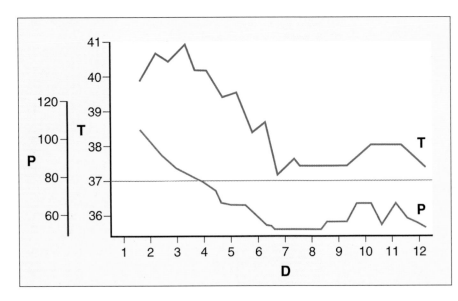

18 Temperature chart of yellow fever case
The increasing slowness of the pulse relative to the temperature (Faget's sign—also seen in typhoid fever, paratyphoid and brucellosis) is of clinical diagnostic value. [D—day of illness; P—pulse; T—temperature (°C).]

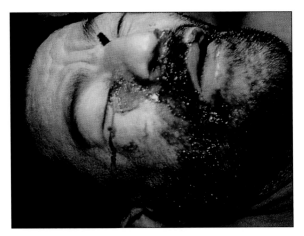

19 'Black vomit' in terminal stage of yellow fever
Despite the name, jaundice is usually not marked in yellow fever. Bleeding from the gut is a grave portent. The Costa Rican patient seen here with severe jaundice vomited material resembling coffee grounds ('black vomit'), as well as fresh blood shortly before dying.

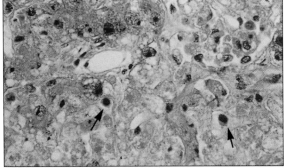

20 Section of liver from fatal yellow fever case
Midzonal necrosis with fatty degeneration and eosinophilic, intranuclear inclusions (Councilman bodies) are characteristic histological features (see arrows). Here the periportal area contains relatively well preserved cells. (*Giemsa* × 800.) (AFIP No. 71–1981)

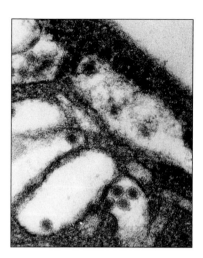

21 Electron micrograph of yellow fever virus
This RNA virus in the genus *Flavivirus* (Togaviridae) is shown here growing in a Vero cell culture. (Original magnification × 80 000.) (Courtesy of Mr Bruce Cropp, Centers for Disease Control, Fort Collins, Colorado.)

DENGUE

22 Dengue temperature chart
Dengue is an *Aedes*-borne disease of wide distribution in the tropics and subtropics and is caused by four serotypes of a species of positive, single-stranded RNA *Flavivirus*. The incubation period is short, on average about five days. The illness is often of short duration with a characteristic 'saddle-back' fever. [D—day of illness; T—temperature (°C).]

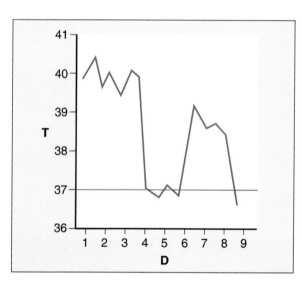

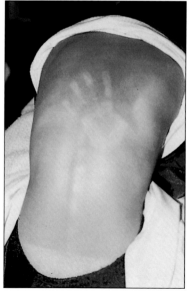

23 Rash of dengue
The figure shows the characteristic blanching rash of dengue fever. The rash is thought to be due to capillary vasodilation in the skin and occurs shortly after defervescence on about day 5 of the infection. The rash lasts one to five days, sparing the palms and soles. It may be followed by a transient morbilliform or scarlatiniform rash that spreads centrally from the extremities during the second bout of fever.

DENGUE HAEMORRHAGIC FEVER

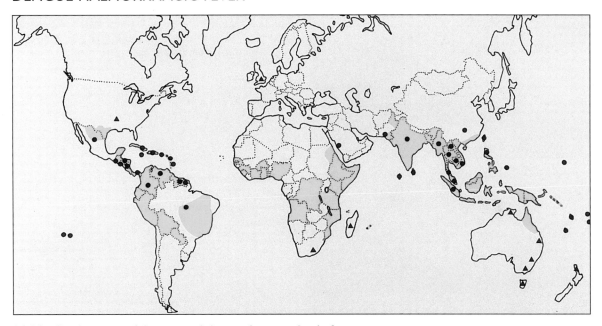

24 Distribution map of dengue and dengue haemorrhagic fever
The distribution of dengue is expanding rapidly. The map indicates the general distribution of the disease (yellow), those countries in which outbreaks of dengue haemorrhagic fever (DHF) were recorded between 1975 and 1996 (●) and localities where imported cases were reported during that period (▲). (During the past two decades, numerous epidemics of DHF have occurred in Southeast Asia and Latin America. All four known serotypes of dengue virus have been isolated in almost all of the countries involved, and *Aedes (Stegomyia) aegypti* has been identified as the main vector. Its peridomestic habits ensure intimate human-vector contact. Strict control of peridomestic breeding sites is the most effective weapon against the spread of infection. In Argentina and Cuba, field trials have shown that the insecticidal fumigant canisters developed for the control of the vectors of Chagas' disease (*see* **205**) are also extremely effective against *Ae. (Stegomyia) aegypti* in human dwellings. As several dengue viruses have been proven to pass transovarially also in *Ae. (Stegomyia) albopictus*, it is likely that epidemics will continue to increase in distribution and number in the future. Monkeys may serve as amplifier hosts in some areas.

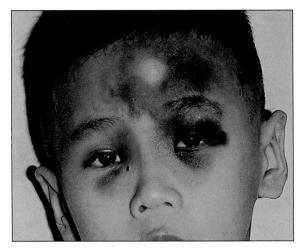

25 Marked ecchymoses in a Chinese boy
Dengue haemorrhagic fever is believed to arise as a result of a second infection, possibly with a different serotype, following an initial attack of uncomplicated dengue via antibody-mediated enhancement. Immune complex formation leads to increased capillary permeability, which may be followed by hypovolaemia and even disseminated intravascular coagulation. Cutaneous haemorrhagic manifestations ranging from petechiae to gross ecchymoses characterise the infection, especially in children. Outbreaks of variable severity occur yearly in Southeast Asia. For example, over 200 patients were admitted daily in an outbreak in Vientiane, Laos, in 1987. The peak age-specific prevalence was 4 to 9 years and the severity of cases ranged from Grade I (fever and positive tourniquet test) to Grade IV (undetectable blood pressure and pulse—dengue shock syndrome). Rapid restoration of plasma volume is mandatory. The case fatality rate can be as high as 15% in the absence of optimal medical management. A tetravalent vaccine is currently undergoing clinical trials but, for the time being, limitation of the infection depends largely on vector control.

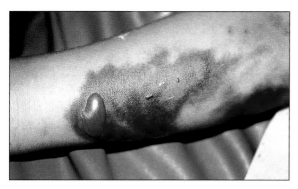

26 Subcutaneous haemorrhage in dengue haemorrhagic fever

This Thai patient had a large haemorrhagic lesion on his upper arm. (Image ID: 9914015, courtesy of Wellcome Trust and WHO, figure WHO/TDR/STI/Hatz.)

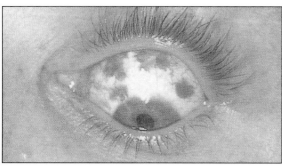

27 Scleral haemorrhage in dengue haemorrhagic fever

Scleral haemorrhages often accompany the skin rash in this condition.

CONGO–CRIMEA HAEMORRHAGIC FEVER

(See **1008–1020** for this and other zoonotic viral infections.)

JAPANESE ENCEPHALITIS

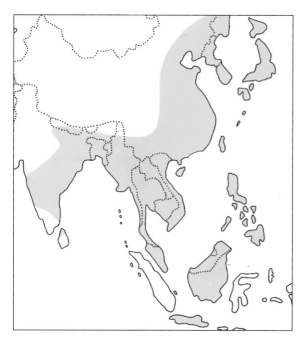

28 Distribution map of Japanese encephalitis

This disease is caused by a flavivirus, which is spread through birds and transmitted by various species of *Culex* and *Anopheles* mosquitoes. These are commonly found breeding in surface water such as flooded paddy fields. Birds form a reservoir for the virus, which is amplified in infected pigs.

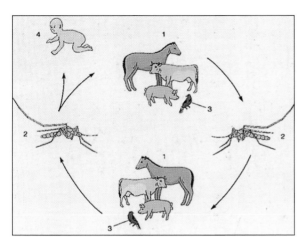

29 Cycle of transmission of Japanese encephalitis
The virus is passed between the amplifier hosts (equines, sheep and, mainly, pigs) (1) and humans (4) by culicine mosquitoes. The amplifier hosts are infected by mosquitoes (2) that have fed on migratory water birds (herons and egrets) (3). Humans (4) are dead-end hosts.

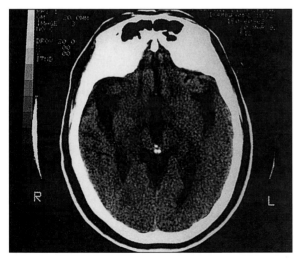

30 Acute Japanese encephalitis
The encephalitis, as seen in this Sri Lankan infant, is severe. He was comatose and had spasms and chorioathetotic movements of all four limbs. The sequelae are serious and may include mental retardation. In Nepal, where a large outbreak occurred in 1986, it is referred to as 'the visitation of the Goddess of the forest.' The incidence of Japanese encephalitis is continuing to increase in the inhibitants of the Nepalese terai. In early 2000, over 10% of more than 1000 infected patients died in spite of a campaign to protect the population by vaccination. (© D.A. Warrell.)

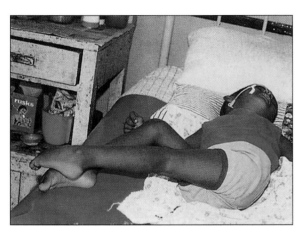

31 Atrophic changes in brain after Japanese encephalitis
This computed tomogram shows marked atrophic changes in the cortex and basal ganglia of a Thai woman seven years after an attack of Japanese encephalitis. Neuronal degeneration and necrosis are commonly seen in many parts of the brain. A striking change is destruction of the Purkinje cells in the cerebellum.

RIFT VALLEY FEVER

32 Virions of Rift Valley fever

Rift Valley fever is a zoonosis acquired either by the bite of infected culicine mosquitoes or from infected domestic sheep or cattle. The virus, which was first identified in 1930, is a *Phlebovirus*, one of the Bunyaviridae. It has caused epizootics from Chad, through the Rift Valley to South Africa, and spread in 1977 to Egypt where it extended to humans, causing massive epidemics. A major outbreak occurred in Kenya and Somalia in 1997–98 and, in 2000, the infection extended for the first time beyond Africa to the southwest of Saudi Arabia and Yemen, possibly imported in sheep from Somalia. Human infection is acquired either by the bites of infected mosquitoes or by direct contact with the infected blood, tissue fluids or organs of viraemic animals. Since the virus can be carried transovarially in the vectors, the latter may serve as amplifiers and maintenance hosts. In 95% of cases, Rift Valley fever gives rise to a self-limiting, febrile condition, but can produce meningoencephalitis, retinitis and haemorrhages typical of the haemorrhagic fevers. In severe cases the liver shows changes similar to those in yellow fever. The virions seen here are attached to the surface of salivary gland cells of *Culex pipiens*, the main vector in Egypt. (*SEM* × 85 000.)

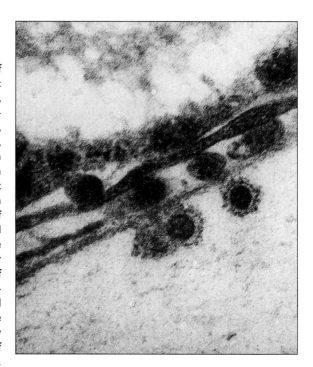

THE RICKETTSIOSES

(See **Table 3**.)

LOUSE-BORNE TYPHUS

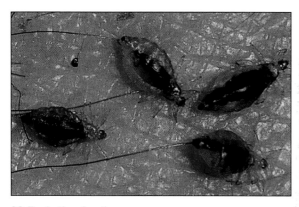

33 Body lice feeding

The body louse, *Pediculus corporis*, transmits typical epidemic typhus, due to *Rickettsia prowazekii*, and trench fever. Rickettsial infection is cosmopolitan. The use of DDT for disinfection of louse-infested communities is a primary control measure in epidemic situations. (Recent studies suggest that a zoonotic reservoir of *R. prowazekii* may exist in flying squirrels in North America.) (× 4.)

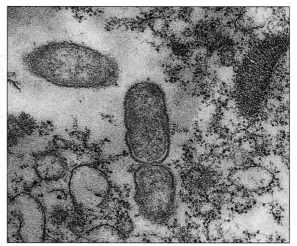

34 Ultrastructure of *Rickettsia prowazekii*

Electron micrographs show that the rickettsial organisms have structural similarities to bacteria. (× 38 500.)

Table 3 The rickettsial diseases[1,6]

Group	Disease	Causative agent	Vector	Animal reservoirs
TYPHUS	Epidemic typhus	*Rickettsia prowazekii*	*Pediculus humanus*	none
	Brill–Zinsser disease	*R. prowazekii*	*P. humanus*	man
	Endemic (murine)	*R. typhi* (= *R. mooseri*)	*Xenopsylla cheopis*	rat
	typhus		*Ctenocephalides felis*	cat, opossum (SW USA)
SPOTTED FEVERS	Rocky Mountain, Eastern, Western, South American	*R. rickettsii*	Various tick spp.[2]	many small mammals
	Fièvre boutonneuse[3]	*R. conorii*	*Rhipicephalus sanguineus*[2]	dog, small mammals
			Haemophysalis leachii	dog
	African tick typhus	*R. africae*	*Amblyomma* spp.[2]	? rodents
	Siberian tick typhus	*R. sibirica*	*Dermacentor* spp.[2]	farm and wild animals
			Haemaphysalis spp.	
	Queensland tick typhus	*R. australis*	*Ixodes holocyclus*[2]	marsupials
	Tasmanian spotted fever	*R. honei*	*I. tasmani*	rodents
	Rickettsial pox	*R. akari*	mites	mice
	Scrub typhus	*Orientia tsutsugamushi*	trombiculid mites	small mammals, rodents, birds
Q FEVER	Q fever	*Coxiella burnetii burnetii*	ticks[4]	cattle, sheep, goats, wild animals
EHRLICHIOSIS	Human monocytic ehrlichiosis (HME)	*Ehrlichia chaffeensis*	*Amblyomma americana*	? white-tailed deer, ? ticks
	Human granulocytic ehrlichiosis (HGE)	Human granulocyte[5] *Ehrlichia*	*Ixodes scapularis*	? white-tailed deer, dogs, rodents
OTHER INFECTIONS	Trench fever	*Bartonella quintana*[6]	*P. humanus*	man, ? long-tailed vole
	Cat scratch disease	*B. henselae*[6]	(mechanical transmission)	cats (especially feral)
	Bacillary angiomatosis	*B. quintana* and *B. henselae*	? cat fleas	? (seen in patients with AIDS)
	Bartonellosis	*B. bacilliformis*[6]	*Lutzomyia* spp.	? man

[1] Identification is usually confirmed by serological typing (e.g. Weil–Felix reaction, *C. burnetii* complement fixation test).
[2] Vertical transmission can occur in vectors.
[3] The most widely distributed species of *Rickettsia*, with numerous vector species.
[4] Transmission is mainly from dairy animals or their products, sometimes by inhaled aerosol.
[5] Human granulocyte *Ehrlichia* may be transmissible by transfusion.
[6] These organisms which were formerly classified in the genus *Rochalimeae* are now included in the genus *Bartonella*.

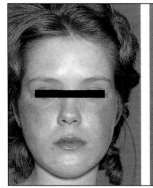 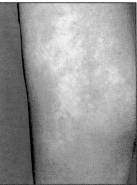

35 Rash of epidemic, louse-borne typhus
The generalised macular or maculopapular rash is similar in all types of rickettsial infections. This woman had a fine, macular erythematous rash on the face and extremities early in the infection.

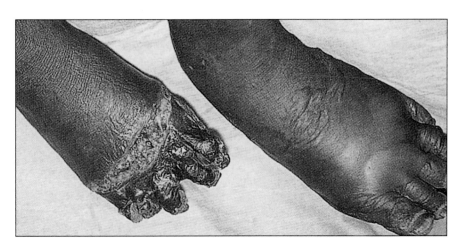

36 Peripheral gangrene in severe typhus
One of the characteristic features of typhus is the severe toxicity of the infection. Gangrene of feet and hands as seen in this Ethiopian patient occasionally occurs.

SCRUB TYPHUS

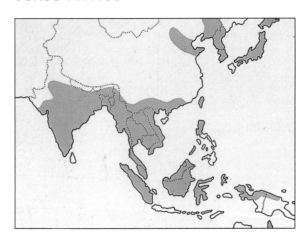

37 Distribution map of scrub typhus
Scrub typhus, or tsutsugamushi disease (from the Japanese name meaning 'noxious bug'), is caused by infection with *Orientia tsutsugamushi* and is transmitted by larval trombiculid mites of the genus *Leptotrombidium* (see **Table 23**). The disease occurs in the Indian subcontinent, Southeast Asia, the Far East and the islands of the Southwest Pacific.

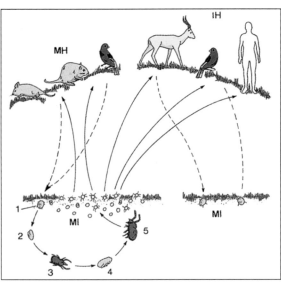

38 Epidemiological cycle of scrub typhus
Orientia tsutsugamushi is present in trombiculid-infested rodents. Not far from Kuala Lumpur, for example, *Leptotrombidium deliensis* is found in the forest, and *L. akamushi* in the grass ('lalang'). The mites occur in colonies known as 'mite islands' that are associated with the nests of the rodents on which they normally feed. They pass through a cycle that includes a parasitic, blood-feeding, hexapod larva (1) and a nymphochrysalis (2), followed by eight-legged, non-parasitic nymphal (3) and adult stages (5), between which is interposed an imagochrysalis (4). The cycle of infection is maintained in the focus, since engorged larvae are returned to the rodent nest where they drop off and complete the rest of their cycle, with the adults finally laying eggs there. Vertical transmission of *O. tsutsugamushi* occurs so that the true reservoir of infection is the mite. Other mammals, humans and occasionally birds may be bitten by the larvae, which cause severe irritation. Thus, scrub typhus, although a zoonosis, can occur in small outbreaks if groups of people (e.g. soldiers in the jungle) rest in the vicinity of a mite island. [MI—mite island; MH—maintenance hosts; IH—incidental hosts; adapted from Audy, 1968.]

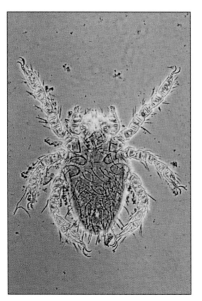

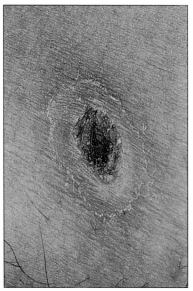

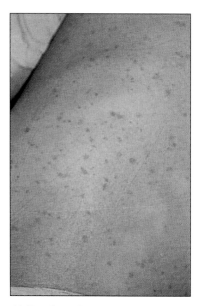

39 Larva of *Leptotrombidium*
Larval mites transmit the infection from rodents to humans when the latter come into accidental contact with mite-infested terrain. The mites act as reservoirs since transovarial transmission of the *Rickettsia* occurs. (× 80.)

40 Eschar of mite bite
A typical 'eschar' forms at the site of the trombiculid bite and precedes the fever. The eschar seen here on the lower abdomen of a Thai patient appeared seven days before the photograph was taken. (© D. A. Warrell.)

41 Scrub typhus rash
The maculopapular eruption which appears on about the sixth or seventh day of the illness, lasts for three or four days. Whereas mainly seen on the trunk, upper arms and thighs, it may also appear on the face, hands and feet.

TICK TYPHUS

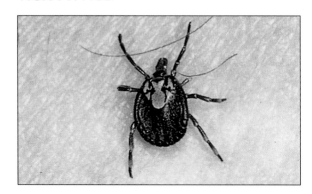

42 Adult female *Amblyomma hebraeum*, a vector of East African tick typhus
Various species of hard ticks transmit a variety of *Rickettsia* species, e.g. *R. africae* in sub-Saharan Africa. Note the characteristic markings of the scutal shield. The immature stages readily feed on humans. (× 3.)

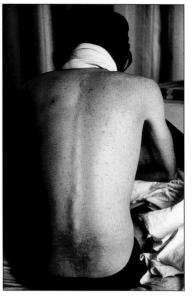

43 Eschar at site of tick bite
As with mite-borne typhus, an 'eschar' forms at the site of the infective tick bite. The distribution of the rash is also seen clearly on the back of this patient infected in South Africa.

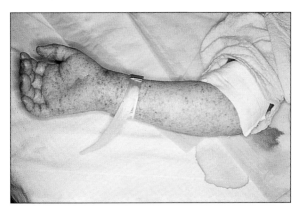

44 Petechial rash of Rocky Mountain spotted fever
Rickettsia rickettsii causes three types of tick-borne infection in the USA. The Western type is transmitted by *Dermacentor andersoni*, the Eastern by *D. variabilis* and the Southern by *Amblyomma americanum* and *Rhipicephalus sanguineum*. Various small rodents, gophers and woodchucks serve as mammalian hosts. This four-year-old child, who was comatose on the eighth day of the illness, recovered fully. An eschar marked the site of the bite. The application of a tourniquet, as seen here, accentuates the haemorrhagic nature of the rash distal to the site of the pressure (Hess test).

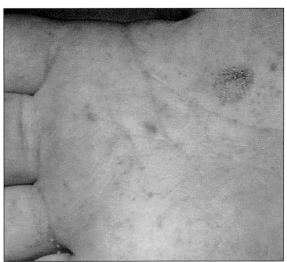

45 Hand of a patient with Rocky Mountain spotted fever
In Rocky Mountain spotted fever the rash is usually seen on the trunk, face and extremities.

Q FEVER

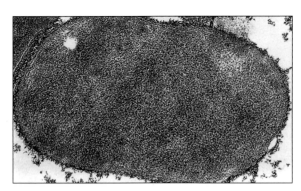

46 Cross section of *Coxiella burnetii*
Q fever due to *Coxiella burnetii* of ruminants, another rickettsial pathogen, is cosmopolitan. It may be spread to humans by ticks but is mainly acquired by direct contact with contaminated milk. This zoonosis is widely distributed in nature, the main reservoirs for infection in humans being cattle, sheep, goats, cats and, occasionally, dogs. (× *38 000*.)

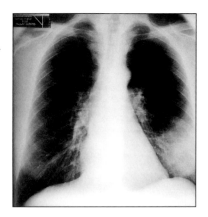

47 Chest radiograph of a patient with Q fever pneumonia
The radiograph shows left lower lobe consolidation in a patient with Q fever pneumonia. The main clinical manifestations include a febrile illness, atypical pneumonia, hepatitis and sometimes endocarditis. Q fever can complicate pregnancy.

48 Male and female *Amblyomma variegatum*
The scutal markings of this vector of *Coxiella burnetii* in Africa are very characteristic. The causative agent of Q fever, *C. burnetii* can be acquired directly by aerosol from dairy animals, which become infected by the bites of various species of ticks that have fed on reservoir mammals such as rodents. Several species of *Hyalomma* and *Haemaphysalis leachi* have been implicated as vectors in the Old World in addition to *Amblyomma variegatum*. In the mammalian host, the organisms develop in the cytoplasm of splenic macrophages and liver Kupffer cells. *A. variegatum* has also been incriminated as a vector of Congo–Crimea haemorrhagic fever (*see* 1008–1011). ($\times$ 5.5.)

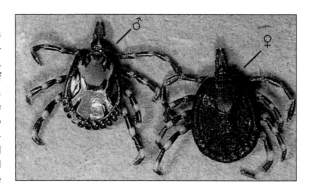

Endemic (murine) typhus may be acquired when fleas from *Rickettsia*-infected rodents harboured, for example, in deserted buildings in the countryside, transmit infection to newcomers who take up residence there.

EHRLICHIOSIS

49 Clusters of *Ehrlichia chaffeensis* cultured in DH82 cells
This recently recognised rickettsial organism causing human monocytic ehrlichiosis (HME) leads to an influenza-like syndrome, which may be associated with a rash in about one third of cases and can result in a severe pancytopenia. Fatalities have included a woman also infected with HIV. The organisms form clusters ('morulae') in the cytoplasm of circulating mononuclear leucocytes, which seem to become infected within the reticuloendothelial tissues. In the USA, *E. chaffeensis* is transmitted by the bite of ixodid ticks. These include *Amblyomma americanum* (probably the nymphal stage), which acquires the infection from the common white-tailed deer of which over 50% may be seropositive. Infection has also been associated with the bites of *Rhipicephalus sanguineus*, which usually feeds on dogs. This zoonosis, which has been identified in humans also in Venezuela, Mali and Portugal, probably has a global distribution and may be distinguished from other rickettsial infections by serology or PCR testing. A closely related organism has been identified in infected humans with so-called 'human granulocytic ehrlichiosis' (HGE) in parts of the USA. This is especially prevalent in areas where Lyme disease occurs. In Connecticut between 1997

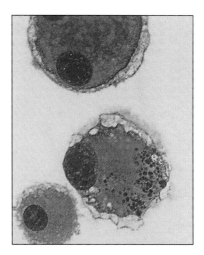

and 1999, positive laboratory findings were obtained in up to 26% of individuals with a history of acute febrile illness and in 50% of *Ixodes scapularis* ticks. Some of the latter were infected, in addition, with *Borrelia burgdorferi*. Human infection with another related organism, *E. sennetsu*, has been reported in Japan and Malaysia. ($\times$ 1500.)

BARTONELLOSIS AND RELATED INFECTIONS

Bartonellosis and related infections are grouped between the rickettsioses and bacterial diseases because of recent work that casts doubt on the taxonomic status of a number of pathogens that are associated with angiomatoses. These include 'Rochalimeae' henselae, which is found in 'cat-scratch disease' (*see* **Table 3**), bacillary angiomatosis (which is also associated with 'Rochalimeae' quintana—usually considered to be the cause of 'trench fever'), as well as *Bartonella bacilliformis*, the agent of Oroya fever (Carrión's disease). The genus *Rochalimeae* is now considered to be a synonym for *Bartonella* on the basis of DNA genotyping. Whereas cat-scratch disease is clearly caused by infection from cats (30–70% of feral cats have been found to be seropositive for *B. henselae* in the USA), bacillary angiomatosis may also follow contact with cats. (The cat flea, *Ctenocephalides felis*, has been found infected with *B. henselae*.) Whereas trench fever (for which the long-tailed vole may be a reservoir host) is transmitted by the body louse, bartonellosis is transmitted by sandflies in certain localities of the Andean highlands. The angiomatosis, Kaposi's sarcoma, has now been found to be due to herpesvirus 8.

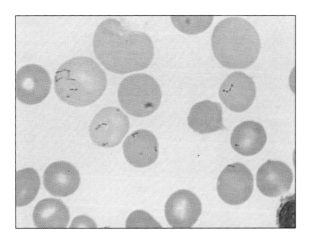

50 Blood film showing *Bartonella bacilliformis* in Carrión's disease

B. bacilliformis is a Gram-negative, intraerythrocytic organism which, in the acute stage, produces fever and acute haemolytic anaemia (Oroya fever), associated with severe bone and joint pains. The infection is fatal in 10–40% of cases within two or three weeks. The organisms also invade reticuloendothelial cells. This disease occurs in Bolivia, Peru, Colombia and Ecuador. (*Giemsa* × *1300*.)

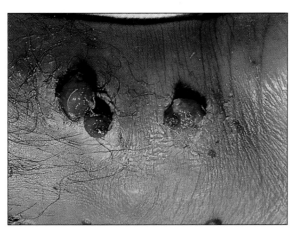

51 Ulcerating lesions of 'Verruga Peruana'

The infection may persist for several months to produce a generalised, verrucous eruption (Carrión's disease), sometimes becoming haemorrhagic in late cases. This figure shows several stages of the lesions, ranging from a very early papilloma to large, ulcerated, angiomatous nodules from which organisms can be cultured. This condition is usually self-healing after two or three months. The disease is transmitted by the sandfly *Lutzomyia verrucarum* at altitudes of 800–3000 m.

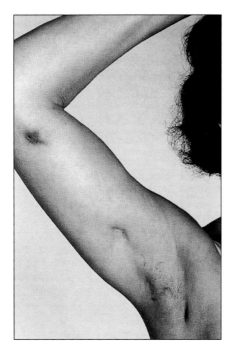

52 Cat-scratch disease

This condition is an exception in that the transmission of the causative organism, *Bartonella henselae*, is by mechanical transmission, usually from feral cats. Numerous sinuses were present in the epitrochlear area and axilla of this patient who presented with a painful lymphadenopathy and lymphangitis.

BACTERIAL INFECTIONS

PLAGUE

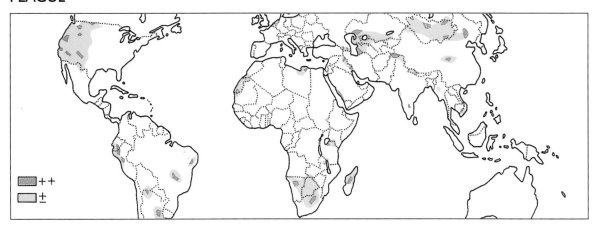

53 Known and probable foci of plague
Plague is a bacterial infection that can be spread through the bites of infected fleas, giving rise to suppurative lymphadenitis ('bubonic plague') or aerosol from humans to humans (causing 'pneumonic plague'). The infection may be epidemic and has been responsible in the past for disastrous pandemics. Plague classically arose when epizootics in *Rattus rattus* and *R. norvegicus* spilled over to humans. However, at the present time infections are usually focal and are associated with enzootic disease that exists in sylvatic rodent species in many areas, including some of the western states of the USA. It has recently been recognised there that cats which prey on infected rodents have, in turn, become infected and served as sources of human infection. In 1992, over 1500 cases of plague were reported from nine countries. Only the deployment of emergency control measures succeeded in cutting short the spread, at national and international level, of an outbreak of plague in the west of India in 1994 that affected at least several thousand of the population. The infection can, however, spread rapidly when social organisation is disrupted, such as in war and other catastrophes, e.g. earthquakes. The collapse of the national surveillance organisation in Eastern Zaire for economic reasons, for example, resulted in an urban outbreak in 1993 that could easily have culminated in a major epidemic. (++—frequent transmission; ±—infrequent or suspected transmission.)

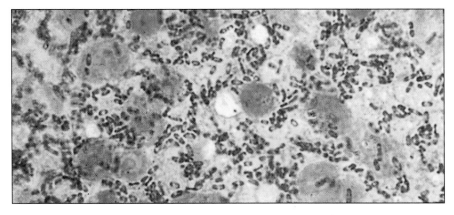

54 *Yersinia pestis* in liver smear
Y. pestis (syn. *Pasteurella pestis*) is a Gram-negative coccobacillus with bipolar staining. It is normally enzootic in rats and is spread to humans by fleas that leave dying rodents. (× 1500.)

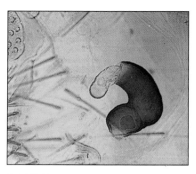
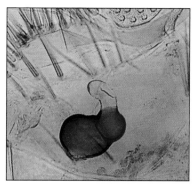
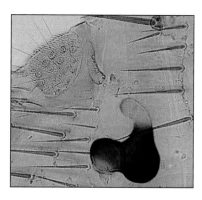

55–57 Spermathecae of female *Xenopsylla* compared

X. cheopis—cosmopolitan (**55**, left); *X. brasiliensis*—Central Africa (**56**, centre); *X. astia*—Oriental region (**57**, right). The rat flea, *X. cheopis*, is the main vector. (× *120.*)

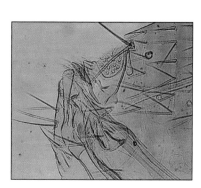
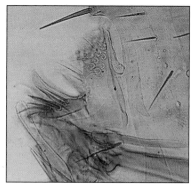
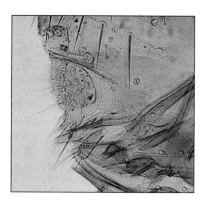

58–60 Male genitalia of *Xenopsylla* compared

X. cheopis (**58**, left) (× *80*); *X. brasiliensis* (**59**, centre) (× *80*); *X. astia* (**60**, right) (× *120.*)

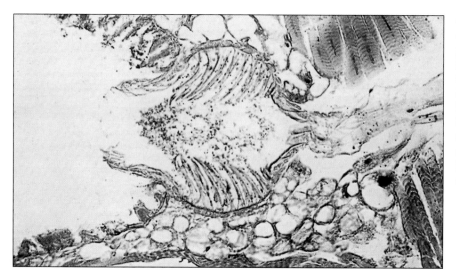

61 Proventriculus of *X. cheopis* blocked by plague bacilli

Hungry fleas abandon dying domestic rats (*R. norvegicus, R. rattus*). The fleas often have their foreguts blocked by bacilli and, in this condition, attempt to feed on any animal. If they bite humans, they transmit the disease. (× *240.*)

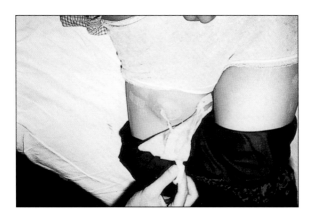

62 Bubonic plague
The organisms pass from the site of the bite to the lymphatics. Fever, and one of the most characteristic clinical features—regional lymphadenopathy with suppuration, especially in the inguinal and axillary regions—commence after an incubation period of less than a week. Infection may proceed to septicaemia with disseminated intravascular coagulation.

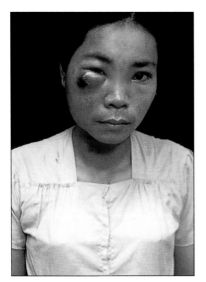

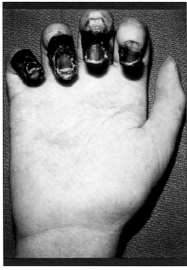

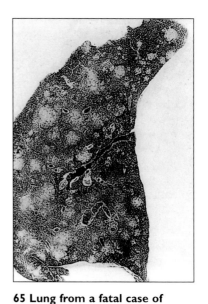

63 Young woman with eschar of an infected flea bite and local facial carbuncle
Such infections yield readily to appropriate antibiotic therapy.

64 Septic plague
This patient with disseminated intravascular coagulation showed cutaneous bleeding and gangrene of the terminal phalanges in a systemic inflammatory response to *Yersinia pestis* septicaemia. (Courtesy of Dr David Dennis, Centers for Disease Control, Fort Collins, Colorado.)

65 Lung from a fatal case of pneumonic plague
Pneumonic infection allows direct spread of bacteria from humans to humans via aerosol. The lower lobe shows intense hyperaemia and haemorrhage with necrotic nodules. The upper lobe contains only necrotic nodules with compensatory emphysemal changes. (AFIP No. 40657.)

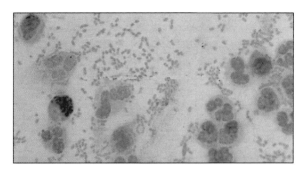

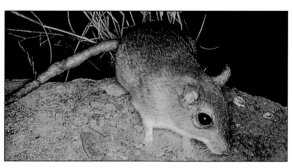

66 *Yersinia pestis* in cerebrospinal fluid
The CSF containing plague bacteria was taken from a patient with meningitis. (*Gram's stain* × *1250*.)

67 *Tatera robusta*
Several gerbils of this genus have been found infected with *Y. pestis* in East and South Africa, as well as in India where they are associated with focal outbreaks in humans.

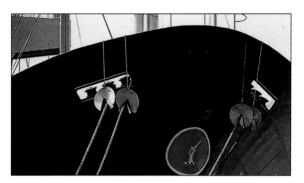

68 Metal guards preventing access of rats along ships' hawsers
Plague control demands strictly enforced rodent control measures and international quarantine regulations, particularly for shipping.

TULARAEMIA

69 Primary ulcer of tularaemia
Francisella (Pasteurella) tularensis is a Gram-negative coccobacillus that affects a wide range of wild rodents but that can also occur in carnivores and some species of birds. Zoonotic infection in man—tularaemia—a plague-like illness, is usually acquired by contact with infected animals, e.g. hunters who prepare animal carcasses, or from the bites of mosquitoes, tabanid flies or ixodid ticks, with infection being trans-stadial in the latter. (The term trans-stadial means that the infection is passed from one stage of the vector's life cycle to the next.) Humans can also become infected by the respiratory or intestinal route. The disease is manifested by ulceration at the site of primary inoculation (as seen here), followed by lymphadenopathy (possibly with suppuration) and fever. Abdominal and pleuropulmonary forms or septicaemia may develop, but the majority of infections seem to remain subclinical. Tularaemia occurs sporadically in North America ('rabbit fever'), parts of Europe, such as Sweden ('lemming fever'), and the former USSR, Central Asia and Japan.

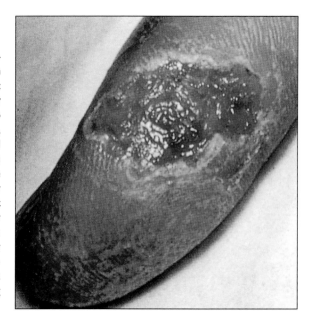

THE RELAPSING FEVERS

(*See* **Table 4**.)

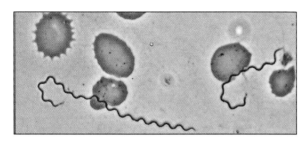

70 *Borrelia duttoni* in human blood film from Tanzania
Endemic relapsing fever—a cosmopolitan disease caused by *B. duttoni*—occurs in rodents and humans. First described in Africa, it occurs also in the Middle East, the Mediterranean basin and the New World. The infection occurs sporadically in the western United States. (*Giemsa—phase contrast* × *1300*.)

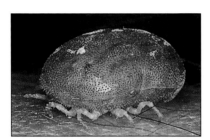

71 Fully engorged *Ornithodorus moubata*
Soft ticks such as *O. moubata* transmit *Borrelia duttoni* from rodents to humans and from humans to humans through infected coxal fluid (seen here between the tick and the skin), which enters skin abrasions. Coxal fluid is the excretory product of the coxal glands resulting from concentration of fluid in the blood meal. As the organism passes from tick to tick by transovarial transmission, the arthropod is itself a reservoir host. In East Africa *O. moubata* lives in soft earth at the base of mudlined walls. (× *5.8*.)

Table 4 Pathogenic spirochaetes of humans

Genus	Species/Serotypes	Mode of transmission	Reservoir	Disease
Leptospira serotype (many other serotypes)	icterohaemorrhagiae canicola	water water	rats dogs, pigs, cattle	leptospirosis, Weil's disease canicola fever
Borrelia	recurrentis duttoni burgdorferi other spp.	*Pediculus humanus* *Ornithodorus* *Ixodes* *Ornithodorus* spp.	none none rodents various mammals, birds etc.	louse-borne relapsing fever tick-borne relapsing fever Lyme disease Asiatic, African, South American relapsing fevers
Treponema	pallidum pertenue carateum vincenti[1]	venereal, congenital endemic contact contact contact	none none none none ? none	syphilis bejel yaws pinta Vincent's angina, secondary infections
Spirillum	minus[2]		rodents, other small mammals	rat-bite fever

[1] Placed by some authors in the genus *Borrelia*.
[2] Not strictly a spirochaete as it is flagellated.

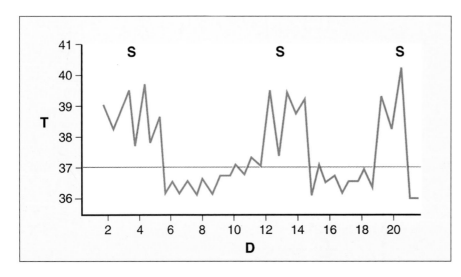

72 Temperature chart of tick-borne relapsing fever
The infection acquires its name from the typical relapsing nature of the fever. *Borrelia duttoni* appears in the blood only during the febrile episodes, which are numerous and of short duration. [D—day of illness; T—temperature (°C); S—spirochaetes in blood.]

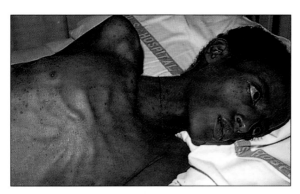

73 Louse-borne relapsing fever in an Ethiopian
Borrelia recurrentis transmitted by body lice occurs in epidemic form in Ethiopia and Eritrea. The febrile periods recur usually on one or two occasions only (up to five in some cases, however). This patient, who presented with fever, jaundice and large petechial haemorrhages on the trunk, was severely emaciated. Mortality in untreated patients may be as high as 40% during epidemics. (© D.A. Warrell.)

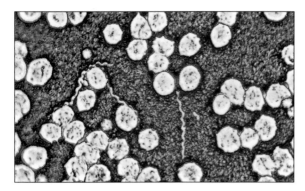

74 *Borrelia recurrentis* in blood film
Infection is acquired from the body fluids of lice crushed on the skin while scratching. The spirochaetal organisms are readily seen in this Indian ink preparation. (× 800.)

LYME DISEASE

Lyme disease is a zoonosis of rodents caused by several species of *Borrelia*, which are spread by the bites of infected ixodid ticks. Human infection is caused by *B. burgdorferi sensu stricto*, *B. afzelii* and *B. garinii*. It is now recognised to be cosmopolitan in distribution. In humans, three stages are recognised: (I) an acute phase often associated with a rash, (II) early disseminated infection involving the circulatory, nervous and skeletal systems and (III) a chronic stage of multiple organ involvement, which may only become apparent months or years after the initial infection.

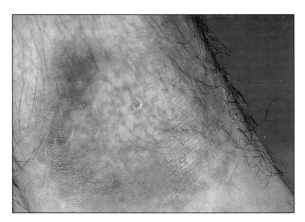

75 Erythema chronicum migrans
This unusual type of chronic rash is associated with the early stage of Lyme disease. It spreads centrifugally in one or two weeks following infection and usually resolves spontaneously within a month or two. In some patients, acrodermatitis chronica atrophicans can develop in the chronic stage III.

76 Arthritis caused by *Borrelia burgdorferi* infection
Acute arthritis and chronic, disabling arthritic lesions (both usually associated with skin lesions) are late sequelae of Lyme disease. Neurological changes such as meningoencephalitis (sometimes with cranial or peripheral radiculopathy) are being increasingly reported. The severity of lesions associated with *B. burgdorferi* may be related to host genetic

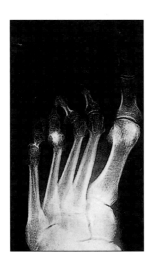

factors. The infection, in fact, seems to produce protean manifestations, and the diagnosis is probably missed in many cases. If the diagnosis—which may be confirmed by culturing the organisms from skin or other tissues and by serology—is made sufficiently early, the disease is usually cured rapidly by chemotherapy.

77 Adult female *Ixodes dammini*
The larvae and nymphs of *I. dammini* feed mainly on rodents but occasionally on humans, to whom they pass the spirochaetes from the rodent reservoirs. This species is responsible for the transmission of Lyme disease in the northeast of Canada and the USA,

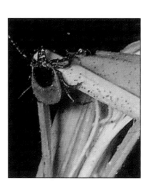

where it is also the vector of *Theileria microti*. The organisms are transmitted trans-stadially (see **69**). (× 2.5.)

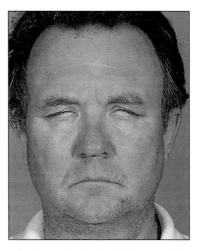

78 Bilateral Bell's palsy lesion in Lyme disease
Meningoradiculitis leading to bilateral, peripheral, facial palsy (Bannwarth's syndrome), was caused by Lyme borreliosis (confirmed serologically) in this 50-year-old German patient. The majority of neurological lesions improve spontaneously with time. In this case, the right facial palsy recovered completely after chemotherapy but the left only partially.

79 *Peromyscus leucopus*: the white-footed mouse—permethrin-impregnated acaricide for control of *Ixodes dammini*.

P. leucopus is the most important maintenance host for *Borrelia burgdorferi* on the eastern seaboard of the USA. Other rodent species harbour the organisms in other countries, e.g. species of *Apodemus* and *Clethrionomys* in Europe where *Ixodes ricinus* is an important vector. Careful ecological observations revealed that this rodent likes to line its nest with soft materials such as cotton wool. When the wild rodents are provided with a ready source of this material in the form of cotton wool balls impregnated with a synthetic pyrethroid, they convey the acaricide into their nests where it kills the rodents' ticks, thus interrupting the cycle of transmission both of Lyme disease and *Theileria microti* (see **83**).

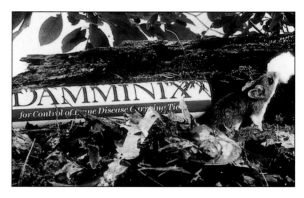

This is a prime example of the importance of good field work and its practical application.

80 Female blackbird (*Turdus merula*) infested with larvae and lymphs of *Ixodes ricinus*

Two thirds of the ticks found on birds in surveys in Switzerland were larvae and one third nymphs, among which 25% were infected with *Borrelia burgdorferi*.

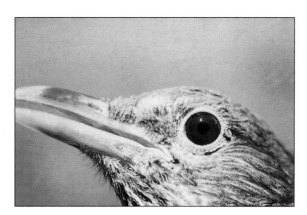

RAT-BITE FEVER ('SODOKU')

81 A patient with 'Sodoku' following a rat bite

Infection with *Spirillum minus* in this young Brazilian woman following a rat bite resulted in a local ulcerative lesion associated with high fever and cervical lymphadenopathy. The spirochaete-like organisms were detected by dark field examination of material from the ulcer. This patient's infection responded to antibiotic therapy, but untreated infections may cause death in over 10% of cases. *Streptobacillus moniliformis* is another infection associated with rat bites.

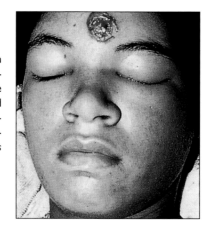

PROTOZOAL INFECTIONS

(*See* **Table 5**.)

PIROPLASMOSIS IN HUMANS

The piroplasms in humans have been reclassified into several genera (*see* **Table 5**). Whereas most piroplasmosis is rare and usually occurs in immunocompromised (e.g. splenectomised) individuals, zoonotic infection with *Theileria microti* is relatively common in parts of North America. The infections are transmitted by various species of ticks from animal reservoir hosts.

82 *Microbabesia divergens* in human blood
Human infection with species of piroplasms from cattle is a rare occurrence. Infection in normal people with other piroplasms may give rise to a self-limiting fever and parasitaemia, e.g. the rodent parasite *Theileria microti* on the eastern seaboard of the USA. Heavy red-cell infection may develop, however, in splenectomised patients, leading to fatal haemolytic

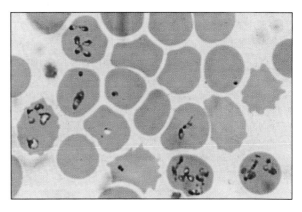

anaemia. This patient died from an infection acquired from the cattle parasite, *M. divergens*, in Scotland. (*Giemsa* × *700*.)

Table 5 Protozoa (phylum Apicomplexa) of medical importance

Phylum	Subclass	Order	Family	Genus and Species
SARCOMASTIGOPHORA (see **Tables 17** and **18**)				
CILIOPHORA (see **Table 17**)				
MICROSPORA (see **Table 19**)				
APICOMPLEXA				
	PIROPLASMASINA		Theileriidae[1]	*Theileria microti*
			Babesiidae[1]	*Microbabesia bovis*
				M. divergens
				Babesia spp.
				Entopolypoides sp.
	COCCIDIASINA			
		EUCOCCIDIORIDA		
		Suborder HAEMOSPORORINA	Plasmodiidae	*Plasmodium (Plasmodium) vivax*
				P. (P.) ovale
				P.(P.) malariae
				P. (Laverania) falciparum
		Suborder EIMERIORINA	Sarcocystidae	*Toxoplasma gondii*
				Sarcocystis hominis[2]
				S. suihominis[3]
				Sarcocystis spp.[4]
			Eimeriidae	*Isospora belli*
				Cyclospora cayetanensis
			Cryptosporidiidae	*Cryptosporidium* spp.

[1] All rare in human.
[2] Human definitive; cattle intermediate, hosts.
[3] Human definitive, pig intermediate, hosts.
[4] '*Sarcocystis lindemanni*' consists of a number of unidentified species for which humans are the intermediate host.

83 *Theileria microti* in human blood
This blood film was made from a German forest worker who had earlier been bitten by a nymphal ixodid tick, probably *Ixodes ricinus*. The patient had a mild, self-limiting fever only. There is an interesting parallel between zoonotic infection with *Th. microti* and *Borrelia burgdorferi* in several countries. (*Giemsa* × 2600.)

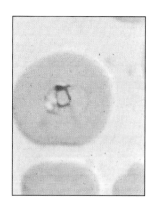

84 Unfed adult female *Ixodes ricinus* (sheep tick)
This common tick of cattle and sheep is widely distributed throughout Europe and the former Soviet Union. It is responsible for the transmission not only of piroplasmosis but also of European tick encephalitis and other arboviruses, including louping-ill of cattle, which occasionally affects humans. (× 4.5.)

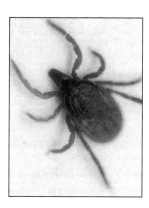

MALARIA

(See **Tables 5, 6.**)

Table 6 *Anopheles* mosquitoes known to transmit malaria

| Geographical zone[1] | Species in subgenera | | | |
	Anopheles	*Cellia*	*Nyssorhynchus*	*Kerteszia*
North American	freeborni[2] quadrimaculatus[2]		albimanus[2]	
Central American	aztecus punctimacula		albimanus[3] albitarsis allopha aquasalis[3] argyritarsis[3] darlingi[3]	
South American	pseudopunctipennis[3] punctimacula		albimanus[3] albitarsis[3] aquasalis[3] argyritarsis[3] braziliensis darlingi[3] nuneztovari s. l.[3]	bellator cruzii
North Eurasian	atroparvus[2 3] messeae[2] sacharovi sinensis	pattoni		
Mediterranean	atroparvus[3] claviger labranchiae[2] messeae sacharovi[2]	hispaniola pattoni		
Afro-Arabian		hispaniola multicolor pharoensis s. l.[3] sergentii[3]		

Table 6 *Continued*

Geographical zone[1]	Species in subgenera			
	Anopheles	**Cellia**	**Nyssorhynchus**	**Kerteszia**
Afrotropical		*arabiensis*[3]		
		funestus[3]		
		gambiae[3]		
		melas[3]		
		merus		
		moucheti		
		nili		
		pharoensis s.l.		
Indo-Iranian	*sacharovi*	*annularis*		
		culicifacies s.l.[3]		
		fluviatilis[3]		
		pulcherrimus		
		stephensi		
		superpictus		
		tesselatus		
Indo-Chinese hills	*nigerrimus*	*annularis*		
		culicifacies s.l.		
		dirus s.l.[3]		
		fluviatilis[3]		
		maculatus s.l.		
		minimus[3]		
Malaysian	*campestris*[3]	*aconitus*[3]		
	donaldi[3]	*balabacensis*[3]		
	letifer[3]	*dirus* s.l.[3]		
	nigerrimus[3]	*leucosphyrus*[3]		
	whartoni	*ludlowae*[3]		
		maculatus s.l.[3]		
		minimus[3]		
		philippinensis		
		subpictus s.l.		
		sundaicus		
Chinese	*anthropophagus*	*pattoni*		
	sinensis			
Australasian	*bancrofti*	*annulipes* s.l.		
		farauti s.l.[3]		
		karwari		
		koliensis[3]		
		punctulatus[3]		
		subpictus s.l.		

[1] Equivalent to 'malariological zone' as defined by Macdonald (1957) *Epidemiology and control of malaria*, Oxford University Press, London.

[2] Species no longer of importance as vectors in this zone.

[3] Most important species in this zone.

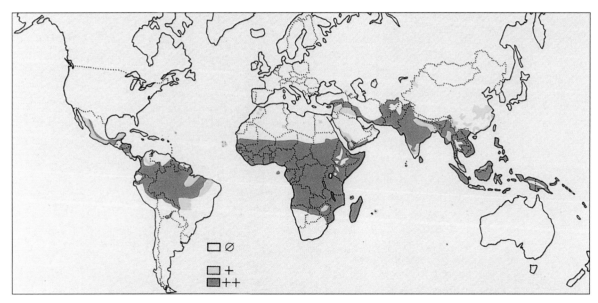

85 Distribution map of malaria
Despite intensive control measures over the past 50 years, malaria is still widely distributed in the tropics and subtropics. The breakdown of large scale vector control operations and the emergence of multiple drug resistance in some of the parasites has led even to an actual increase in the incidence of malaria in some regions. [Ø—areas where malaria has disappeared, been eradicated or never existed; +—areas with limited risk; ++—areas where malaria transmission occurs; (adapted from WHO, 1999, *Map No. WHO 99419 EF.*)

86 Generalised life cycle of a malaria parasite
The diagram is based on the life cycle of *Plasmodium vivax* and *P. ovale*. The invertebrate cycles of all malaria species of humans and other mammals are similar and take place in female anopheline mosquitoes only. The sexual stages (1), male (micro-) gametocytes and female (macro-) gametocytes are taken (2) into the stomach of a female *Anopheles* when it feeds. Within the blood meal (which is surrounded by a peritrophic membrane secreted by the mosquito gut cells), the gametocytes mature to the microgametes and macrogametes, which fuse (3); the resulting zygote forms a motile ookinete (also known as a 'travelling vermicule') (4). This ookinete penetrates the peritrophic membrane and then the midgut wall and comes to rest between the outer membrane of the midgut and the midgut epithelial cells. There it develops into an oocyst (5) within which develop several thousand sporozoites. When mature (after about seven to 20 days—depending on the host and parasite species and the environmental temperature), the sporozoites escape into the body cavity by rupturing the oocyst wall; they then migrate through the body cavity and penetrate into the acini of the salivary glands (6). After a further, brief period of maturation there, they enter the salivary ducts from where they are passed into a new vertebrate

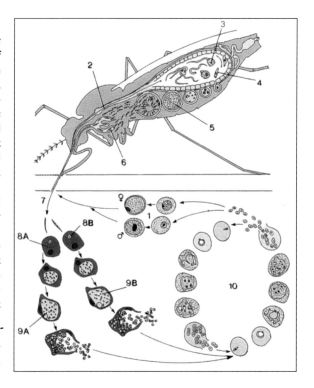

host (7) when the mosquito next feeds. In humans, the sporozoites pass via the blood stream into parenchymal cells of the liver (8A) where they form large, pre-erythrocytic schizonts (9A) in which form several thousand daughter cells, called merozoites. After about seven to 21 days (depending on parasite species), these merozoites enter red blood cells within the hepatic sinusoids to start the asexual intraerythrocytic cycle (10) and to form new gametocytes

(1). The asexual red cell stages are responsible for the pathological changes that occur in malaria. In the true relapsing species of *Plasmodium* (i.e. *P. vivax* and *P. ovale* in humans), some sporozoites remain latent as rounded, unicellular hypnozoites (8B) that only start the process of pre-erythrocytic schizogony (9B) several months after they first arrive in the hepatocytes. This stage does not exist in *P. falciparum* or *P. malariae*. (See **89–95, 122, 128–132** *and* **137**.)

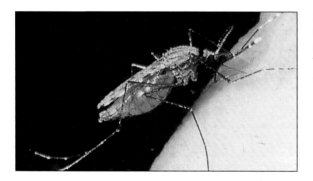

87 *Anopheles gambiae* biting
Malaria is transmitted by female *Anopheles* mosquitoes. Most species bite indoors at night but some are outdoor feeders. The adults are recognised by the antennae and palps. (*See also* **9** *and* **11**.) (× 4.)

88 Breeding site of *Anopheles gambiae* in West Africa
A. *gambiae* and closely related species are the most dangerous malaria vectors in tropical Africa. A. *gambiae* breeds in small temporary collections of fresh surface water exposed to sunlight and in such sites as residual pools in drying river beds. The majority of important vectors in other parts of the world are also surface-water breeders. Malaria control operations since the early 1950s were based mainly on the destruction of house haunting anopheline vectors by DDT or other insecticides sprayed on the interior walls where mosquitoes usually rest before and/or after feeding; larviciding played a relatively minor role. Some South American vectors of the subgenus *Anopheles (Kerteszia)* breed in the axils of bromeliads, the destruction of which is possible only on a very limited scale in most endemic areas. The adults bite out-

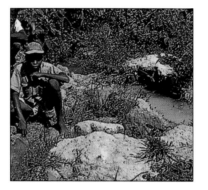

doors rather than indoors. Consequently, the control of these vectors by insecticides is often extremely difficult.

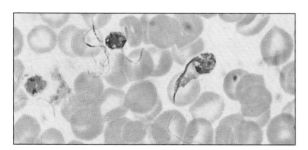

89 Development of male gametes
Male gametes develop by a process of flagellar extrusion, known as exflagellation, from microgametocytes contained in the blood meal in the midgut of the female anopheline (× 950.)

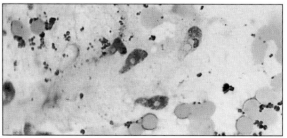

90 Ookinetes in midgut
Male and female gametes fuse to produce motile ookinetes, which enter midgut epithelial cells. (× 950.)

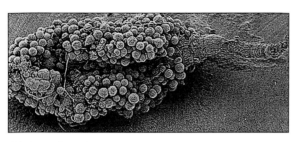

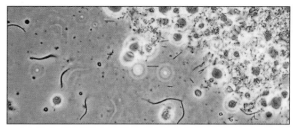

91 Scanning electron micrograph of oocysts outside anopheline midgut
Infective stages (sporozoites) develop in oocysts, which lie on the outside of the mosquito's midgut. (× 65.)

92 Living infective sporozoites
Bow-shaped sporozoites emerge from the oocysts and enter the insect's salivary glands. They are passed into the small vessels of the skin with saliva when the mosquito next takes a blood meal. (× 370.)

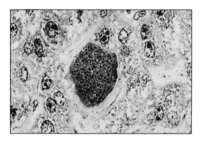

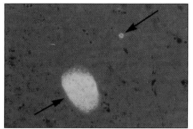

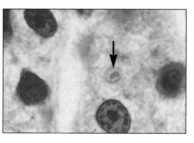

93 Exoerythrocytic schizont of *Plasmodium malariae* in liver
Within 30 minutes the sporozoites enter the parenchymal cells of the host's liver where they may form large pre-erythrocytic (PE) 'tissue' schizonts or, in *P. vivax* and *P. ovale*, hypnozoites (see **89** and **90**). The PE schizonts mature in six to 14 days according to the species, before liberating daughter cells ('merozoites') into the hepatic circulation. (*Giemsa– colophonium technique* × 350.)

94 Hypnozoite and pre-erythrocytic schizont in liver biopsy
The unicellular, dormant hypnozoite (arrowed, right) stands in sharp contrast to the maturing pre-erythrocytic schizont (left) in this fluorescent antibody-stained section of rhesus monkey liver containing *Plasmodium cynomolgi*—a relapsing species with the same life cycle as *P. vivax*. (× 270.)

95 Hypnozoite of *Plasmodium cynomolgi*
Enlarged view of a single hypnozoite. (*Giemsa–colophonium technique* × 2000.)

96 Tertian and quartan fever patterns
The asexual blood stages of *Plasmodium falciparum*, *P. vivax* and *P. ovale* require 48 hours to complete their schizogony. Fever is produced when the schizonts mature, i.e. at 48-hour intervals. This gives the classic tertian periodicity, which is, however, uncommon in a primary attack of *P. falciparum* malaria. *P. malariae* requires 72 hours and is associated with quartan fever, i.e. 72 hours between paroxysms. [D—day of illness; T—temperature (°C).]

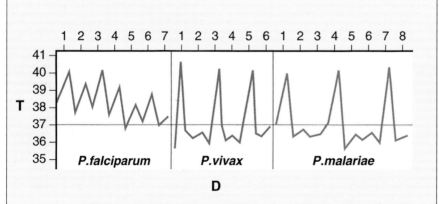

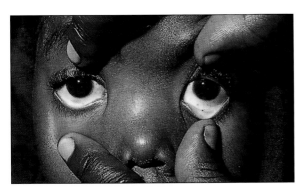

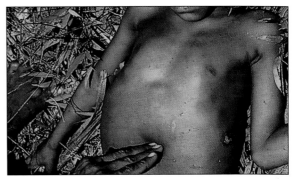

97 Malarial anaemia
The pathogenesis of malarial anaemia is multifactorial, involving destruction of parasitised cells, haemolysis of uninfected cells, dyserythropoiesis and iron sequestration. In parts of Africa, malarial anaemia is an important cause of death in children under two years of age. This young Kenyan boy with *Plasmodium falciparum* parasitaemia had profound anaemia, with a haemoglobin concentration of 12 g/l. (*See also* **1037**.) (© D.A. Warrell.)

98 Child with grossly enlarged liver and spleen
Haemolysed red cells and parasite debris are phagocytosed by macrophages, particularly of the spleen and liver (which become enlarged). This child was seen on a field survey in a holoendemic area of northern Papua New Guinea.

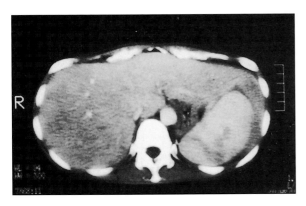

99 Massive hepatosplenomegaly in a patient with severe malarial anaemia
Computed tomogram of the abdomen of a traveller from West Africa who presented with a haemoglobin concentration of less than 50 g/l. The tomogram shows a massively enlarged liver, the left lobe of which is encircling an enlarged spleen.

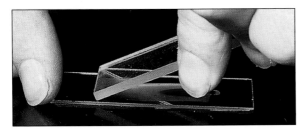

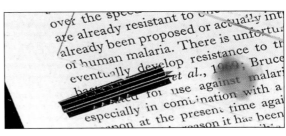

100 & 101 Preparation of thick and thin blood films
Although a number of rapid diagnostic tests such as those figured in **102, 103** as well as polymerase chain reaction are becoming widely available, the 'gold standard' diagnosis of malaria is still based primarily on the recognition of parasites in well prepared thick and thin blood films stained with a Romanowsky-type stain (Giemsa, Leishman, Field, etc.) at pH 7.2–7.4. A small drop of blood from a finger or ear is placed on a clean slide. The thin film is made by pulling a second slide away from the drop (**100**, left). A thick film is made by spreading two or three larger drops on a slide, then spreading them out with the corner of a second slide. The thick smear should still be sufficiently transparent to see print through it, as shown here (**101**, right). Sophisticated diagnostic tools such as *Plasmodium*-specific DNA probes are of value mainly for epidemiological surveys but are of little value in diagnosing malaria in individual patients.

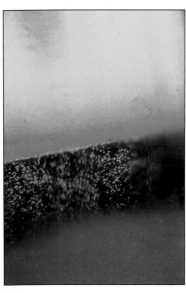

102 Diagnostic test based on fluorescent staining of centrifuged blood

In this technique a fluorescent stain (green in this case) is used to stain malaria parasites in blood containing anticoagulant, which is centrifuged in a special capillary tube containing a float. With ultraviolet epi-illumination, the parasites can readily be seen just beneath the buffy coat and in a thinned-out layer of red cells. The procedure can also be used to detect other parasites such as trypanosomes (*see also* **184**) and microfilariae. (Figure of QBC test[R] by courtesy of Becton Dickinson, Tropical Diseases Diagnostics, Sparks, Maryland, USA.) (× 40.)

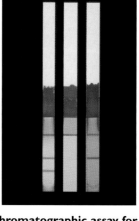

103 Immunochromatographic assay for *Plasmodium falciparum* and *P. vivax*

To aid the rapid diagnosis of *P. falciparum* and other species of malaria in individual patients and for ease and speed of diagnosis as an alternative to microscopy in field surveys, a simple immunochromatographic assay has been devised, which is based on the use of monoclonal antibodies. These recognise the presence, in very small quantities, of isoforms of lactate dehydrogenase (pLDH) that differ from the LDH of the host erythrocytes. The paper-like dipstick, which is impregnated with antibodies and dye-containing microcapsules, is reported to detect as few as 100–200 parasites/µl of blood, i.e., a parasitaemia of 0.002%. In this figure the left-hand strip shows a positive reaction for *P. falciparum* and the right-hand strip a positive reaction for *P. vivax, P. ovale* or *P. malariae*. The centre strip is a negative control. (Figure of OptiMAL[R] Rapid Malaria Test by courtesy of Dr D Bashforth DiaMed, Cressier, Switzerland.)

Plasmodium falciparum

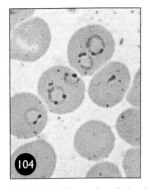

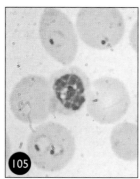

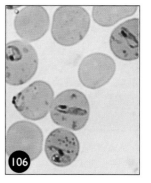

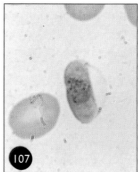

104–108 Life cycle of the blood stages (thin blood films)

Fine rings (**104**) predominate, with mature trophozoites and schizonts (**105**) appearing uncommonly in the peripheral circulation because parasites bind (cytoadhere) to the post capillary venules of the internal organs. Host cells are not enlarged. Basophilic clefts and spots of irregular shape and size (Maurer's clefts and dots) may be seen in erythrocytes containing more mature parasites. They are thought to be aggregates of parasite proteins that are being exported from the parasite to the surface of the red cell (**106**). Crescent-shaped male (**107**) and female gametocytes (**108**) are diagnostic. Infection with *Plasmodium falciparum* gives rise to 'malignant tertian malaria,' so-called because severe, often lethal complications such as those figured later can develop; such cases must be treated as medical emergencies. (*Giemsa* × 1500.)

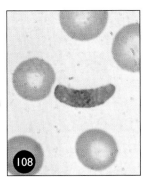

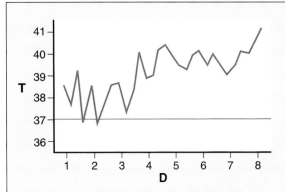

112 Temperature chart in falciparum malaria

In first infections the fever is usually irregular rather than tertian. Thrombocytopenia is commonly found. Relapses do not occur after adequate treatment with blood schizontocides because there are no hypnozoites and hence no secondary tissue schizogony (*c.f. P. vivax* and *P. ovale*). Recrudescences, as opposed to relapses, occur when treatment is inadequate and asexual parasites are not cleared from the blood. [D—day of illness; T—temperature (°C).]

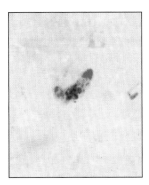

109 & 110 Thick blood films

Usually only young rings (**109**, left) are seen in acute infections, although sometimes in very large numbers. Heavy parasitaemia leads to severe haemolytic anaemia. Gametocytes (**110**, right) appear about a week after the onset of the illness. (*Field* × 1500.)

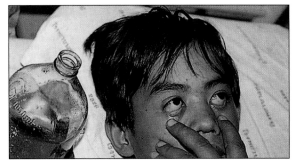

113 Malarial haemoglobinuria, 'Blackwater fever'

This condition may be due to severe intravascular haemolysis and is mainly seen in semi-immune patients. More commonly, however, haemoglobinuria is due to haemolysis developing in patients deficient in the enzyme glucose-6-phosphate dehydrogenase, in response to oxidant antimalarials, e.g. primaquine, quinine or other drugs. Note the small quantity of very dark urine passed by this Thai patient and the pale conjunctivae. (© D.A. Warrell.)

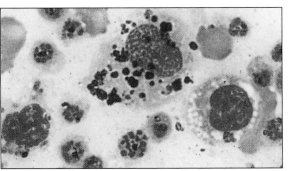

111 Macrophages from spleen of a patient with acute falciparum malaria

Parasitised erythrocytes and malaria pigment (haemozoin) are segregated from the peripheral circulation in reticuloendothelial organs. Pigment in macrophages and falciparum schizonts are seen in this spleen smear. (*Giemsa* × 1500.)

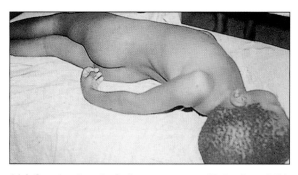

114 Cerebral malaria in a comatose Malawian child with opisthotonus

In holoendemic areas of Africa, cerebral malaria commonly occurs in children between six months and three years of age—often older than those with severe malarial anaemia. The opening pressures of cerebrospinal fluid are often raised in children when measured at lumbar puncture. About 10% of children who survive cerebral malaria have neurological sequelae. These include hemiparesis, cerebellar ataxia, cortical blindness, severe hypotonia, mental retardation, generalised spasticity, and aphasia.

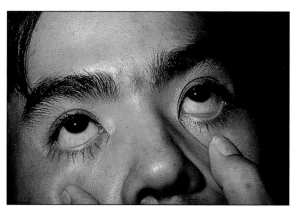

116 Severe malarial jaundice

Deep jaundice, which is clearly seen in this Vietnamese man who had severe falciparum malaria, is much more common in adults than in children. Liver failure, however, occurs only in individuals in whom a concurrent viral hepatitis is present. (© D.A. Warrell.)

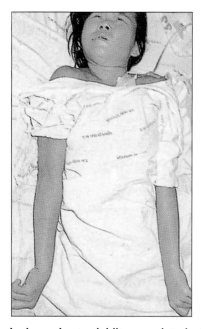

115 Classic decerebrate rigidity associated with hypoglycaemia

This Thai woman with cerebral malaria displays classic decerebrate rigidity, which was almost certainly due to a profound quinine-induced hypoglycaemia. The latter is more common during pregnancy, when the warning signs are fits, abnormal behaviour and a change in the level of consciousness. (© D.A. Warrell.)

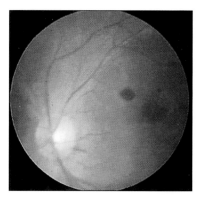

117 Retinal haemorrhage in severe falciparum malaria

Examination of the fundus is an important part of the physical examination of a patient with falciparum malaria. In this Thai patient with cerebral malaria, the haemorrhage is near the macula. Such haemorrhages have been found in as many as 18–30% of patients with cerebral malaria and are an indication for parenteral therapy. In children, papilloedema and extramacular retinal oedema predict a poor prognosis. (© D.A. Warrell.)

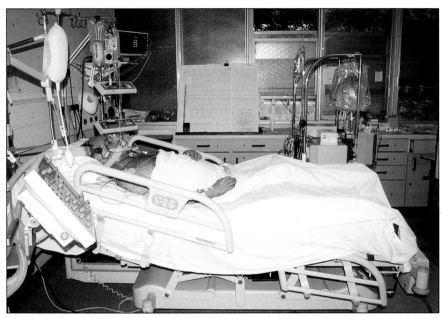

118 Multiorgan failure in severe falciparum malaria
This patient in an intensive therapy unit presented with renal failure and is being haemdiafiltered. In addition he developed Gram-negative septicaemia with hypotension and metabolic acidosis ('algid malaria'). These complications developed without signs of cerebral malaria.

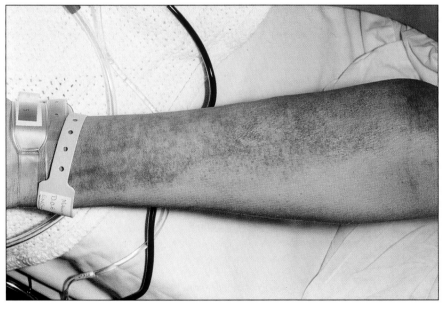

119 Disseminated intravascular coagulation in falciparum malaria
Bleeding into the skin seen in a patient who demonstrated disseminated intravascular coagulation with thrombocytopenia, a prolonged prothrombin time, increased fibrinogen degradation products and hypofibrinogenaemia. He had no signs of cerebral malaria.

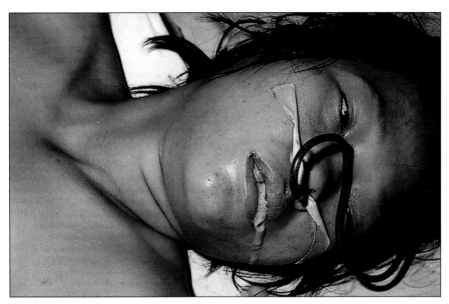

120 Acute pulmonary oedema
Two types of pulmonary oedema occur in severe falciparum malaria. The first, due to overhydration, is preventable with good management of the patient. The second, acute respiratory distress syndrome occurs during the fourth or fifth day of the illness when the patient seems to be improving; its causation is not clearly understood. This Vietnamese woman in addition had cerebral malaria complicated by hypoglycaemia.
(© D.A. Warrell.)

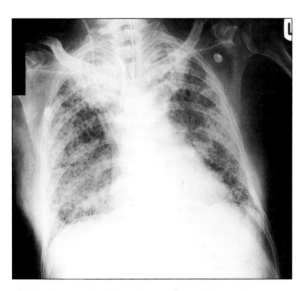

121 Radiograph of the chest of a patient with acute respiratory distress syndrome
The radiograph shows new, bilateral, diffuse, homogeneous pulmonary infiltrates without evidence of cardiac failure, fluid overload or chronic lung disease in an adult with severe falciparum malaria. This condition is rare in children.

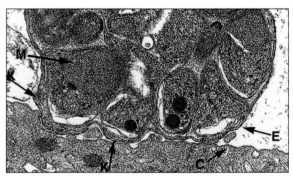

122 Electron micrograph of mature *Plasmodium falciparum* schizont in a red cell
The merozoites (M) form asexual parasites, which grow inside erythrocytes to form the trophozoites. These ingest haemoglobin, producing insoluble pigment (haemozoin) as a waste product. When growth is complete, the parasites undergo cell division (schizogony) and the daughter cells (merozoites), after rupture of the host erythrocyte membrane (E), invade new red cells. Note the small protrusions ('knobs', K) on the surface of the host cell. These are associated with the cytoadherence of *P. falciparum*-parasitised erythrocytes to the endothelium of post capillary venules (C) in the brain and other deep organs. (× *9000*.)

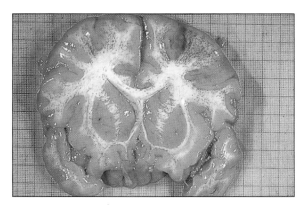

123 Gross section of brain in cerebral malaria

Cerebral malaria results when cerebral capillaries are blocked by erythrocytes containing developing falciparum schizonts (*see also* 124). The blockages lead to petechial haemorrhages around many of the capillaries, as seen in this section. Cerebral malaria is a medical emergency, which demands immediate treatment by intravenous administration of suitable antimalarials. Rehydration is also often required, but careful attention must be paid to avoiding overhydration, which may result in pulmonary oedema. It is now recognised that other factors such as the over-production of certain cytokines (e.g. tumour necrosis factor), are involved in the pathogenesis of cerebral malaria.

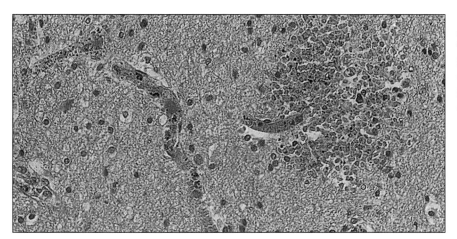

124 Microscopic section of brain

The blockage of a capillary has led to its disruption and the formation of a microhaemorrhage.
(*H&E* × *200.*)

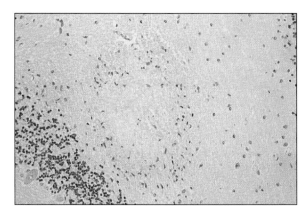

125 Dürck's granuloma

This histological section of a post mortem specimen from a patient with cerebral malaria shows focal areas of necrosis with lymphocytic infiltration. Dürck's granulomata are probably the sequelae of what, at the time of acute malaria, would appear as small microhaemorrhages around the small vessels in the brain.

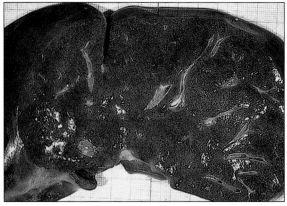

126 Liver in chronic malaria

In chronic infection, accumulation of malaria pigment (haemozoin) in the macrophages produces a dark brown colouration of liver and spleen.

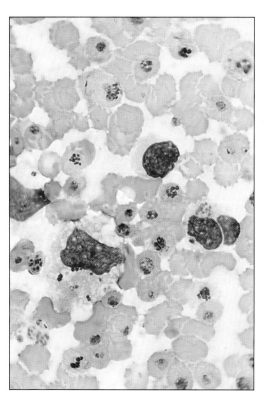

127 Placental smear with falciparum schizonts and macrophage

The accumulation of falciparum schizonts in the maternal side of the placental circulation may result in the delivery of underweight infants, especially in primigravidae. True congenital malaria is very rare. Note the presence of haemozoin granules in the macrophage. Pigment-loaded macrophages and neutrophils in the peripheral circulation usually indicate that the blood infection has been present for some days. (*Giemsa* × *900.*)

Plasmodium vivax

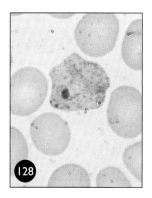

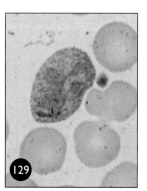

128–132 Life cycle of the blood stages (thin films)

All stages of asexual parasites—from young trophozoites (**128**) to schizonts—appear in the peripheral circulation in vivax malaria together with gametocytes. The parasites are large and amoeboid (**129**) and produce schizonts with about 16 daughter cells (merozoites) (**130**). Pigment is well developed. Host red cells are enlarged and uniformly covered with fine eosinophilic stippling (Schüffner's dots). Gametocytes are round, with the male (microgametocytes) (**131**) being about 7 µm and the female (macrogametocytes) (**132**) 10 µm or more in diameter. (*Giemsa* × *1500.*) (*See also* **86**.)

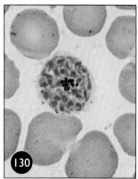

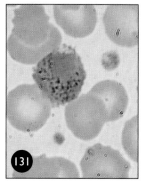

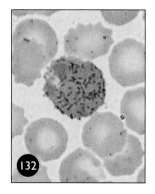

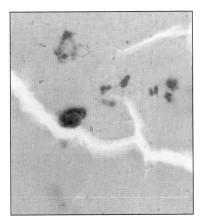
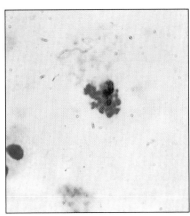
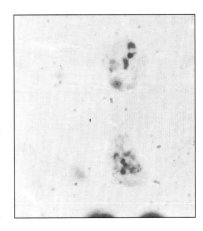

133–135 Thick blood films
All stages of parasites may be present; parasitaemia is often less heavy than in falciparum malaria; thrombocytopenia is commonly found. The parasites seen here are all in a single thick film: in the thicker part are amoeboid trophozoites (**133**, left); in a thinner part, a schizont with centrally clumped pigment (**134**, centre) is visible. Two young trophozoites are seen in **135** (right). Sometimes, as in this film, the Schüffner's dots can be seen as 'ghost cells' in the thinner parts of the film where the host cell has been haemolysed. (*Field* × *1500*.)

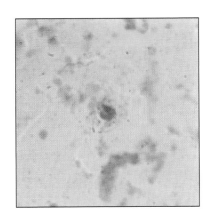

136 Thick film of *Plasmodium ovale*
The Schüffner's (James') dots of *P. ovale* also may show up in a thick film as a 'ghost cell,' but the parasite can be distinguished from *P. vivax* by the solid appearance and heavy pigment even of young trophozoites (*c.f.* **139**). (*Field* × *1500*.)

137 Diagram of relapse patterns in vivax malaria
Variations in parasitaemia over time after inoculation are shown. The primary attack (1) arises from the first generation of schizonts in the hepatocytes (pre-erythrocytic (PE) schizogony). One or more recrudescences (2) arise when subpatent intraerythrocytic asexual parasites escape the host immunity. True relapses (3, 4, 5, etc.), as opposed to recrudescences, occur when new generations of merozoites are later released from previously dormant hypnozoites (H) that undergo secondary schizogony in hepatocytes. In tropical areas, the first relapses may arise within three to four months of a primary attack but, in subtropical areas, usually only after nine months or more. The fever threshold (FT) rises with increasing immunity, i.e. the host tolerates the parasitaemia. Also, with increasing immunity, smaller numbers of merozoites survive in the erythrocytes and the infection may become subpatent (i.e. below the microscopic thresh-

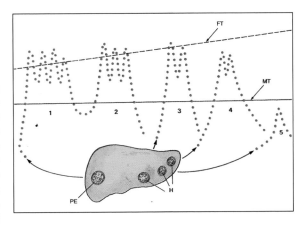

old—MT), although still present. Most *P. vivax* infections will die out within one to three years, even if untreated.

Plasmodium ovale

138–142 Life cycle of the blood stages (thin films)
Like *Plasmodium vivax*, *P. ovale* sporozoites can develop immediately into first generation pre-erythrocytic schizonts or into hypnozoites, which are responsible for long-term relapses. These can occur over many years if untreated. Intra-erythrocytic ring forms (**138**) have a prominent nucleus. The older

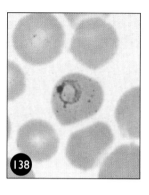
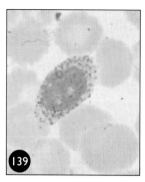
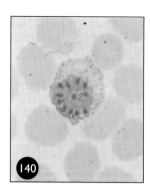

parasites (**139**) differ from *P. vivax* in being more compact and producing about eight merozoites at schizogony (**140**). As with *P. vivax*, the host red cells contain Schüffner's dots (sometimes called James' stippling) and tend to be ovoid and fimbriated. Male (micro-) and female (macro-) gametocytes (**141** and **142**) are smaller than those of *P. vivax*. Relapses occur as with *P. vivax*, but the disease tends to be more chronic (*Leishman* × *1500*). (See **136** *for thick film*.)

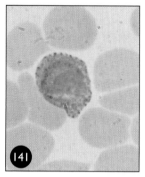
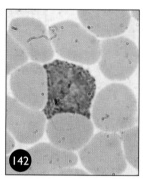
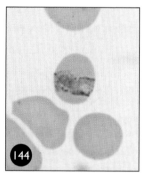
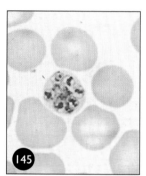

Plasmodium malariae

143–147 Life cycle of the blood stages (thin films)
The sporozoites of this species do not produce a relapsing, hypnozoite stage. All intraerythrocytic stages may appear in the peripheral circulation, from young trophozoites (**143**) to compact schizonts (**145**) with eight merozoites. 'Band forms' (**144**) stretching across the red cell as if in a

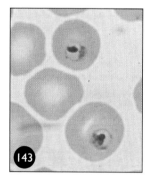
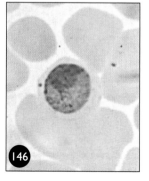
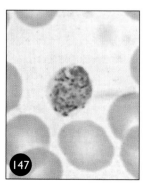

band are common. With special staining, a very fine stippling (Ziemann's dots) is sometimes seen. Host red cells are not enlarged. Gametocytes, no larger than their host cells, are round and compact, with distinct blackish pigment, the females (**146**) usually staining a bluer colour and the males (**147**) somewhat mauvish. (*Leishman* × *1500*.)

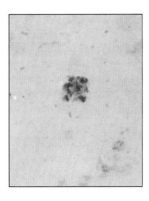
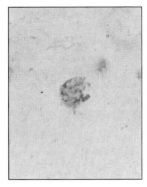

148 & 149 Thick blood films

Younger parasites can be recognised by their heavy pigment, but this may be so heavy that it obscures the other inner structures. Schizonts containing up to eight merozoites with a central mass of pigment (148, left) are characteristic. Gametocytes, such as the female seen in 149 (right), containing large, dark granules of haemozoin, are also distinctive. *Plasmodium malariae* is difficult to differentiate from *P. ovale* in thick films, in which the parasites are easily confused. However, unlike *P. malariae*, *P. ovale* may be seen in 'ghost cells' (*c.f.* 136). (*Field* × 1500.)

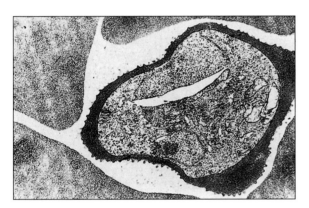

150 Ultrastructure of *Plasmodium malariae* trophozoite

Very small but regular bosses occur on the surface of the host erythrocyte (possibly corresponding to the Ziemann's dots) (*c.f.* 'knobs' on *P. falciparum*-infected red cells 122). (× 11 000.)

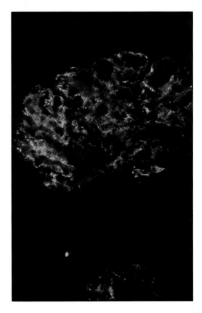

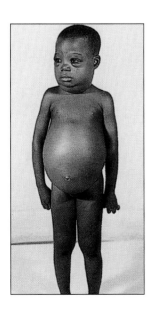

151 Nephrotic child with *Plasmodium malariae* infection

A close association has been established between quartan malaria and the nephrotic syndrome in children. Note the gross oedema and ascites in this West African child.

152 Immunofluorescence of immune complexes in kidney

Immunofluorescent antibody techniques have demonstrated the deposition of immune complexes on the basement membrane of the glomeruli in 'quartan malarial nephrosis.' (× 350.)

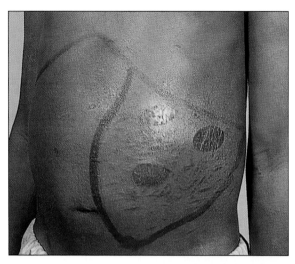

153 Hyperreactive malarial splenomegaly (HMS)

Gross enlargement of the spleen is a characteristic feature of hyperreactive malarial splenomegaly, previously known as 'tropical splenomegaly syndrome' (TSS) or 'big spleen disease.' The syndrome is thought to be due to an abnormal immunological response to malaria infection. High IgM levels are invariably found. Note scars due to application of indigenous medicines.

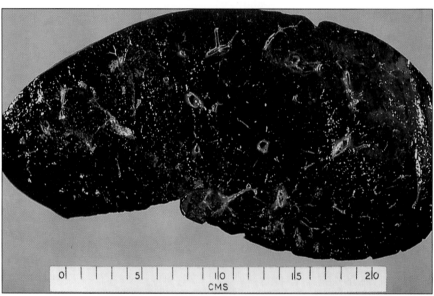

154 Massive spleen in hyperreactive malarial splenomegaly

Regression of the enlarged spleen occurs when long-term antimalarial therapy is given.

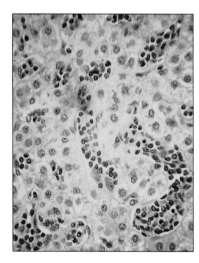

155 Section of liver in hyperreactive malarial splenomegaly

Liver biopsy shows hepatic sinusoidal dilation with marked infiltration of lymphocytes and hypertrophy of the Kupffer cells. (*H&E* × 430.)

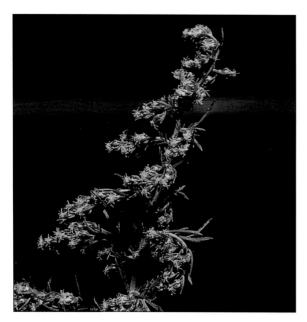

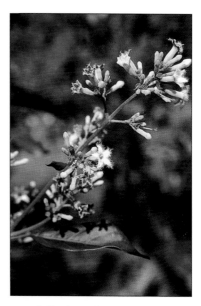

156 'Qinghao': the oldest antimalarial

Resistance of parasites, especially *Plasmodium falciparum*, to antimalarial drugs is one of the biggest problems in the management of malaria. In the search for new drugs with which to combat drug-resistant malaria, attention has focussed away from synthetic chemistry to a search for natural products, some of them used from time immemorial in traditional therapy. Among such remedies is 'Qinghao' (the Chinese wormwood—*Artemisia annua* Linn.), which has yielded one of the most potent compounds available currently: 'Qinghaosu' (artemisinin). Qinghao has been recorded as an anti-fever plant in traditional Chinese medicine for over 2000 years, considerably longer than the Peruvian plant that yields quinine (*see* **157**), the beneficial effects of which were first recorded a mere 400 years ago.

157 Flowers of *Cinchona ledgeriana*, the source of quinine

A young plant growing in a plantation in Madagascar. Quinine and related alkaloids are harvested from the bark of the *Cinchona* tree.

158 The mosquito net: an emerging method for malaria control!

In addition to the widespread problem of multiple drug resistance in *falciparum* malaria, vector control has failed in many countries because of insecticide resistance or other factors, some of them socioeconomic. Protection of the populations of endemic countries remains an elusive target. These obstacles have necessitated a vigorous search for additional, sustainable ways of preventing malaria. Field trials of mosquito nets impregnated with synthetic pyrethroids have given promising results in terms of lowering the rate of infected bites in the community, but are still far from eliminating transmission in most places. The situation is especially challenging in tropical Africa where transmission is very intense.

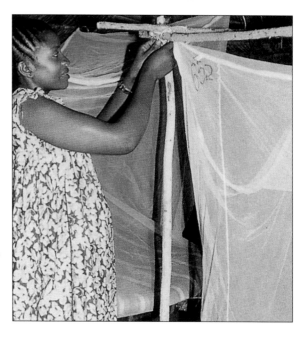

TRYPANOSOMIASIS

(See **Tables 7** *and* **18**.)

AFRICAN TRYPANOSOMIASIS

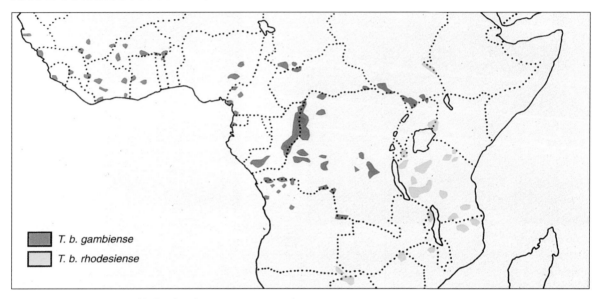

T. b. gambiense

T. b. rhodesiense

159 Distribution map of infection in man
African trypanosomiasis is confined to equatorial Africa, with a patchy distribution depending on detailed topographical conditions. It is caused by two subspecies of *Trypanosoma brucei*: *T. b. gambiense* infection is widespread in West and Central Africa, mainly by riverine species of tsetse flies (*Glossina*), but *T. b. rhodesiense*, transmitted mostly by savannah species, is restricted to the east and east central areas, with some overlaps between the two. Although domestic pigs form an important reservoir for *T. b. gambiense* infection, various wild ruminants are the major sources for *T. b. rhodesiense*. (Adapted from WHO *Map No. 98005*.)

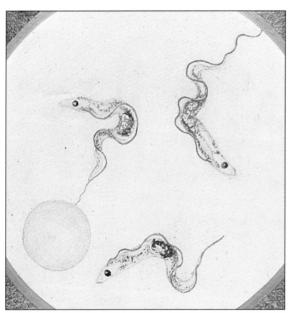

160 Original illustration of *Trypanosoma (Trypanozoon) brucei gambiense* in human blood by J. Everett Dutton.
Polymorphic trypanosomes were first discovered a century ago, in 1895, by David Bruce, an Australian-born pathologist in the British Army Medical Service. While on a posting to Zululand in South Africa he discovered the parasites in the blood of domestic cattle suffering from a wasting disease known as 'Nagana'. The first observation of these protozoa in humans was by R.M. Forde, who noted, in 1902, 'small worm-like, extremely active bodies' in the blood of a sick European seaman in the Gambia. The parasites seen here in a Romanowsky-stained thin blood film, which were described and named by Dutton in the same year, are responsible for sleeping sickness in West Africa. (Reproduced by kind permission of the Director, Liverpool School of Tropical Medicine.)

Table 7 Trypanosomes of medical and veterinary importance

Section	Genus (Subgenus)	Species	Host Species	Disease
Africa SALIVARIA	Trypanosoma (Duttonella)	vivax	antelopes, ruminants, equines, dogs	souma
		uniforme	antelopes, ruminants	(pathogenic)
	T. (Nannomonas)	congolense	antelopes, ruminants, equines, pigs, dogs	(pathogenic)
		simiae	pigs, warthogs, camels	(pathogenic)
	T. (Trypanozoon)	brucei brucei	antelopes, domestic mammals	nagana
		b. rhodesiense	antelopes, humans	sleeping sickness (acute form)
		b. gambiense	humans, pigs	sleeping sickness (chronic form)
		evansi[1]	bovines, equines, camels, dogs, etc.	surra
		equiperdum[2]	equines	dourine
	T. (Pycnomonas)	suis	domestic and wild pigs	(pathogenic)
South America SALIVARIA	T. (Duttonella)	vivax[3]	bovines	(pathogenic)
	T. (Herpetosoma)	rangeli[4]	many wild animals, humans	(non-pathogenic)
STERCORARIA	T. (Schizotrypanum)	cruzi[4]	humans, armadillos, opossums, dogs, etc.	Chagas' disease

All species transmitted by tsetse flies except:
[1] by tabanid flies.
[2] by coitus.
[3] by various biting flies.
[4] by reduviid bugs.
See **Table 5** for general systematic position in protozoa (Sarcomastigophora).

161 Life cycle of African trypanosomes in humans and reservoir hosts

There are three phases in the life cycle of African trypanosomes: i, in the reservoir host; ii, in the tsetse fly; iii, in humans. Metacyclic trypomastigotes (1) pass from the fly's proboscis into the mammalian host's skin. There, the parasites reproduce, forming long flat trypomastigotes (2A), and (in humans) a chancre develops. The trypomastigotes enter the blood and circulate to the tissues. Some, in the liver, seem to form multinucleate giant forms (3) from which arise sphaeromastigotes (4) and further long flat forms (2A) or very long slender trypomastigotes (5). Some of the long flat forms develop into short stumpy forms (2B), but these degenerate trypomastigotes, although taken up by the tsetse fly (6), are not infective. The slender forms, directly or via the crop, enter the midgut in which they reproduce by binary fission (7). Most of the progeny exit via the terminal part of the peritrophic membrane and pass back from the ectoperitrophic space, through the hypopharynx, to reach the salivary ducts and thence, in reverse direction to the salivary flow, to the glands themselves where they become attached and reproduce further as epimastigotes (8). These convert back to metacyclic trypomastigotes (1), which pass back down the salivary ducts to enter a new mammalian host when the fly bites again. (See also **161, 162, 164, 165** and **173**.)

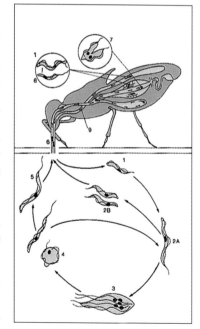

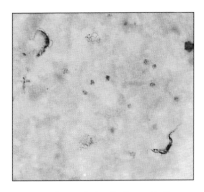

162 *Trypanosoma brucei rhodesiense* in human blood
T. b. brucei parasitises wild and domestic animals but does not
infect humans. The different subspecies can be distinguished
with certainty only by biochemical techniques, such as elec-
trophoretic typing of their isoenzymes (*see also* **210 *and***
610) or by the use of DNA probes. *T. b. gambiense, T. b. rhodesiense* (and *T. b. brucei* of animals) are virtually indistinguishable in blood films. Note the small kinetoplast and free
flagellum. Both subspecies from humans will infect guinea
pigs, but only *T. b. rhodesiense* is infective to rats, in which the
parasites are polymorphic, i.e. long, thin, intermediate and
short stumpy forms of trypomastigotes may coincide.
(*Giemsa* × *900.*)

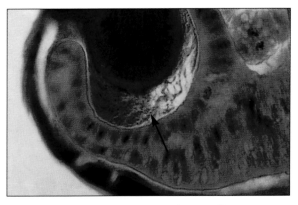

164 Trypanosomes in section of tsetse fly
After ingestion by the tsetse fly, the trypomastigotes pass to
the midgut. After asexual reproduction, the parasites migrate
forward between the peritrophic membrane and gut wall to
re-enter the pharynx and proboscis. They migrate back into
the salivary glands where they transform first into epimastigotes (*see also* **161**), then to the infective stage (metacyclic
trypomastigotes) (**165**). The section shows trypomastigotes
(arrow) massed at the entrance to the midgut ready to enter
the proventriculus. (× *90.*)

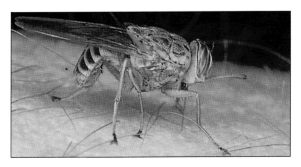

163 Tsetse fly feeding
The common vectors of *Trypanosoma brucei gambiense* in
West Africa are *Glossina palpalis* and *G. tachinoides*. *T. b. rhode-
siense* is associated with *G. morsitans*, *G. swynnertoni* and
G. pallidipes. Other, secondary, vectors have more localised
distributions. (× *5.5.*)

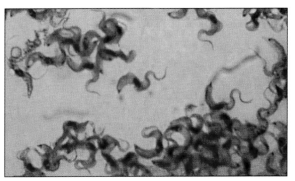

165 Metacyclic trypanosomes in salivary 'probe'
The infective stages are passed into the bite together with
the saliva when the fly next feeds. They may be observed in
saliva expressed from the proboscis of the fly onto a microscope slide. (× *900.*)

166 Larva, pre-pupa and pupa of *Glossina morsitans*
A single larva develops inside the female tsetse fly and is
deposited when mature in dry soil. Here it pupates and
metamorphoses to the adult. (× *3.2.*)

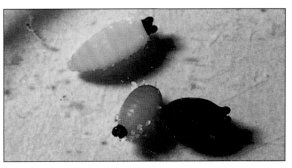

167 Ecology of gambiense infection

Gambiense trypanosomiasis is transmitted by riverine species of *Glossina*, requiring optimum shade and humidity— shady trees near lakes, rivers and pools of water are ideal habitats. The figure shows a typical site for transmission by *G. tachinoides*, one of the *G. palpalis* group, which transmit human trypanosomiasis over a wide geographical area. Man–fly contact is intimate when villagers congregate around pools for collecting water or washing, as at this riverside near Kampala in Uganda. Domestic pigs are an important reservoir of infection with *Trypanosoma brucei gambiense* in West African villages. *G. tachinoides* is second in importance to *G. palpalis* as a vector of this parasite. In contrast to gambiense trypanosomiasis, the rhodesiense form is transmitted by *G. morsitans* and its subspecies, whose habitat is scrubby savannah woodland. These flies are less dependent on moisture. Moreover, in such terrain, wild animals and domestic cattle provide alternative feeding opportunities for the fly. Trypanosomiasis due to other species is a serious

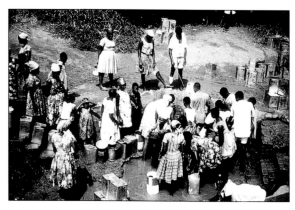

disease of domestic animals, causing great economic loss and depriving human populations of much needed protein. *T. b. brucei*, *T. vivax* and *T. congolense* are the commonest parasites involved. Pigs may also be decimated by other species such as *T. suis* or *T. simiae*.

168 Blood sample being taken from a Roan antelope

The reservoir of *Trypanosoma brucei rhodesiense* was long suspected to be wild animals; the first species found infected with this trypanosome was the bushbuck (*Tragelaphus scriptus*), but other species of game animals have since been found to harbour these parasites. This antelope was immobilised with an anaesthetic dart for a blood sample to be collected.

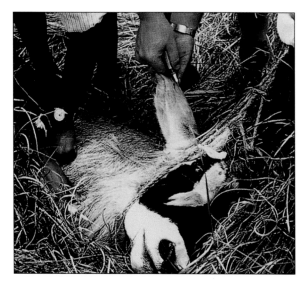

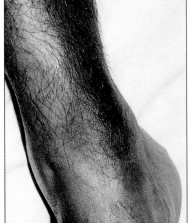

169 Trypanosomal chancre

The bite reaction, the earliest clinical lesion, is known as a 'trypanosomal chancre.' It resembles a boil but is usually painless. Fluid aspirated from the nodule contains actively dividing trypanosomes. This reaction is seen more commonly in rhodesiense than in gambiense infection.

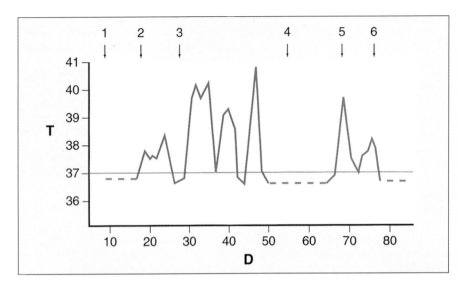

170 Temperature chart in a patient with trypanosomiasis
Episodes of pyrexia that occur irregularly are often associated with the rash. Trypanosomes appear in the blood one to three weeks after infection. They may be scanty in gambiense but are commonly numerous in rhodesiense infection, which is usually a more fulminating disease. [D—day of illness, T—temperature (°C); 1—headache; 2—trypanosomal chancre; 3—oedema of left eyelid; 4, 5, 6—rash.]

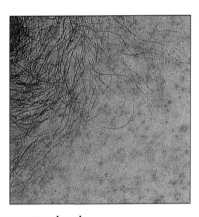

171 Trypanosomal rash
In fair-skinned individuals, each peak of fever may be accompanied by a remarkable skin eruption in the form of annular patches of erythema. In other cases, the rash may be more generalised, as seen here on the sixth day of an infection with *Trypanosoma brucei rhodesiense*.

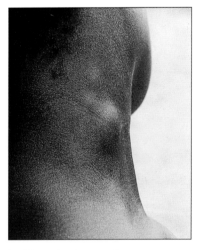

172 Cervical lymphadenopathy
Enlargement of lymphatic glands, especially in the posterior triangle of the neck ('Winterbottom's sign'), is an important clinical feature of infection with *Trypanosoma brucei gambiense* infection and calls for diagnostic gland puncture. Examination of a needle aspirate from the glands is a valuable and simple means of providing an early diagnosis, especially in Gambian trypanosomiasis.

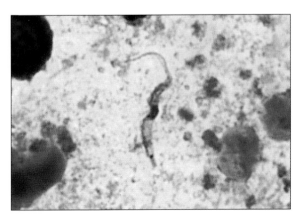

173 Trypanosome in gland fluid
The trypanosomes are easily identified as actively motile organisms in the wet preparation of aspirated gland juice. Their identity can be confirmed by staining. (*Giemsa* × *1650*.)

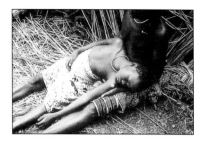

174 Nigerian child with early sleeping sickness due to *Trypamosoma brucei gambiense*
Involvement of the central nervous system is first manifested by non-specific neurological symptoms, partly due to meningeal irritation, followed by a classic reversal of the sleep rhythm and daytime somnolence, as seen in this child.

175 Sleeping sickness
In the absence of treatment, the patient with gambiense infection becomes progressively more wasted and comatose, finally showing the classic picture of sleeping sickness as the central nervous system (CNS) becomes further involved. Although infection with *Trypanosoma brucei rhodesiense* often leads to

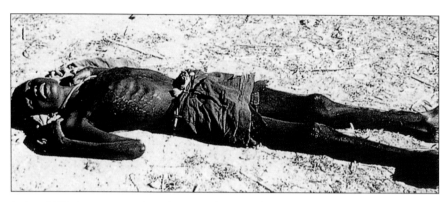

death from toxic manifestations before CNS changes are evident, this man, who was infected in Juba, southern Sudan, displayed early cerebral manifestations.

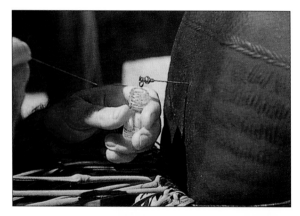

176 Lumbar puncture
This procedure should be carried out to determine whether the central nervous system (CNS) has been invaded. In such instances, the cerebrospinal fluid will reveal a lymphocytic pleocytosis, and an increased protein content, and trypanosomes may be found in stained films of the centrifuge deposit. In infection with *Trypanosoma brucei rhodesiense*, invasion of the CNS may occur very early, whereas several months or years usually elapse before meningoencephalitis develops in gambiense disease. (Note: this procedure should be carried out with full sterile and other precautions that are not shown in this figure.)

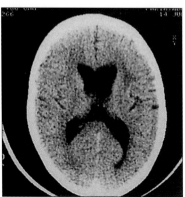

177 Cerebral changes in *Trypanosoma brucei rhodesiense* infection
Computed tomography may show evidence of cerebral involvement prior to treatment. Atrophic changes with hydrocephalus are seen in the tomogram of this young child, nine months after clinical cure.

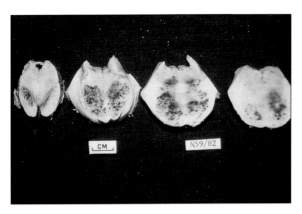

178 Acute haemorrhagic leucoencephalopathy

Numerous small haemorrhagoc foci, some of them confluent, are seen in these sections of the brain stem from a fatal case of African trypanosomiasis. (Original figure from the Department of Neuropathology, Southern General Hospital, Glasgow, reproduced by courtesy of WHO. ID: 9204178, WHO/TDR.)

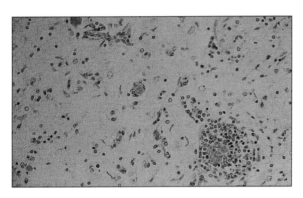

179 Microscopic changes in brain

The leptomeninges are congested, there may be oedema, and small haemorrhages are commonly present. The basic pathological change is a meningoencephalitis in which perivascular cuffing with round cells is often pronounced. (*H&E × 200.*)

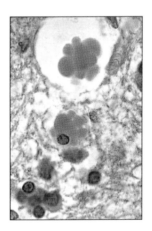 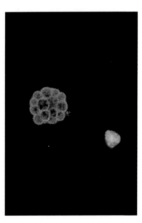

180 & 181 Morula cells in brain

Scattered irregularly through the brain substance, there occur large eosinophilic mononuclear cells (**180**, left) with eccentric nuclei known as morula cells of Mott (*H&E × 1500*). These are IgM-producing plasma cells, as shown in this preparation (**181**, right) treated with fluorescent anti-IgM antibody. (× 1500.)

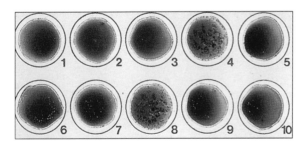

182 Card agglutination test for (gambiense) trypanosomiasis (CATT)

Anti-trypanosomal IgM, which is raised both in the blood and the cerebrospinal fluid in trypanosomiasis, can be detected by this simple test, which is invaluable for rapid diagnosis, especially in field surveys. Other useful serological aids are the complement-fixation test, quantitative IgM radial immunodiffusion assay and fluorescent antibody test staining. In the CATT test card shown here, the presence of blue granular deposits in wells 4 and 8 are indicative of infection.

183 'Minicolumn' separation of trypanosomes

The Sephadex 'minicolumn,' which permits the detection of very small numbers of trypanosomes in specimens of blood or cerebrospinal fluid, can be an invaluable diagnostic aid in individual patients and has been employed in field surveys. Once eluted from the base of the column, even a single parasite is readily identified under the microscope.

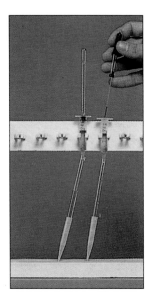

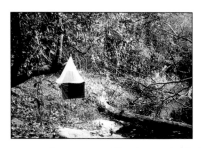

185 Vavoua trap in use at a *Glossina palpalis*-infested riverine site in West Africa

This is a cheap and simplified version of the Lancien trap. Note the alternating black and blue cloth that provides a colour attractant for this species of tsetse. The trap contains a liquid bait at the apex of the cone. It is used extensively in West Africa. Impregnating the material from which it is constructed with a synthetic pyrethroid such as deltamethrin improves its performance.

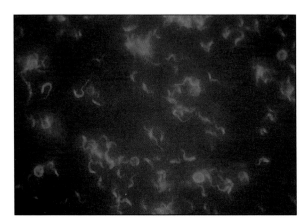

184 Acridine orange-stained *Trypanosoma brucei rhodesiense* in centrifuged blood

The examination of centrifuged blood to detect trypanosomes is facilitated by the use of the QBC[R] technique with fluorescent staining, as seen here. The method is highly sensitive and simple to use. (*See also* **102**.) ($\times$ 200.)

186 Target trap with an odour attractant

The control of African trypanosomiasis is based mainly on the destruction of vectors. One of the most successful methods currently employed is the use of various types of target traps treated with long-lasting, synthetic pyrethroids. The attractant

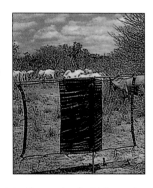

in this model is placed in a bottle, the neck of which can be seen near the central pivot. Based on observations of the attractiveness of cattle odour to tsetse, a number of compounds were discovered (including octenol and various phenols), the use of which with acetone or butanone greatly enhances the efficiency of colour-baited and screen traps. Cattle can themselves be used as a bait for tsetse control. A synthetic pyrethroid such as deltamethrin, applied either in a cattle dip or as a simple pour-on preparation, can be extremely effective in reducing the population of tsetse and other biting flies for weeks or months without having any harmful effects on the animals.

CHAGAS' DISEASE (AMERICAN TRYPANOSOMIASIS)

187 Distribution map of Chagas' disease

Two species of trypanosome infect humans in the New World. The most prevalent is *Trypanosoma (Schizotrypanum) cruzi*, the causative agent of Chagas' disease. The second, which is probably a harmless commensal, is *Trypanosoma (Herpetosoma) rangeli*. *T. cruzi* is transmitted by large blood-sucking Hemiptera belonging to the family **Reduviidae** which, because of their notorious tendency to bite the exposed face of sleeping people, are also known as 'kissing bugs.' The species of major importance in the transmission of Chagas' disease are *Rhodnius prolixus*, *Triatoma infestans*, *T. brasiliensis*, *T. dimidiata* and *Panstrongylus megistus*. The long-standing confusion about the relationship between specific vector species, infection of *T. cruzi* in humans and the same parasite in animal reservoirs, has been resolved to a large degree by the use of biochemical techniques (mainly the characterisation of trypanosome isoenzymes) to differentiate closely related, but biologically and epidemiologically distinct 'zymodemes' of *T. cruzi*, some of which are now known to be non-pathogenic to humans. Those triatomid species that are vectors of pathogenic zymodemes readily colonise human and animal dwellings, where they feed, often indiscriminately, on humans, their domestic animals and birds, as well as house-visiting wild mammals such as opossums and armadillos. The latter are important reservoirs of the zoonotic infection that is transmitted to humans. Individuals who survive the acute stage are often left with chronic and progressive neuronal and smooth muscle lesions in the heart and gastrointestinal tract. Human infection is endemic in parts of Central and South America, from the Andes to the Atlantic coast and as far south as the latitude of the River Plate (Río de la Plata). Two major intergovernmental programmes were started in 1991 to eliminate domestic vectors by a combination of spraying residual

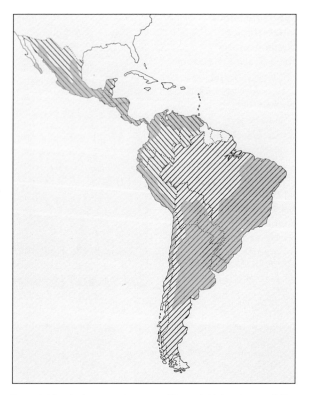

insecticides in houses, the use of insecticidal paints and the deployment of fumigant canisters. The countries covered in the two initiatives, the second of which started in 1997, are shown in the figure. In less than a decade remarkable progress has been made. Transmission (by the major vector, *Triatoma infestans*) was eliminated in Uruguay by 1997, in Chile by 1999 and was expected to cease in Brazil during 2000. Major reductions in transmission have also been reported from other endemic countries. [▨ 'Southern Cone Initiative' area; ▨ 'Andean and Central American Initiative' area.]

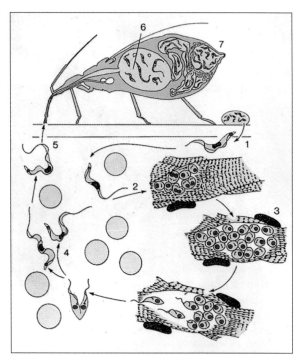

188 Life cycle of *Trypanosoma cruzi* in humans and triatomid bugs

(1) Infective, metacyclic trypomastigotes passed with the faeces enter the body either through the site of the bite or by direct penetration of mucosal surfaces such as that of the eye; some enter reticuloendothelial cells of the subcutaneous tissues near the site of entry to produce a local swelling known as a 'chagoma.' (2) Other trypomastigotes reach the circulatory system from which they penetrate smooth muscle in organs such as the heart, the walls of the gastrointestinal tract or skeletal muscle. Associated ganglion cells of the autonomic system may also be invaded. (3) In these organs, they convert to amastigotes, which reproduce by binary fission to form pseudocysts. (4) Some amastigotes later revert to sphaeromastigotes and epimastigotes, which form trypomastigotes that re-enter the circulation. (5) Circulating trypomastigotes, which are taken up when another triatomid feeds, enter the bug's midgut. (6) In the gut, the flagellates change to short epimastigote and rounded sphaeromastigote forms in which they multiply profusely by binary fission. (7) After one or two weeks, longer epimastigotes enter the rectum, where they form metacyclic trypomastigotes that are passed when the bug again defaecates (*adapted from Geigy and Herbig, 1955*). (*See also* **189, 192** *and* **196**.)

189 *Trypanosoma cruzi* in human blood film

The causative agent occurs in blood films characteristically as short 'C' or 'S'-shaped trypomastigotes with a prominent kinetoplast. It is otherwise monomorphic. (*Giemsa* × 950.)

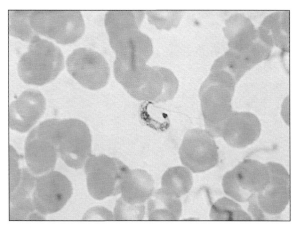

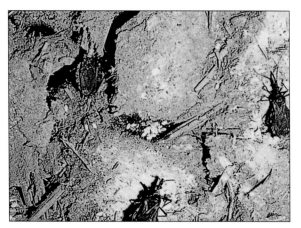

190 Ecology of triatomid vectors

The favourite habitats of the reduviid bugs are cracks in the walls of mud huts in poor rural areas; here, the insects shelter and breed. Transmission occurs predominantly at night. Adults and clusters of eggs can be seen here.

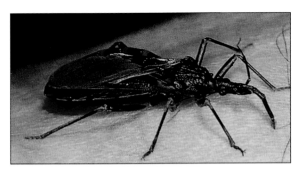

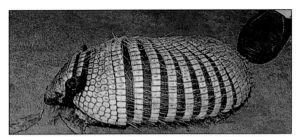

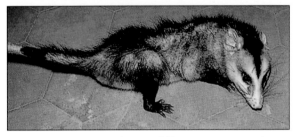

191 Male *Triatoma infestans* feeding on a human arm

This is one of the most widely distributed species. Note the position of the proboscis. Reduviid bugs (also known as 'assassin' or 'kissing' bugs), particularly in the genera *Triatoma*, *Rhodnius* and *Panstrongylus*, transmit *Trypanosoma cruzi* while feeding, not by inoculation but by faecal contamination. Both sexes are similar and feed on blood, with the male having a small, ventral abdominal swelling. The insects normally hide in the walls during the daytime and emerge after dark to feed on the sleeping inhabitants. The bite is remarkably painless even though the bug may take from 10–20 minutes to become fully engorged. (× 1.6.)

193 & 194 Reservoir hosts of *Trypanosoma cruzi*

Chagas' disease is a zoonosis. *T. cruzi* has an extensive mammalian reservoir in both wild hosts (especially armadillos, such as the *Dasypus novencinctus* seen here—**193**, top) and opossums (*Didelphis* species—**194**, bottom), as well as some domestic animals.

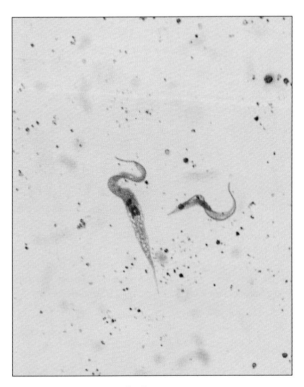

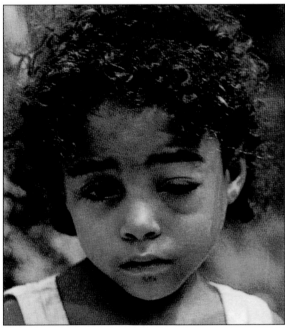

192 Metacyclic stage in faeces

Infection is through contamination by parasites in bug faeces produced on the skin. These may invade the site of the bite or adjacent mucosa (e.g. the conjunctiva). (*Giemsa* × 1500.)

195 Romaña's sign

The infection often begins with a local lesion, the chagoma. It causes marked local oedema which, should it occur in the region of the eye or within the conjunctival sac, is accompanied by swelling of the lids and chemosis. These unilateral periorbital changes constitute Romaña's sign.

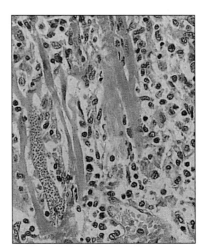

196 Amastigotes in heart muscle
After a stage of initial parasitaemia associated with fever (often unrecognised), trypomastigotes pass to the cardiac muscle and the smooth muscle lining the intestinal tract. Here, they transform to the amastigote stage (Leishman–Donovan bodies) in which they multiply to form pseudocysts. In the heart, this is associated with severe myocarditis, especially in the early stages of the infection. The severity of the acute myocarditis seems to seal the eventual fate of the sufferer from chronic cardiac changes. These can be reactivated in patients with AIDS. (*Giemsa* × *350*.)

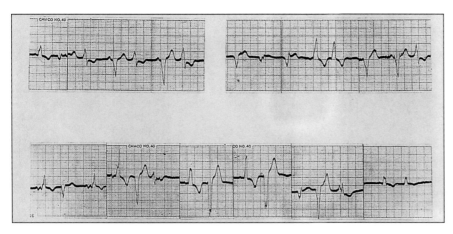

197 Electrocardiogram showing heart block
Dysrhythmias of various types and degrees are a characteristic feature of Chagas' disease; complete heart block with Stokes–Adams attacks can occur and may result in sudden death.

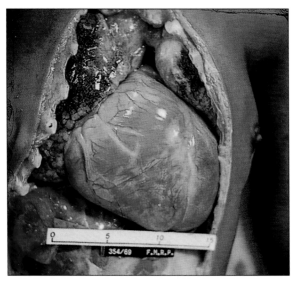

198 Cardiomegaly
The heart shows gross enlargement and dilation. The dilation of the right atrium and both ventricles is marked in this specimen. The pathogenesis seems to be associated with a loss of autonomic control due to destruction of the ganglionic plexuses. Autoantibodies are probably involved in this process. (*See also* **200**.)

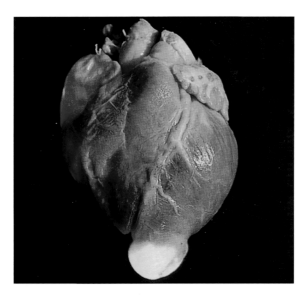

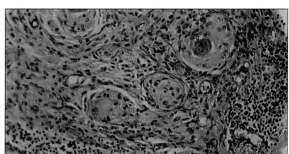

200 Sympathetic ganglion in wall of atrium
Degenerative changes in neuronal cells from a ganglion in the heart of a patient with Chagas' disease who died of sudden cardiac failure. Mononuclear cellular infiltration is conspicuous, especially around the capsule of the ganglion. Central nervous system involvement may present as diffuse meningoencephalitis with necrosis in individuals who develop AIDS. (*H&E × 130.*)

199 Apical aneurysm of heart
Mural thrombi may be present at the apex of the left ventricle, with marked thinning of both ventricular walls. Apical aneurysm formation is commonly seen.

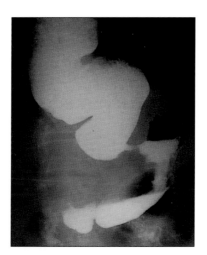

201 Radiograph of megaoesophagus
Muscular degeneration and denervation of segments of the alimentary tract through destruction of the cells of Auerbach's plexus cause megaoesophagus, megastomach and megacolon, etc., which can be detected radiologically.

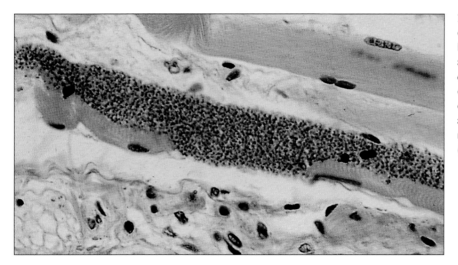

202 Amastigotes in oesophageal muscle
Pseudocysts containing amastigotes of *Trypanosoma cruzi* can rarely be demonstrated in ganglion cells of the intestinal tract, although the smooth muscle is often invaded. (× *480.*)

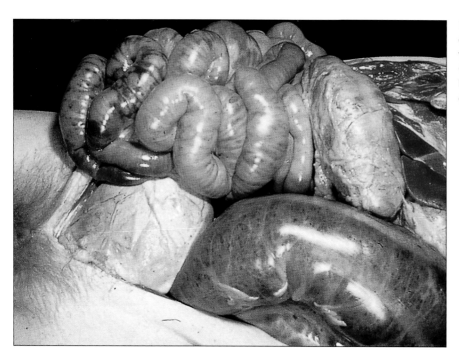

203 Post mortem examination of patient with megacolon
Gross megacolon is shown here in a woman who died of chronic Chagas' disease.

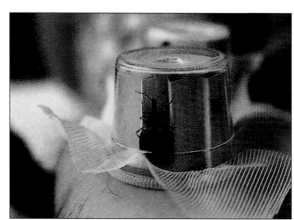

204 Xenodiagnosis
Absolute confirmation of active infection is obtained by demonstrating that the patient can infect the vector (xenodiagnosis). Laboratory-bred, clean reduviid bugs are fed on patients suspected of having trypanosomiasis. Two weeks later the hindgut is dissected out and is examined for metacyclic trypanosomes.

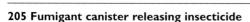

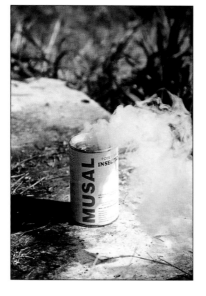

205 Fumigant canister releasing insecticide
This type of canister was especially designed to kill domestic insects. When lit, it releases a cloud of insecticide that is very effective in killing the triatomine vectors of Chagas' disease, as well as other insect pests (*see also* **24**). The large scale deployment of such canisters has made a large contribution to the reduction or arrest of transmission of Chagas' disease in a major part of the endemic areas. (Figure by courtesy of WHO, ID: 9905250, WHO/TDR/Crump.)

206 Enzyme-linked immunosorbent assay
An ELISA employing antigen from epimastigotes of *Trypanosoma cruzi* cultivated *in vitro* is widely used and is one of the most sensitive means of diagnosis. It can indicate past or present infection and does not necessarily imply the presence of parasites. Five positive reactions are shown in this microtitre plate in which an immunoperoxidase procedure was followed. Fluorescent antibody tests may also be employed, using whole cultured epimastigotes as the

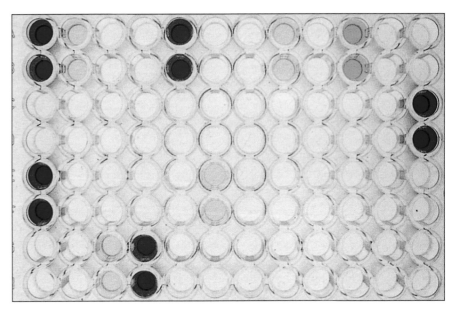

antigen. The exquisitely sensitive polymerase chain reaction technique, which is capable of detecting the DNA from a single parasite, is invaluable in the control of blood for transfusion in endemic countries, as well as for the diagnosis and follow-up of individual patients in whom few parasites may be accessible for detection by other methods. The screening of all blood donors to reduce transmission is an integral part of the 'Southern Cone Initiative' because chemotherapy of established infection remains unsatisfactory.

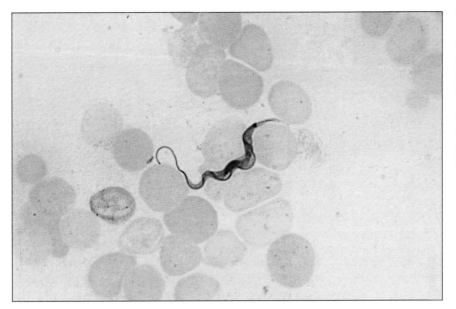

207 *Trypanosoma rangeli*
T. rangeli is a long, slender trypanosome also transmitted by reduviid bugs from wild animals to humans. It is readily distinguished by its shape from *T. cruzi* in blood films, and seems to be non-pathogenic to humans. (*Giemsa* × *1200*.)

LEISHMANIASIS

(*See* **Tables 8** *and* **9**.)

208 Life cycle of *Leishmania*

(1) Infective, flagellated promastigotes pass from the proboscis with the saliva into the subcutaneous tissues when a sandfly feeds. (2) The promastigotes penetrate local tissue macrophages, becoming rounded amastigotes (also known as Leishman–Donovan bodies) as the flagellae degenerate. (3) The amastigotes multiply by asexual binary fission to form 'cell nests,' which rupture the host cells—the progeny are taken up by other local or circulating macrophages. (4) Depending on the species of parasite, some amastigotes remain in the superficial tissues where the reproductive cycle continues, whereas others settle in macrophages in the deep organs of the reticuloendothelial system such as lymph glands, bone marrow, spleen and liver. (5) When another sandfly takes a blood meal, some amastigotes in macrophages (either in the skin or in the peripheral circulation) are taken into the midgut where they convert to promastigotes within the peritrophic membrane. (6) The promastigotes reproduce further, mainly by binary fission, and escape into the midgut when the peritrophic membrane breaks down; some possibly undergo a form of sexual conjugation. (7) Promastigotes of *Leishmania (Leishmania)* move forward to the oesophagus and proboscis, attaching for some time *en route* to the stomodaea valve (situated between the thoracic midgut and oesophagus) where some species continue to divide. Species of *Leishmania (Viannia)* move posteriorly to

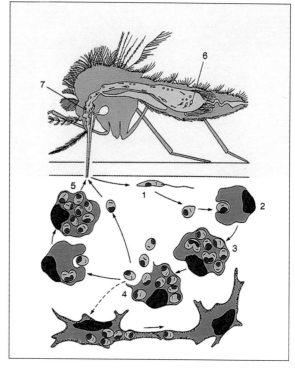

the pylorus and ileum of the hindgut where they reproduce further before once again moving anteriorly to the proboscis. (*See also* **209**, **211**, **216**, **217**, **234**, **235**, **252** *and* **271**.)

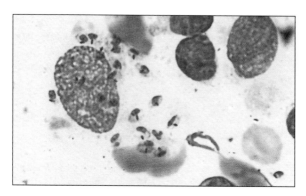

209 Amastigotes of *Leishmania infantum* in a macrophage from dog skin

The amastigotes of different species are very similar on light microscopy (apart from their sizes) and can be distinguished—even by experts—to a limited degree only. (*Giemsa* × *1250*.)

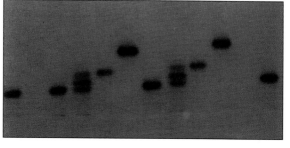

210 Isoenzyme electrophoresis: a tool for biochemical taxonomy

A widely used method for identifying species of *Leishmania* (which is also of considerable value for other parasites, e.g. trypanosomes, amoebae, schistosomes and their molluscan hosts) is the characterisation of isoenzymes by electrophoresis on starch gel or other bases. This figure of duplicate specimens of five *Leishmania* isolates illustrates banding of glucose phosphate isomerase in four distinct patterns, each of which indicates a different species; two of the pairs are identical. This technique has now largely been superseded by the use of specific DNA probes and polymerase chain reaction to identify isolates from vertebrate or invertebrate sources (*see also* **231**, **256**).

Table 8 The genus *Leishmania* and the leishmaniases—systemic disease[1,2]

Type of disease	Species	Localities	Main vectors	Main reservoirs
Kala-azar (60% 10–20 years old)	*L. (Leishmania) donovani*	India	*Phlebotomus argentipes*	humans
		China (north of Yangtze)	*P. chinensis*	dog, ? jackal
	L. (L.) donovani?	Kenya	*P. martini*	? humans
	L. (L.) archibaldi	Sudan	*P. orientalis*	serval cat, genet
Infantile kala-azar (80–90% under 10 years old)	*L. (L.) donovani* complex	Saudi Arabia	?	*Rattus* spp.
		Yemen	?	?
		Ethiopia	?	?
	L. (L.) infantum	Former USSR	*P. major*	fox, wolf, dog
		China	?	'raccoon dog'
		Iraq	*P. major*	? jackal
		France and Italy	*P. ariasi*	dog, fox
			P. perfiliewi	*Rattus rattus*
		Mediterranean basin	*P. perniciosus*	dog
			P. major	
		Egypt	*P. langeroni*	
		Saudi Arabia	?	dog
	L. (L.) chagasi[3]	Brazil, Colombia	*Lutzomyia longipalpis*	fox, dog
		Venezuela, Mexico	*Lu. longipalpis*	dog
		Paraguay, Ecuador	?	?
		Honduras, El Salvador	?	?
		Bolivia, Guatemala	?	?
		Colombia	*Lu. evansi*	?
Oronasal kala-azar	*L. (L.) infantum*	France	(as classic kala-azar)	
Post kala-azar dermal leishmaniasis (PKDL)	*L. (L.) donovani*	India	(as classic kala-azar)	
		China		
	L. (L.) donovani?	Kenya		
Atypical, adult kala-azar	*L. (L.) tropica* complex	Northeast Saudi Arabia	?	?

[1] This genus has been divided into *Leishmania* (*Leishmania*) type species *L. donovani* and *Leishmania* (*Viannia*), type species *L.* (*V.*) *braziliensis*.
[2] See **Table 18** for general systematic position in the Protozoa
[3] Now generally accepted to be synonymous with *L.* (*L.*) *infantum*.

Table 9 The genus *Leishmania* and the leishmaniases—cutaneous and mucocutaneous disease[1]

Type of disease	Species	Localities	Main vectors	Main reservoirs
CUTANEOUS LEISHMANIASIS (OLD WORLD)				
Oriental sore and recidiva	*Leishmania (L.) tropica*	India	*Phlebotomus sergenti*	dog
		Former USSR (urban)[2]	*P. sergenti*	humans
		Iran	*P. ansarii*	dog
		Mediterranean basin	*P. sergenti*	humans
			P. perfiliewi	
		Saudi Arabia	*P. sergenti*	?
Oriental sore and oronasal	*L. (L.) major*	Former USSR (rural)[2]	*P. papatasi*	gerbils
		Saudi Arabia, Central Asia	*P. papatasi*	gerbils, merions
		Mediterranean basin	*P. papatasi*	gerbils, merions
		Sudan	*? P. papatasi*	rodents
		Senegal	*P. duboscqi*	rodents
		India	*P. saheli*	rodents
	L. (L.) tropica complex	Namibia	*P. rossi*	hyrax
		Kenya	*P. guggisbergi*	?
Oriental sore	*L. (L.) infantum*	Mediterranean basin, Italy	?	? dog ? *Rattus rattus*
	L. (L.) donovani	Kenya	?	?
Single sore and diffusa	*L. (L.) aethiopica*	Ethiopia	*P. longipes*	hyrax
		Kenya	*P. pedifer*	hyrax, *Cricetomys*
NEW WORLD CUTANEOUS AND MUCOCUTANEOUS				
Simple cutaneous and diffusa	*L. (L.) mexicana*	Mexico, Guatemala, Belize	*Lutzomyia olmeca*	forest rodents
	L. (L.) mexicana complex	Belize	?	?
		Trinidad	*Lu. flaviscutellata*	forest rodents
		São Paulo State	?	?
		Dominican Republic	?	?
		Texas	*? Lu. anthropophora*	*Neotoma micropis*
	L. (L.) pifanoi	Venezuela	*? Lu. flaviscutellata*	?
	L. (L.) amazonensis	Brazil (Amazon basin)	*Lu. flaviscutellata*	forest rodents
	L. (L.) venezuelensis	Venezuela	*? Lu. olmeca bicolor*	?
	L. (L.) garnhami	Venezuela	*? Lu. townsendi*	opossum
	L. (V.) naiffi	Brazil (Pará)	*? Lu. paraensis, anduzei*	armadillo
	L. (V.) lainsoni	Brazil (Pará), Peru	*Lu. ubiquitalis*	paca
	L. (V.) spp.	Belize	*? Lu. ovallesi*	?
		Central America	*? Lu. crucians*	?
Espundia	*L. (V.) braziliensis*	Brazil[3]	*Lu. wellcomei*	forest rodents
		Brazilian Amazon	*Lu. wellcomei*	
			Lu. squamiventris	
			Lu. complexus	
		Bolivian lowlands	*Lu. carrerai*	?
		Venezuela, Peru	?	?
		Paraguay, Ecuador	?	?
		Colombia	?	?
Pian bois	*L. (V.) guyanensis*	Guyanas	*Lu. umbratilis*	sloths, ant-eaters
		Northern Brazil	*Lu. whitmani*	? rodents
			Lu. anduzei	
Simple sore or pian bois	*L. (V.) panamensis*	Panama	*Lu. trapidoi*	sloths
		Costa Rica	*Lu. ylephiletor*	monkeys
		Colombia	*? Lu. gomezi*	kinkajou
			? Lu. panamensis	olingo
	L. (V.) colombiensis	Colombia	*Lu. hartmanni*	sloths
	L. (V.) shawi	Brazil (Pará)	*Lu. whitmani*	sloths, monkeys, coatimundi
Uta	*L. (V.) peruviana*	Peru (west of Andes),	*Lu. verrucarum*	dog
		Argentina	*Lu. peruensis*	?

[1] See footnote [1] to **Table 8**.

[2] USSR = Turkmenia, Uzbekistan of former USSR.

[3] Forested areas east of the Andean chain.

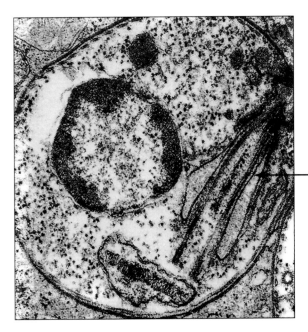

211 Ultrastructure of amastigotes
Leishmanial amastigotes within a parasitophorous vacuole in the host cell. The short flagellum (or mastigote, F) does not extend beyond the outer cell membrane in this stage. (× 37 500.)

F

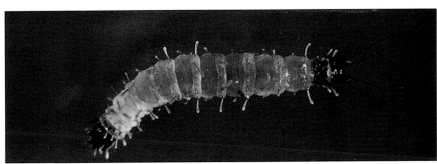

212 Third instar larva of *Phlebotomus perfiliewi*
Leishmania are transmitted by sandflies of the genus *Phlebotomus* in the Old World and Far East, and by *Lutzomyia* in the New World. The photograph shows the larva of *P. perfiliewi*, which is a vector of leishmaniasis in southern Europe. In dry areas, the larvae occupy cracks and crevices, which provide a humid, cool microclimate; forest species possibly prefer leaf mould on the forest floor. (× 10.)

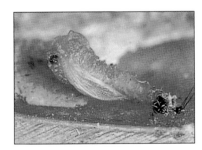

213 Pupa of *Lutzomyia longipalpis*
Lu. longipalpis transmits visceral leishmaniasis in Brazil. (× 13.7.)

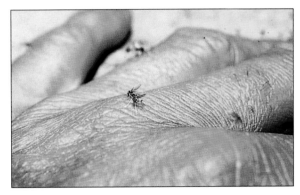

214 Adult female *Lutzomyia longipalpis* biting
This figure gives an impression of the small size of these flies. (× 2.)

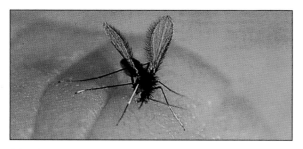

215 Close-up view of *Lutzomyia longipalpis*. (× 10.)

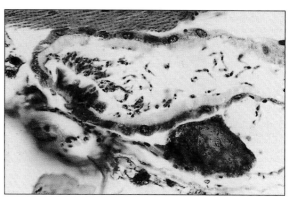

217 Promastigotes in vector midgut
In the midgut of the poikilothermic vector, amastigotes transform to promastigotes, which then divide asexually. (*Giemsa* × 1150.)

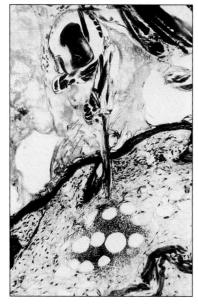

216 Cross section through *Phlebotomus argentipes* in the process of feeding
The female feeds from the pool of capillary blood that accumulates at the tip of the proboscis. (*Haematoxylin* × 100.) (Photographed from a specimen prepared by the late Colonel H. E. Shortt, FRS.)

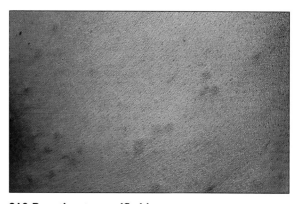

218 Reaction to sandfly bites
A persistent macule appears at the site of each bite, even from an uninfected fly; this may be the starting point of the lesion in simple cutaneous leishmaniasis. Multiple primary lesions occur when the sandfly probes repeatedly in the course of feeding.

VISCERAL LEISHMANIASIS (KALA-AZAR, DUM-DUM FEVER, BLACK SICKNESS)

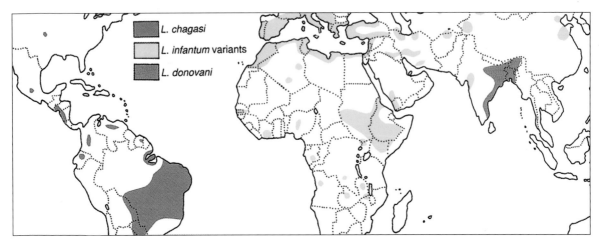

219 Distribution map of visceral leishmaniasis
Visceral leishmaniasis caused by parasites of the *Leishmania donovani–L. infantum* complex occurs in the Mediterranean littorals, the Middle East and adjacent parts of the former USSR, the Sudan, East Africa, the Indian subcontinent and China, and South America ('*L. chagasi*') (*see* **Table 8**). An arid, warm environment provides ideal ecological conditions for the breeding of many species of sandflies. Zoonotic kala-azar due to *L. infantum* and *L. chagasi* is commonly associated with dry, rocky, hill country where cases are typically scattered. In India, *L. donovani* is essentially an anthroponosis. This type of kala-azar may occur in severe epidemic fashion, as can kala-azar in The Sudan.

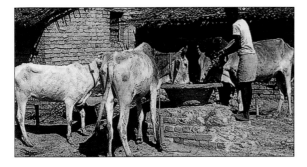

220 Ecology of kala-azar in India
In parts of India (e.g. North Bihar) new epidemics of kala-azar have occurred in recent years. The close association between humans and their domestic animals in this Bihari village favours the growth of populations of *Phlebotomus argentipes,* the local vector of *L. donovani.*

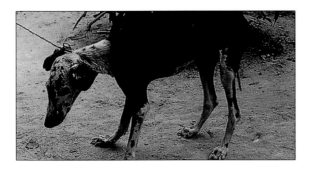

221 Reservoirs of zoonotic *Leishmania infantum*
The massive loss of hair, overgrowth of nails and generally poor condition of this dog found in Colombia are typical of chronic infection with *L. infantum*. Several varieties of this parasite that occur in the Old World are distinguishable by isoenzyme typing; these varieties can give rise to different clinical syndromes in humans—e.g. cutaneous or mucocutaneous lesions rather than kala-azar. In addition to dogs, wild carnivores and various species of rodents may serve as reservoirs for the different varieties (zymodemes) (*see* **Table 8** *and* **9**).

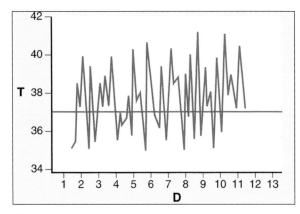

222 Temperature chart in kala-azar
The temperature chart shows a double peak every 24 hours. Despite the high temperature, the patient often looks remarkably well and has a good appetite. A leucopenia with a relative lymphocytosis is often present. Kala-azar should be suspected if this picture is seen in a patient who is a HIV positive. [D—day of illness; T—temperature (°C).]

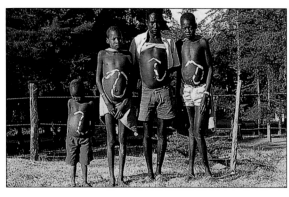

223 Clinical picture of kala-azar in Kenya
Increasing enlargement of the spleen and liver is a characteristic feature, whereas, in dark-complexioned subjects, deepening skin pigmentation is seen—hence the synonym kala-azar, the 'black sickness.' Generalised lymphadenopathy is common in African kala-azar; the parasite in this area is considered to be in the *Leishmania donovani* complex.

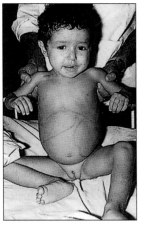

224 Infantile kala-azar
Children present with chronic, irregular fever, anaemia, leucopenia and thrombocytopenia, a moderately enlarged, non-tender liver and a greatly enlarged firm spleen. If left untreated, the infection is often fatal, commonly from secondary infections. This infant was infected in the northeast of Brazil with *Leishmania chagasi* (regarded by some to be synonymous with *L infantum* of the Old World).

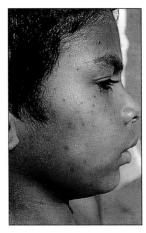

225 Purpura in kala-azar
The condition may present as a petechial rash if the thrombocytopenia is severe as in this Indian boy with *Leishmania donovani, sensu stricta*. Petechial haemorrhages of the retina also occur not infrequently.

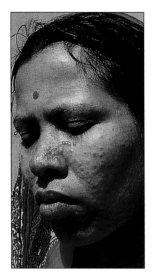

226 Post kala-azar dermal leishmaniasis
This syndrome is a sequel to visceral leishmaniasis that may arise several years after successful treatment of the primary *Leishmania donovani* infection, as in this Indian woman. Dermal lesions vary greatly in appearance and may contain amastigotes in large numbers. Some patients with hypopigmented macules may serve as reservoirs for fresh epidemics if conditions occur that favour sandfly breeding and transmission.

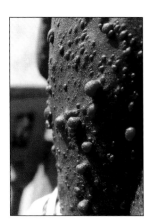

227 Post kala-azar dermal leishmaniasis nodules in an Indian patient
Nodules of various sizes, some pedunculated, are seen in this patient who had been treated for kala-azar over a period of six months, 20 years previously.

228 Post kala-azar dermal leishmaniasis in a Chinese patient

The patient was completely cured by chemotherapy. This response differentiates the condition from the anergic, 'diffusa' type of leishmaniasis (see **270**).

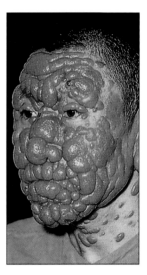

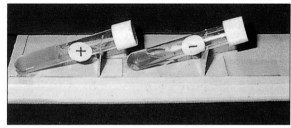

229 Formol-gel test

Large quantities of IgG are produced by patients with kala-azar, and the albumin/globulin ratio is reversed. This may be demonstrated by electrophoresis or by a simple test such as the addition to serum of a drop of 30% formalin. The formation of a gel after standing at room temperature for about 20 minutes indicates the presence of a high proportion of globulin in the sample—the formol-gel test. The complement-fixation test becomes positive later than the fluorescent antibody test ($\times$ 1250.)

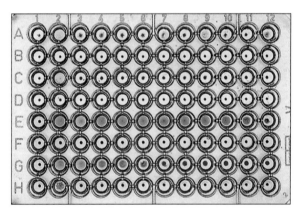

230 Direct agglutination test

This procedure, which has largely replaced the fluorescent antibody test, is now considered to give the most reliable and specific diagnosis of kala-azar, and detects circulating antibodies. The plasma samples in rows E and G of this picture are strongly positive. (See also **206**.)

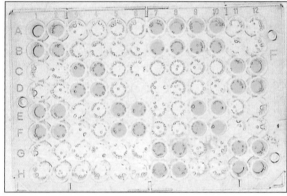

231 Polymerase chain reaction in the diagnosis of leishmanial infection

This exquisitely sensitive technique—it is capable of detecting the DNA from a single parasite—is invaluable in the diagnosis of subclinical or cryptic infection from a blood sample. This slide illustrates the technique as used with *Leishmania donovani* in experimentally infected mice. Each block of four yellow wells indicates the presence of parasites in a single infected animal, samples from negative control animals remaining uncoloured.

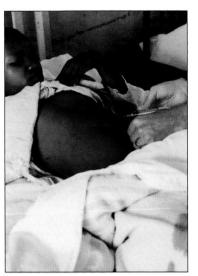

232 Splenic puncture in the diagnosis of visceral leishmaniasis

The most direct means of diagnosis of kala-azar is the detection of amastigotes in bone-marrow, spleen or blood; the organisms are recognised in dried smears of material stained with a Romanowsky-type stain by their characteristic morphology. When performing splenic puncture the needle must be inserted at an angle that permits the spleen to move up and down the needle on inspiration or expiration to avoid tearing the capsule. As soon as the needle has penetrated the skin and before entering the spleen, the plunger is withdrawn to apply suction. The needle is then inserted into and withdrawn from the spleen very rapidly. The aspirated material can be placed into culture and used to make a thin smear that is then stained with Giemsa or another Romanowsky-type stain.

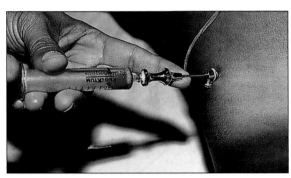

233 Iliac crest puncture of bone marrow

This procedure is less commonly used than splenic aspiration. In general the newer serological techniques shown above avoid the necessity for these more invasive procedures, which are not always necessary.

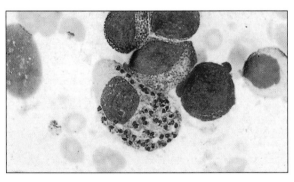

234 *Leishmania infantum* in a macrophage from bone marrow

Although typically found in macrophages, as shown here, isolated extracellular amastigotes from disrupted host cells are commonly seen in such preparations. (*Giemsa* × *810*.)

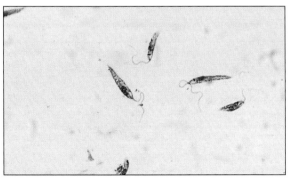

235 Promastigotes in Novy-Nicolle-MacNeal (NNN) culture

After inoculation of aspirated material into appropriate media such as blood agar (NNN medium) and incubation at 28°C for 1–4 weeks, promastigotes may appear in the fluid overlay. *Leishmania donovani* is more readily isolated in culture than *L. infantum*, which sometimes grows better in Schneider's insect tissue culture medium than in NNN. The parasites may also be isolated by intrasplenic inoculation into hamsters; after 4–6 weeks, characteristic visceral lesions are seen macroscopically, and amastigotes are found in large numbers in smears of the liver and spleen. (*Giemsa* × *950*.)

OLD WORLD CUTANEOUS LEISHMANIASIS (ZOONOTIC CUTANEOUS LEISHMANIASIS)

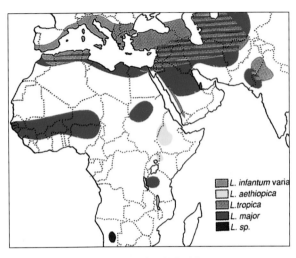

236 Distribution map of Old World cutaneous leishmaniasis
Cutaneous leishmaniasis in the Old World is caused by *Leishmania major*, *L. tropica*, *L. aethiopica* and certain zymodemes of the *L. infantum* complex (see **Table 8**). With the possible exception in some localities of *L. tropica*, these infections are essentially zoonoses that occur in scattered foci throughout the tropical and subtropical belts. Depending on the area, cutaneous leishmaniasis is known as Oriental sore, Aleppo button, Bouton de Biskra, Baghdad boil, Delhi sore, etc.

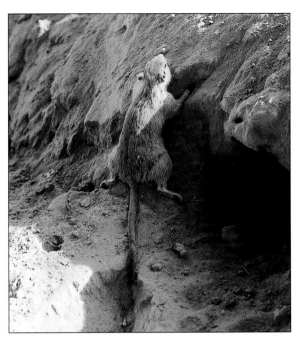

238 Animal reservoirs of *Leishmania major*
Various rodent species such as this 'great gerbil,' *Rhombomys opimus*, of eastern Iran and neighbouring parts of the former USSR, and the 'fat-tailed sand rat,' *Psammomys obesus* (see **239**), of Libya, Israel and Saudi Arabia, are important reservoirs of *L. major*.

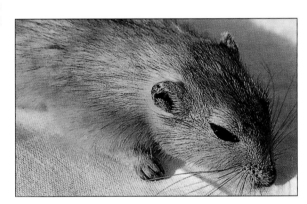

239 Ear lesion on *Psammomys obesus*
These rodents and the sandflies that rest in their burrows are responsible for outbreaks of zoonotic cutaneous leishmaniasis (ZCL) in newly urbanised areas that intrude on their normal habitat—arid or even semi-desert terrain. The burrows provide ideal breeding and resting sites for sandfly vectors such as *Phlebotomus papatasi* that transmit *Leishmania major*, the species causing ZCL. Sandflies also rest during the day in cool deep crevices in the ground, between rocks, in caves, cellars and house walls, etc. Although the eroded ear seen here is typical of *L. major* in its natural host, many infected animals have no obvious skin lesions.

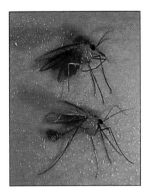

237 Male and female *Phlebotomus (Ph.) papatasi*
This is the most important vector of *Leishmania major* from north Africa, through the Middle East to Mongolia. The female (upper figure) has a fully engorged midgut. Note the contrast between the terminal abdominal segments of the two sexes of this pale sandfly. (× 9.)

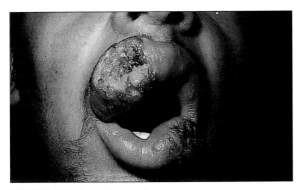

240 'Wet' lesion of mouth

Leishmania major occurs most commonly in rural areas, causing moist, ulcerative lesions that may be extensive and sometimes involve the epithelium of lips and nose.

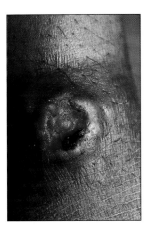

241 Nodulo-ulcerative lesion of *Leishmania major*

These are the commonest types of lesion caused by *L. major*. The prominent 'rolled' edge of the lesions is the best area in which to demonstrate the parasites, which are present in macrophages or are free in surrounding tissue, often in small numbers.

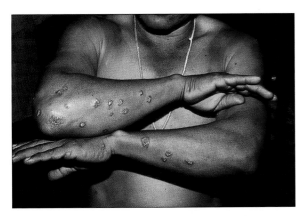

242 Multiple lesions of *Leishmania major* in a non-immune man

This Thai builder received multiple bites by infected *Phlebotomus (Ph.) papatasi* through sleeping outdoors without protection in a highly endemic area of eastern Saudi Arabia.

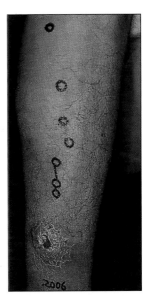

243 Lymphatic spread of *Leishmania major*

The ink marks indicate a line of subcutaneous nodules along the lymphatic, passing proximally from the lesion on the lower part of this man's arm. Readily palpated, the lymphatic is sometimes referred to as a 'beaded cord.' The nodules usually resolve without complications when the primary lesion heals with or without specific therapy.

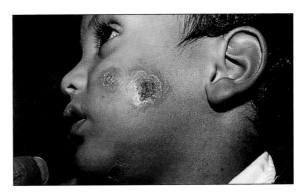

244 Simple 'dry' lesion of *Leishmania tropica*

This parasite often produces dry, usually self-healing lesions which, unlike the infection seen here, are generally single. This form is commonly seen in and around towns from North Africa and the Middle East to the former USSR, Afghanistan and western states of India, especially in mountainous areas. The lesions often contain very large numbers of parasites.

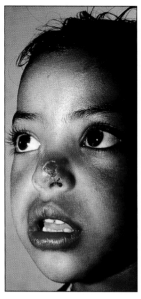

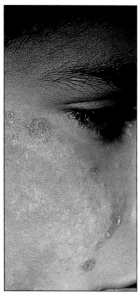

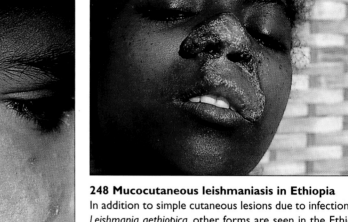

248 Mucocutaneous leishmaniasis in Ethiopia
In addition to simple cutaneous lesions due to infection with *Leishmania aethiopica*, other forms are seen in the Ethiopian highlands, where rock hyraxes are the reservoirs. It has not yet been ascertained whether the mucocutaneous condition seen here is due to *L. aethiopica* or another species of *Leishmania* (see also **240, 247**). Mucocutaneous lesions in Sudanese patients are probably associated with *L. major*.

245 Cutaneous leishmaniasis due to *Leishmania tropica* transmitted by *Phlebotomus sergenti* in an Arabian child
The lesions caused by this parasite are commonly found on the head or neck and may become chronic, leading to the condition known as leishmaniasis recidivans.

246 Leishmaniasis recidivans
Infection with *Leishmania tropica* may become very chronic, with a hyperallergic reaction leading to lupus-like lesions such as seen in this child in Israel. Amastigotes may be very difficult to find in the lesions.

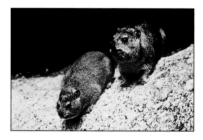

249 *Procavia capensis*
Widely distributed in Africa and Arabia, this hyrax is the reservoir of cutaneous leishmaniasis in Namibia. An unnamed species of *Leishmania* similar to *L. major* causes cutaneous leishmaniasis in parts of Namibia where *Phlebotomus (Synphlebotomus) rossi* is the probable vector.

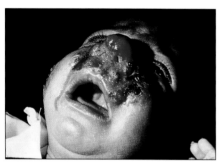

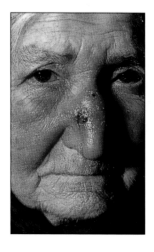

250 Dry lesion on nose of woman in southern France
This lesion proved to be due to a zymodeme of the *Leishmania infantum* complex.

247 Infant with mucocutaneous lesions caused by *Leishmania major*
In some cases, especially in young infants or older individuals whose cellular immune responses are impaired, zoonotic cutaneous leishmaniasis may proceed to involve mucous tissue, much as occurs in the New World disease known as espundia (see **265**). This infant was seen in eastern Saudi Arabia but the condition is also reported from The Sudan and Ethiopia (see **248**) where it may also be associated with *L. major*.

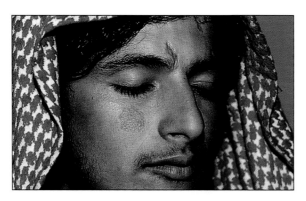

251 Typical healed cutaneous lesion
An atrophic, papery, slightly depressed scar results when healing occurs. This man was probably infected with *Leishmania tropica*, which resolved spontaneously.

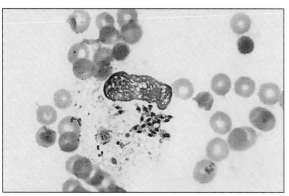

252 Amastigotes in macrophages from skin
The diagnosis is confirmed by demonstrating amastigotes in smears made from the cutaneous lesions (*see* **244** *and* **245**). Various simple techniques such as biopsy by dental broach or skin-slit and scrape can be used. (*Giemsa* × *950.*)

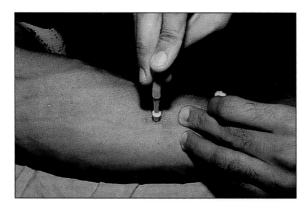

253 Punch biopsy
A piece of tissue may be removed under local anaesthetic with a disposable skin punch for histology, culture and the direct demonstration of amastigotes.

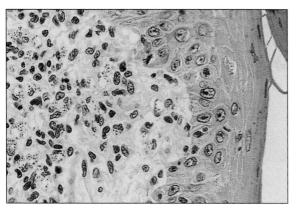

254 Parasitised macrophages in skin section
Many parasitised macrophages can be seen in this section from an acute lesion caused by *Leishmania major*. (*H&E* × *220.*)

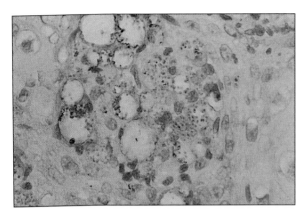

255 Immunoperoxidase staining of *Leishmania*
This procedure is very useful to demonstrate small numbers of amastigotes in tissue sections in which H&E staining is often unsatisfactory. The section shown here has many brown-staining amastigotes in parasitophorous vacuoles within mauve-staining macrophages. ($\times$ *260.*)

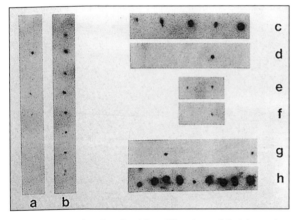

256 DNA probe for the identification of *Leishmania major* in *Phlebotomus papatasi*
Highly specific DNA probes have been developed not only for detecting *Leishmania*, but also for sandflies; their combined application can be invaluable in epidemiological studies. Sandflies collected in the field are squashed onto special papers and are then hybridised sequentially with probes against the parasite and suspected vector species. This permits both the numbers of the vector in the collection and the proportion of those vectors that are infected to be determined in parallel in a short time, thus avoiding the need for laborious and time-consuming dissections and subsequent cultivation and identification of the parasites. The figure shows autoradiographs of *Ph. papatasi*, some of which are infected with *L. major*. [a—positive hybridisation to an *L. major* probe in 3/8 flies found positive on dissection; b—positive responses to a *Ph. papatasi* probe in 8/8 flies; d, e, f, g—positive responses to *L. major*; c, h—positive responses to both probes.]

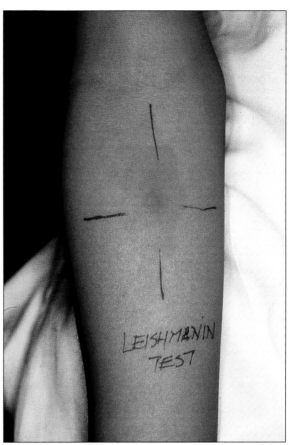

257 Leishmanin (Montenegro) test
The diagnosis may be assisted by the injection of an intra-dermal antigen prepared from cultured promastigotes of *Leishmania major* or other species. This produces a typical cell-mediated, delayed hypersensitivity response in most cases of active cutaneous disease within one to two months of its onset; the test usually gives positive results for life. It gives negative results in the active stages of kala-azar, but may give faintly positive results during the course of treatment, especially in East African patients. The reaction shown in the antigen site is maximal after 48 hours; it should be measured by first feeling and marking the limits of the induration, as shown. The size is then compared with that of a control injection (not shown here).

NEW WORLD CUTANEOUS LEISHMANIASIS

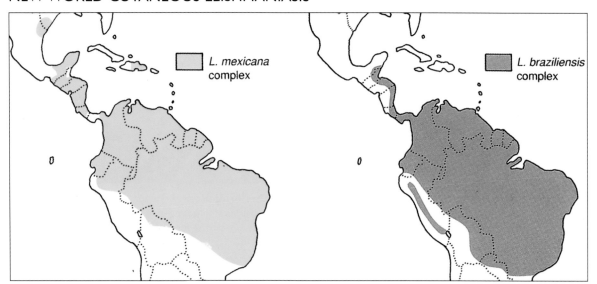

258 Distribution map of New World cutaneous and mucocutaneous leishmaniasis (including Espundia)
New World cutaneous and mucocutaneous leishmaniasis ('Espundia') occur focally from Texas (USA) and Mexico south-wards throughout Central America and South America as far south as São Paulo State of Brazil. The disease is limited by the Andean chain to the west except in Peru where a special form of cutaneous disease, 'Uta,' is found on the western slopes of the Andes. (*See* **Table 9**.)

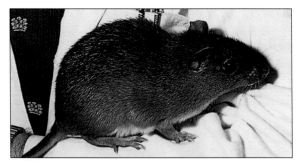

259 Rodent reservoir of *Leishmania amazonensis* in the Brazilian rain forest
Most cutaneous leishmaniases in the New World are zoonoses associated with rodents of the rain forest. *L. amazonensis* has been isolated from this species of rodent, *Proechimys guyanensis*, in the Amazon basin of Brazil.

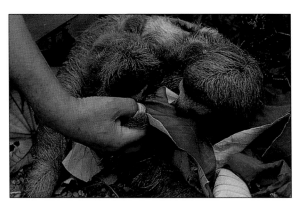

260 Arboreal animals as reservoirs
In other areas, e.g. Panama, Brazil and the Guyanas, a wide variety of arboreal animals serve as reservoirs for *Leishmamia panamensis* and *L. guyanensis*. The hosts include species of monkeys, marmosets and ant-eaters and such bizarre animals as the three-toed sloth (*Bradypus variegatus*), shown here in Panama.

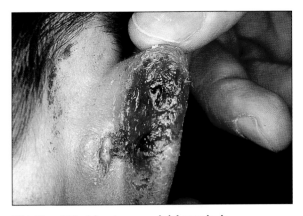

261 New World cutaneous leishmaniasis
The early stage of a lesion caused by *Leishmania mexicana* is seen on the back of the ear of a man infected in the jungle near Belize.

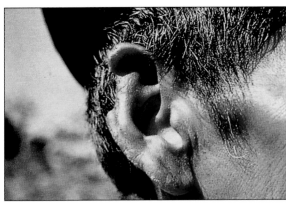

262 Chiclero's ulcer
Forest workers collecting gum from wild chicle trees commonly sleep near the forest floor and are bitten on exposed parts of the head by vectors that normally maintain transmission of *Leishmania mexicana* among the forest rodents. Lesions leading to erosion of the auricular cartilage are known as 'chiclero's ulcers.'

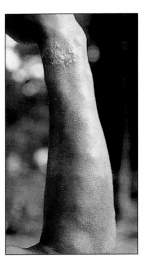

263 'Sporotrichoid' dissemination
As noted for *Leishmania major* (see **243**), lymphatic spread may also occur with New World species. This patient was infected with *L. guyanensis*, the agent of 'Pian bois.' In such infections the lymphatic nodules may ulcerate, resulting in chains of 'sporotrichoid' lesions.

MUCOCUTANEOUS LEISHMANIASIS

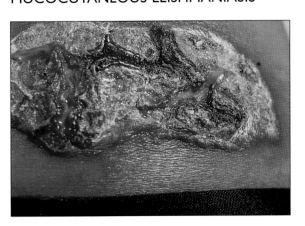

264 Cutaneous lesion caused by *Leishmania braziliensis*
Chronic cutaneous ulceration as seen on the lower abdomen of this man living in the town of Coarí along the River Amazon often precedes the development of the nasopharyngeal lesions of Espundia.

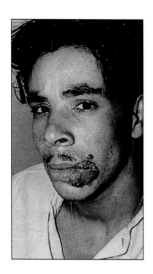

265 Early lesion of Espundia

The lesions of mucocutaneous leishmaniasis due to infection with *Leishmania braziliensis* may first become evident as ulcers involving the mucocutaneous junctions of the mouth and nose. This condition often follows a primary cutaneous lesion, which may have healed with or without specific therapy some years earlier.

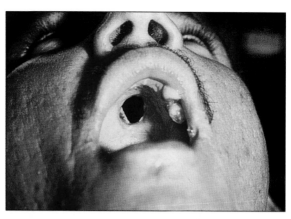

266 Pharyngeal involvement

Ulceration often extends to the pharynx and soft palate, and the first symptoms may be related to tissue destruction in this area. This man from Pará, Brazil, had a large, destructive lesion of the hard palate.

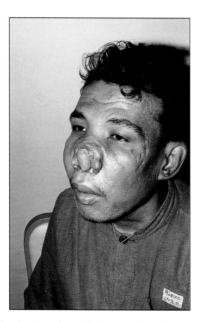

267 Early destruction of the nasal septum

The progress of the disease in this man seen in Belo Horizonte, Brazil, was arrested by intensive chemotherapy leaving him with the need for reconstructive surgery.

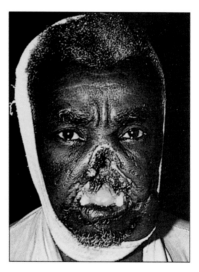

268 Destructive Espundia

Gross destruction of the nose, including the septum and palate, may follow inadequate treatment of *Leishmania braziliensis* infection. Many patients with this disease respond very poorly if at all to any form of chemotherapy, and reconstructive plastic surgery is called for. The tissue destruction is probably due to cytotoxic immune complexes formed in this hyperallergic response.

DIFFUSE CUTANEOUS LEISHMANIASIS

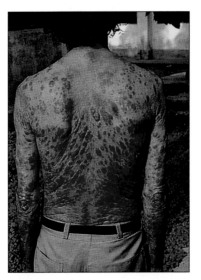

269 Diffuse cutaneous leishmaniasis in the New World

In some individuals, a rare failure of specific cell-mediated immunity may result in the development of chronic disseminated disease, 'Leishmaniasis diffusa,' resembling lepromatous leprosy, after infection with parasites of the *Leishmania mexicana* complex. In such cases chemotherapy, at best, produces only a temporary remission, and complete cure to date is unknown. This Brazilian patient first developed lesions due to *L. amazonensis* more than 20 years before this picture was taken. A similar syndrome occurs in Ethiopia and western Kenya in patients infected with *L. aethiopica*. Diffuse cutaneous leishmaniasis never affects the mucosae and is thus readily distinguished from post kala-azar dermal leishmaniasis or Espundia (*c.f.* **227**, **268**).

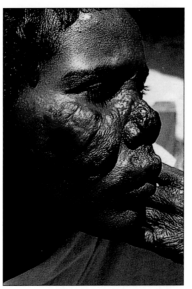

270 Diffuse cutaneous leishmaniasis in the Old World

This Ethiopian patient who was infected with *Leishmania aethiopica* was treated for years in a leprosarium with no improvement, in the mistaken belief that he was suffering from lepromatous leprosy (*c.f.* **228**).

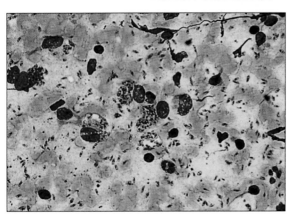

271 Skin smear in diffuse cutaneous leishmaniasis

This smear from a skin biopsy from another Ethiopian patient with diffuse cutaneous leishmaniasis shows large numbers of amastigotes. Parasites are rarely so numerous in biopsies from patients with other forms of cutaneous leishmaniasis. (*Giemsa* × *390.*)

NEMATODES—THE FILARIASES

(See **Tables 10** *and* **11**.)

WUCHERERIA BANCROFTI, BRUGIA MALAYI AND BRUGIA TIMORI

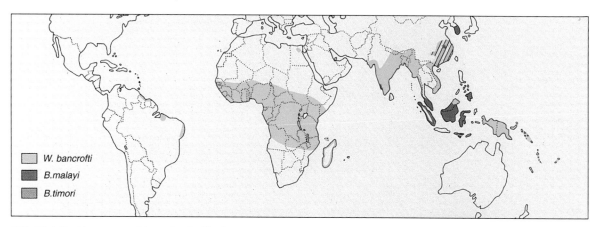

272 Distribution map of lymphatic filariases
It is estimated that about 78 million of the 750 million people living in areas endemic for lymphatic filariasis are infected, mainly with *Wuchereria bancrofti*. Throughout most of its range this species is nocturnally periodic, i.e. the microfilaria reach a maximal density in the peripheral blood at night. The non-periodic or diurnally subperiodic forms are found in some islands of the eastern Pacific. In most of its endemic area of Southeast Asia, China and Korea, *Brugia malayi* is nocturnally periodic, but a subperiodic form occurs in parts of West Malaysia, Thailand, southern Vietnam, Sabah and the Philippines, where it is probably a zoonosis with monkey, cat and dog reservoirs. *B. timori* is found only in Indonesia, where it is transmitted by *Anopheles barbirostris*. The shaded area indicates that part of China where *W. bancrofti* has been greatly reduced in incidence or eradicated. (Adapted from WHO *Maps Nos. 92354 and 92353*.)

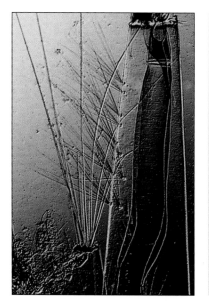
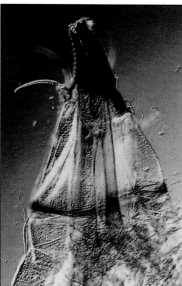
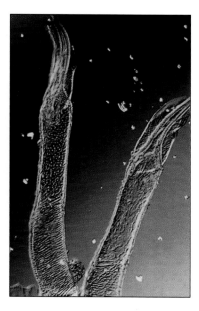

273–275 Aquatic stages of *Culex* and *Mansonia*
Unlike *Anopheles* mosquitoes (*see* **9**) or those of *Culex* (**273**, left), *Mansonia* larvae (**274**, centre) and pupae (**275**, right) are attached by their breathing tubes (siphons) to underwater roots, stems and leaves of aquatic plants. Note the saw-edged tips of the siphons that are used to penetrate the plants. Their ideal breeding habitats are open swamps, with *Pistia stratiotes*, water lilies and other aquatic plants. (× *60*.) (*See also* **5–11**.)

Table 10 Microfilariae occurring in humans[1]

Location	Sheath +/−	Structure	Main characters	Species
Blood (all tropics)	+	TAIL HEAD BODY SHEATH	nuclei not to tip nuclei almost to tip 244–296 μ, smooth curves stains pale mauve with Giemsa	*Wuchereria bancrofti*
(Southeast Asia)	+	TAIL HEAD BODY SHEATH	2 tiny nuclei in terminal thread clear cephalic space 177–230 μ, kinked stains bright pink with Giemsa	*Brugia malayi*
(Timor, Lesser Sunda islands of Indonesia)	+	TAIL HEAD BODY SHEATH	2 tiny nuclei in terminal thread longer cephalic space 265–323 μ, kinked unstained with Giemsa	*Brugia timori*
(African forest areas)	+	TAIL BODY SHEATH	nuclei to tip, often bent on body 250–300 μ, kinked unstained with Giemsa	*Loa loa*
(New World, Caribbean)	−	TAIL BODY	nuclei not to tip, pointed 200 × 5 μ	*Mansonella, ozzardi*
(all tropics)	−	TAIL BODY	nuclei to tip, rounded 200 × 5 μ	*Mansonella perstans*
Skin (West Africa)	−	TAIL HEAD BODY	nuclei to tip, crooked single column 10–12 nuclei, then double column 180–240 μ × 5 μ	*Mansonella streptocerca*
(Africa, Yemen Central and South America)	−	TAIL HEAD BODY	nuclei not to tip, crooked spatulate 285–368 μ × 8 μ 150–287 μ × 8μ	*Onchocerca volvulus*

[1] See **Table 11** for prevalence of the various species.

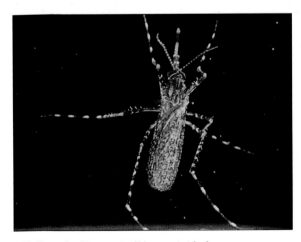

276 Female *Mansonia* (*Mansonioides*) spp.
In the Far East and southwest Pacific, several species of this subgenus (all of which are common swamp breeders) are the main vectors of *Brugia malayi*. (× 6.)

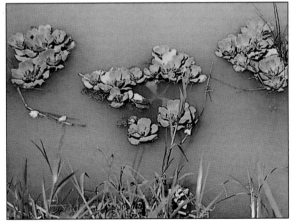

277 *Mansonia* breeding site
Pistia stratiotes growing at the edge of a swamp. The roots and leaf veins of this widely distributed water plant are commonly used as attachment sites by larvae and pupae of these mosquitoes, which acquire oxygen from them.

Table II Nematodes of medical importance and their prevalence[1]

Subclass	Order (Suborder)	Superfamily	Genus and species	Probable prevalence in humans
ADENOPHOREA	ENOPLIDA	Trichuroidea	*Trichinella spiralis*	49 million
			Trichuris trichiura	500 million
			Capillaria hepatica	rare
			C. philippensis	thousands
SECERNENTEA	RHABDITIDA	Rhabditoidea	*Strongyloides stercoralis*	70 million
	STRONGYLIDA	Ancylostomatoidea	*Ancylostoma duodenale* ⎫ *Necator americanus* ⎭	700–900 million
			Ancylostoma caninum	thousands
			A. braziliense	thousands
			A. ceylanicum	rare
			Ternidens deminutus	thousands
			Oesophagostomum bifurcus	> 250 000
			Syngamus laryngeus	rare
		Trichostrongyloidea	*Trichostrongylus* spp.	10 million
		Metastrongyloidea	*Metastrongylus elongatus*	rare
			Parastrongylus cantonensis	thousands
			Parastrongylus costaricensis	thousands
	OXYURIDA	Oxyuroidea	*Enterobius vermicularis*	400 million
	ASCARIDIDA	Ascaridoidea	*Ascaris lumbricoides*	800–1000 million
			Toxocara canis	thousands
			T. cati	thousands
			Lagochilascaris minor	rare
			Baylisascaris procyonis	rare
			Anisakis spp.	rare
			Pseudoterronova decipiens	thousands
	SPIRURIDA (SPIRURINA)	Spiruroidea	*Gongylonema pulchrum*	rare
		Gnathostomatoidea	*Gnathostoma spinigerum*	thousands
		Thelazoidea	*Thelazia callipaeda*	rare
		Filarioidea	*Wuchereria bancrofti*	70–75 million
			Brugia malayi ⎫ *B. timori* ⎭	6 million
			Loa loa	33 million
			Onchocerca volvulus	<17 million[2]
			Mansonella perstans	65 million
			M. streptocerca	2 million
			M. ozzardi	15 million
			Dirofilaria spp.	rare
	SPIRURIDA (CAMALLANINA)	Dracunculoidea	*Dracunculus medinensis*	<3 million[2]

[1]The estimated prevalences of helminthic infections vary greatly. These figures and the figures in **Table 12** are based on estimates by the WHO (1993).
[2]As a result of ongoing eradication campaigns these numbers are falling drastically each year.

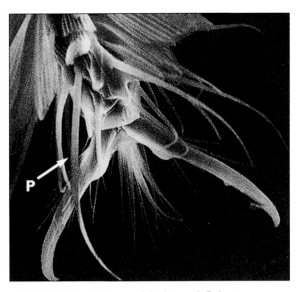 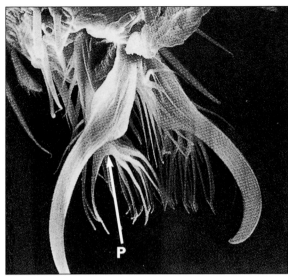

278 & 279 Tarsal claws of *Aedes* and *Culex*
The tarsal claws of *Aedes* (**278**, left) have strong hooks and a simple pulvillus (P), (× *1000*.) *Culex* (**279**, right) has fleshy pulvilli and no hooks. (× *1300*.) (The hooks are not seen in the *Aedes* in these scanning electron micrographs; the contrast between the simple pulvillus of *Aedes* and the complex pulvillus of *Culex* is clearly demonstrated.)

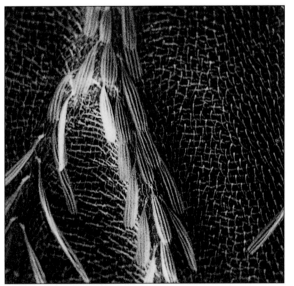 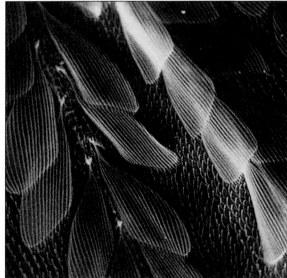

280 & 281 Wing scales of *Culex* and *Mansonia*
The adults of *Mansonia* are distinguished from other culicines by the typical, large wing scales. *Culex* (**280**, left); *Mansonia* (**281**, right). (× *370*.)

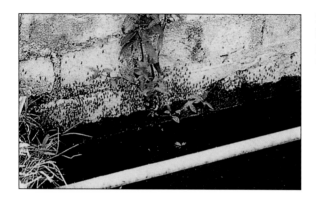

282 Peridomestic culicine breeding site near Delhi
Septic pits and drains containing stagnant water are ideal breeding grounds for *Culex quinquefasciatus*—a peridomestic vector of bancroftian filariasis.

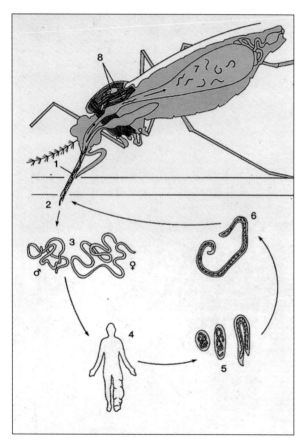

283 Life cycle of *Wuchereria bancrofti* and *Brugia malayi*
Third stage infective larvae (1) from the mouthparts of the mosquito enter the hole made by the proboscis in the skin when the mosquito feeds (2). The larvae pass through the lymphatics where they mature to thread-like adults, 4–8 cm long (3), and pass to regional lymphatic glands (4). After mating, they remain in the glands where the females develop eggs (5) and larvae (6), which they release as microfilariae into the peripheral circulation. Picked up with the blood meal of another mosquito (7), the larvae penetrate the insect's gut wall to enter the thoracic muscles (8), where they moult to produce sausage-shaped, second stage larvae, and then long, thin, infective third stage larvae (1), which migrate to the proboscis. (*See also* **286–289, 299, 300, 301**.)

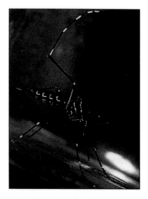

284 Female *Aedes (Stegomyia) polynesiensis*
Night-biting *Culex quinquefasciatus* and various species of *Anopheles* are the main vectors of the nocturnal periodic form of *Wuchereria bancrofti*. Day-biting *Ae. polynesiensis* transmits the subperiodic form of *W. bancrofti* in various Pacific islands. Compare the hump-backed stance with that of *Anopheles* (see **87**). (× 4.2.)

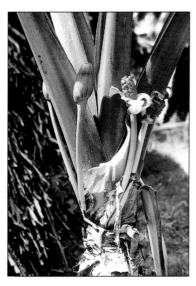

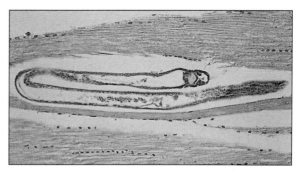

286 Larvae in mosquito thorax
Ingested microfilariae exsheath, migrate from the midgut and penetrate the thoracic muscles, where they mature to sausage-shaped first stage and second stage larvae. (× 170.)

285 Taro plants, breeding sites for vectors of the *Aedes (Stegomyia) scutellaris* group in the southwest Pacific
Rain water accumulating in leaf axils such as those of taro, banana and pineapple is readily colonised by many species of mosquitoes and *Culicoides* in forested areas. Rainwater collecting in holes in bamboos as well as in coconut husks, old tyres and other small receptacles also serve as breeding sites for this group of vectors.

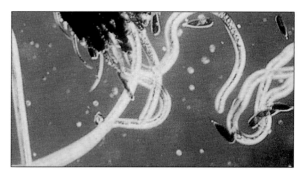

287 Infective larvae emerging from the proboscis of *Culex quinquefasciatus*
After about two weeks, the larvae develop into third stage, filariform larvae, which enter the mosquito's proboscis. These infective larvae later penetrate the skin of a new host through the puncture wound made when the mosquito bites. (*Interference optics* × 250.)

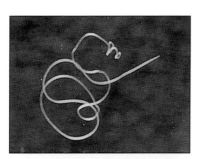

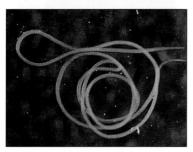

290 Lymphangitis
Acute involvement of lymphatic vessels is common, especially in the extremities. In association with lymphangitis, there is almost always some local lymphadenitis and fever.

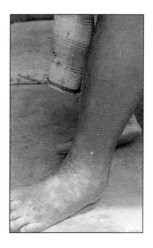

288 & 289 Male and female *Wuchereria bancrofti* adults
On maturation, the infective larvae copulate and the adult filariae become localised in lymph glands (e.g. in the groin). Adult male *W. bancrofti* (**288**, top) are about 4 cm long; females (**289**, bottom) are about 8–10 cm long. (× 9.)

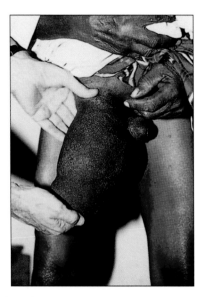

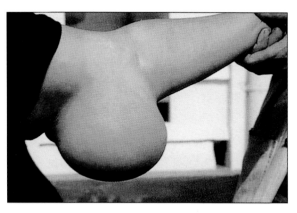

292 Elephantiasis of right epitrochlear gland in a Fijian

A feature that is unusually common in the South Pacific and is also due to *Wuchereria bancrofti* is gross enlargement of the epitrochlear lymph node.

291 Hydrocele

Orchitis may occur in the acute stage; it is commonly associated with hydrocele, and microfilariae may be found in the hydrocele fluid. This is a relatively late lesion seen in a Tanzanian patient.

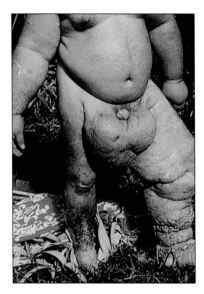

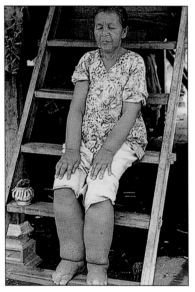

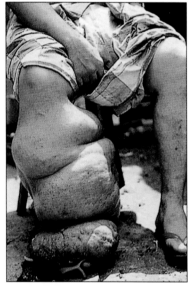

293 Elephantiasis of the leg and scrotum due to *Wuchereria bancrofti* in Tahiti

Gross elephantiasis of the scrotum may produce gross and incapacitating deformity that requires radical surgery to remove the surplus tissue.

294 Early elephantiasis due to *Brugia malayi*

Lymphatic obstruction (especially in the leg) progressing in chronic cases to elephantiasis may occur in regions of high endemicity. Lymphatic obstruction may also arise in the arm, breast or scrotum. By this late stage, microfilariae are rarely found in blood films.

295 Massive elephantiasis due to *Brugia malayi*

As in that caused by *Wuchereria bancrofti* (see **293**), the enlargement is commonly unilateral.

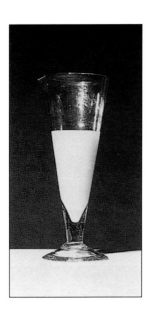

296 Urine containing lymph
The dilated lymph vessels rupture and discharge chyle into the urinary tract, thus producing the milky appearance known as chyluria.

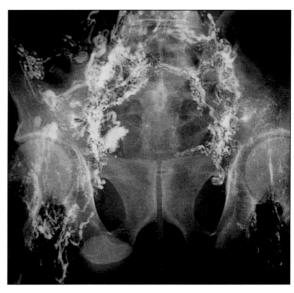

297 Lymphogram in patient with chyluria
Obstruction of the cisterna chyli or its tributaries may occur, giving rise to chyluria.

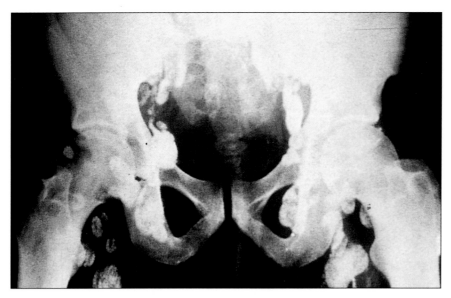

298 Calcified lymph nodes
Numerous calcified inguinal lymph nodes and ducts are seen in this radiograph of a patient with chronic *Wuchereria bancrofti* infection.

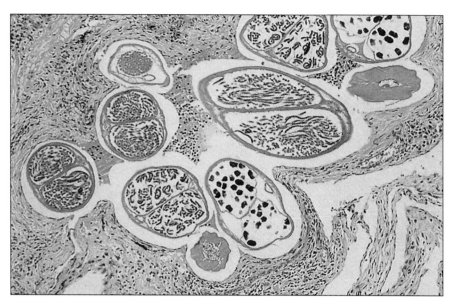

299 *Wuchereria bancrofti* in an occluded lymphatic vessel
Note the marked cellular reaction surrounding the microfilaria-containing female worms, seen here in cross section. (*H&E × 20.*)

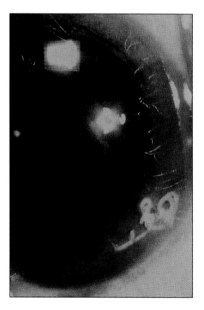

300 Male *Wuchereria bancrofti* in the anterior chamber of the eye
A motile nematode was removed from the anterior chamber of the eye of this 20-year-old Indian man who had soreness of the eye and diminished vision of one week's duration. The worm, which measured about 20 × 0.1 mm, was identified as a male *W. bancrofti*. The patient made a complete recovery following surgery, which is the treatment of choice for this rare condition.

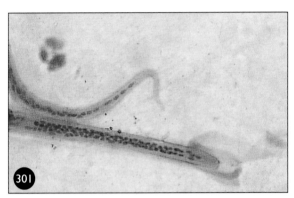

301–307 Microfilariae in blood films

Identification of microfilariae and parasite counts per unit quantity of blood are necessary for the epidemiological evaluation of filariasis (although not for individual diagnosis). Twenty μl pipettes are commonly used to make a thick blood film of specific size. If microfilariae are present in the peripheral circulation, they can usually be found by examining a fresh preparation of blood that has been taken between 10 pm and midnight. The worms may be seen in a wet preparation, but morphological differentiation is only possible after suitable staining with a Romanowsky-type stain (Leishman or Giemsa), or haematoxylin. *Wuchereria bancrofti* (**301**); *Brugia malayi* (**302** *and* **303**); *Loa loa* (**304** *and* **305**); *Mansonella ozzardi* (**306**); *M. perstans* (**307**) (× 920.) (*See* **Table 10** *and* **352** *and* **353** *for skin-snip technique for other species.*)

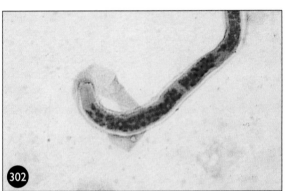

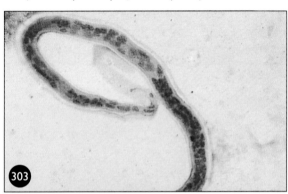

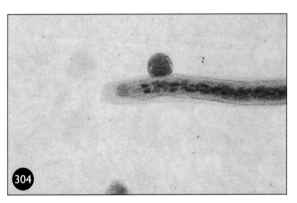

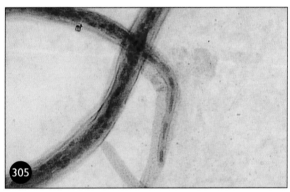

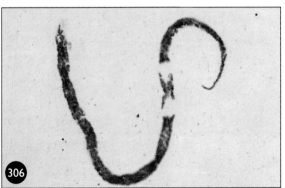

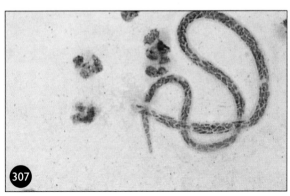

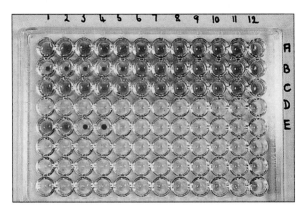

308 Serological diagnosis of filariasis

The complement-fixation test using *Dirofilaria immitis* of the dog as antigen will confirm a diagnosis of filariasis, but it does not distinguish between the different species of filaria. [Row A—negative control serum; row B—positive titre of 1/64; row C—negative reaction from another patient; E—complement control.] An enzyme-linked immunosorbent assay based on the use of a monoclonal antibody to detect filarial antigen has proved to be very sensitive but is not yet in widescale use. DNA probes are being developed.

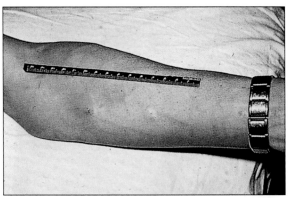

309 Positive skin test with *Dirofilaria* antigen

A similar antigen to that used in the complement-fixation test may also be used to demonstrate delayed cutaneous hypersensitivity.

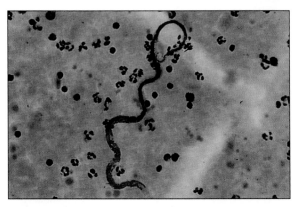

310 Giemsa-stained microfilariae

The sheathed microfilaria of *Brugia timori* is easily distinguished from that of *B. malayi* and *Wuchereria bancrofti* by its large size, the lack of staining of the sheath of *B. timori* in Giemsa stain and the distribution of the nuclei in the posterior end. *B. timori*, as with *B. malayi*, has two distinct nuclei in the tail (*c.f.* **301** *and* **303**). In *B. timori*, as in *B. malayi* or typical *W. bancrofti* infection, parasite counts reveal a marked nocturnal periodicity. (In the diurnal, subperiodic type of *W. bancrofti*, microfilariae are readily seen in blood taken during the day.) (× *310*.)

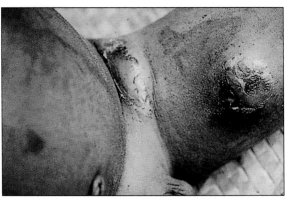

311 Abscesses in groin and thigh due to *Brugia timori*

Both this species and *Wuchereria bancrofti* are found in some Indonesian islands (see **272**) where up to 25% of village populations have been found infected with *B. timori*. The clinical disease resembles that caused by *B. malayi*, except that abscess formation is fairly common in the early stages along the line of the great saphenous vein in the upper thigh (as seen here), whereas chronic lymphoedema is more common rather than frank elephantiasis in later cases. This parasite is transmitted by *Anopheles barbirostris*.

MANSONELLA PERSTANS

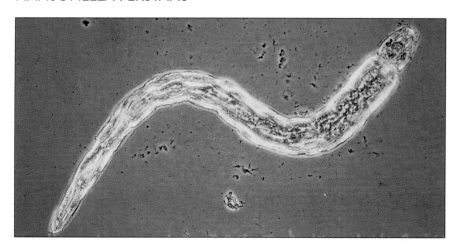

312 Larva of *Culicoides*
Manonella perstans is found in tropical Africa and in coastal regions of Central and South America. The vectors of *M. perstans* are small, speckled-wing flies of the genus *Culicoides*, of which *C. austeni* and *C. grahami* seem to be the main vectors in West Africa. The aquatic stages are commonly found in tree holes, leaf axils (**285**) and other small natural water containers. (× 24.)

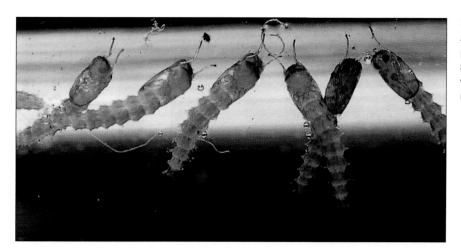

313 Pupae of *Culicoides*
As in mosquito pupae, the pupae of *Culicoides* obtain air by piercing the surface water film with their respiratory siphons. (× 15.)

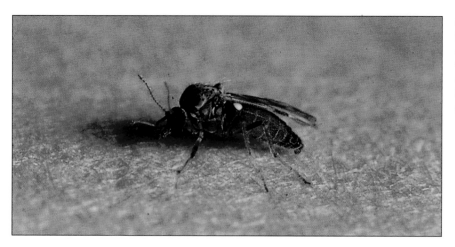

314 Adult *Culicoides* female
Although these flies are very small, their bites can cause severe irritation. The biting mouthparts are clearly visible here. (× 30.)

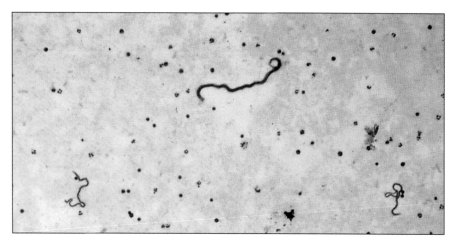

315 *Mansonella perstans* and *Loa loa* in blood film
The unsheathed microfilaria of *M. perstans* is readily distinguished (even at a fairly low magnification) from the sheathed microfilaria of *L. loa* (or that of *Wuchereria bancrofti*) in blood films by its smaller size. Multiple infections with several species of blood-dwelling microfilariae are common. *M. perstans* infection is usually asymptomatic and may last for many years. Males measure about 45 mm in length and females about 70–80 mm. (*Giemsa* × *150.*)

LOAIASIS

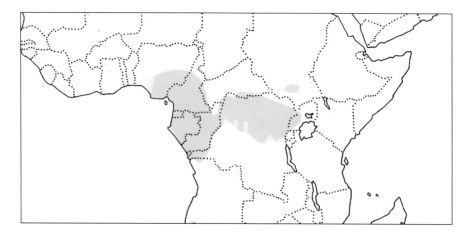

316 Distribution map of loaiasis
Loaiasis is confined to Africa, extending from the Gulf of Guinea in the west to the Great Lakes in the east. Infection with an almost identical parasite is common in these areas in certain monkeys (such as the mandrill), and some infections may be zoonotic.

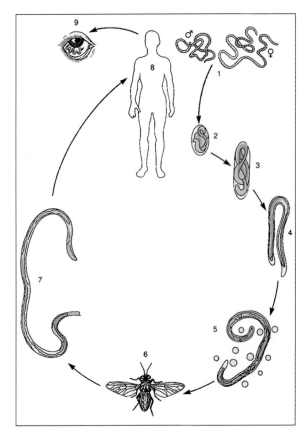

317 Life cycle of *Loa loa*

The adult worms (1) live in man for 4–12 years. The females (about 7 cm long) migrate through the subcutaneous tissues and may cross the front of the eye under the conjunctiva (9). Microfilariae (5) develop from larvae (2–4) in the female and circulate in the blood, in which they are picked up by a *Chrysops* (6). In the gut of the fly, the microfilariae exsheath and enter the fat bodies in which they mature first to sausage-like forms, then to infective third stage larvae (7). These larvae infect a new host (8) when the *Chrysops* takes another bloodmeal and mature to adult worms within about one year.

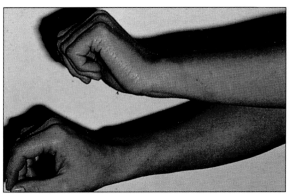

319 Calabar swelling in left forearm

Recurrent large swellings lasting about three days are characteristic and indicate the tracks of the migrating adults in the connective tissue. They are most often seen in the hand, wrists and forearm. A marked eosinophilia (60–90%) accompanies this phase of the infection.

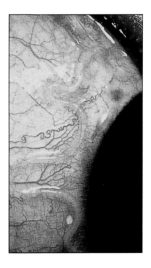

320 Adult *Loa loa* in the eye

The movement of the adult worm under the conjunctiva causes considerable irritation and congestion.

318 Female *Chrysops silacea* (top) and *C. dimidiata* (bottom)

Tabanid flies of the genus *Chrysops* transmit loaiasis. *C. silacea* and *C. dimidiata* are the most important vectors in Nigeria, the Cameroons and the Congo highlands. (× 3.0.)

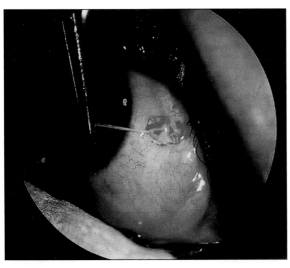

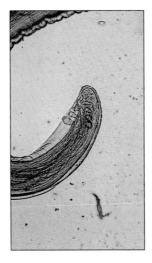

322 Tail of male *Loa loa*
The spicules at the posterior end of the male worm are typical of this species. (× *90.*)

321 Extraction of worm
The adult worm can be extracted with fine forceps after anaesthetising the conjunctiva.

ONCHOCERCIASIS

323 Distribution map of onchocerciasis
Onchocerca volvulus is a tissue-dwelling nematode, the microfilariae of which are found predominantly in the skin and eye. Onchocerciasis has a focal distribution in Africa and South America. In Africa, onchocerciasis is mainly a disease of riverine country—e.g., of the extensive ramifications of the Niger and Volta in West Africa, and of mountainous regions in Zaire, Ethiopia and East Africa. In addition, small foci of transmission exist in the mountainous country of Yemen and possibly southwest Saudi Arabia. In the New World, onchocerciasis, once believed to be restricted to Central America, is now known to be endemic in large foci in Colombia, Ecuador and northern Venezuela, as well as in an important area of southern Venezuela bordering Amazonian Brazil. The incidence of new infections in West Africa has been considerably reduced in the past decade thanks to a mass campaign to destroy the larvae of the vectors with insecticides and the infective pool of filariae in the human hosts with chemotherapy. The shaded area in West Africa indicates the region in which the Onchocerciasis Eradication Programme is operative (see **351**). (Adapted from WHO *Maps Nos. 94910 and 94911.*)

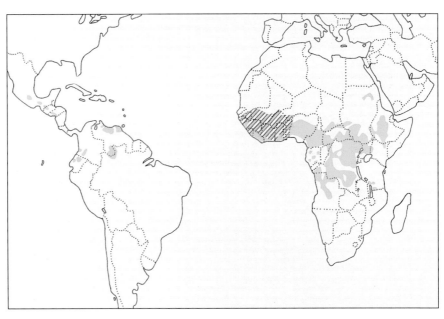

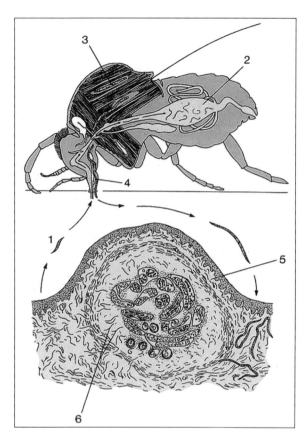

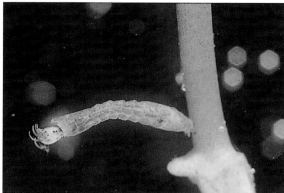

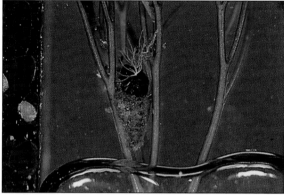

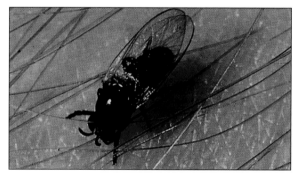

324 Life cycle of *Onchocerca volvulus*
(1) Microfilariae in the subepidermis are taken up with blood when the *Simulium* bites. From the midgut (2), the larvae pass into the haemocele, then enter the thoracic muscles where they grow and undergo two moults. In the process, they pass through the second ('sausage') stage (3), then become long, thin, infective third stage larvae (4); the whole process takes f6–12 days depending on the ambient temperature. The infective larvae make their way to the proboscis through which they enter the skin when the fly again feeds. Infective larvae mature into adults as they migrate through the subcutaneous tissues, with males and females mating and becoming encapsulated by fibrous tissue in prominent subcutaneous nodules (5). Within the nodules, the females produce larvae and these microfilariae (6) migrate into the nearby subepidermal tissues, with those in the head region reaching the tissues of the eye. (*Adapted from Geigy and Herbig, 1955.*) (*See also* **333–335** *and* **353–356.**)

325 & 326 Aquatic stages of the vectors
The filarial worm is transmitted by biting flies of the genus *Simulium*. The larvae (**325**, top) and the pupae (**326**, bottom) of *Simulium* are attached to submerged objects in fast-running water, from which they extract oxygen through head filaments ($\times$ 5). (*See also* **329–331.**)

327 Adult *Simulium damnosum*
Because of their hump-backed stance, these insects are commonly known as 'buffalo flies' in some areas. *S. damnosum* is now recognised to be a large complex of sibling species of which at least 10 are proven vectors in different parts of Africa. In East Africa, the *S. naevei* complex used to be an important vector in some highland areas. *S. ochraceum* and *S. metallicum* are important vectors in Central and South America. ($\times$ 10.)

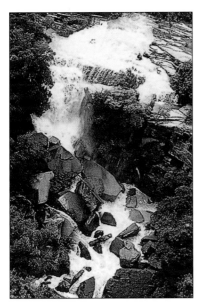

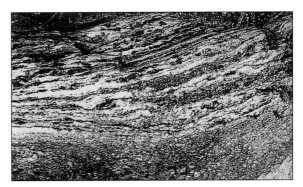

330 *Simulium* larvae and pupae attached to rocks
Rapidly moving water in a river in the dry season showing stone boulders in the bed of the stream which, by causing eddies in the water, provide enough oxygenation to permit the *Simulium* to survive while the river level is low.

328 Typical locality of *Simulium* in West Africa
Fast-moving, highly oxygenated water in streams, rivers, waterfalls, etc. provides the essential ecological environment for *Simulium*. The figure shows a branch of the Upper Volta River. In some hyperendemic villages in West Africa, a third of all adults may be blinded by onchocerciasis.

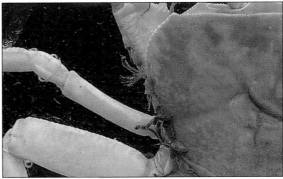

331 *Simulium* larvae and pupae on a crab
In East Africa, larvae and pupae of the *S. neavei* complex are attached to freshwater crabs. Several of each stage of *S. nyasalandicum* can be seen on this preserved specimen of *Potamonautes pseudoperlatus*, which inhabits small hill streams in Tanzania.

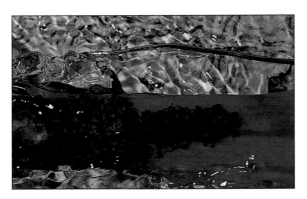

329 Eggs of *Simulium*
The black eggs are seen attached to a narrow leaf just below the surface of rapidly flowing water.

332 *Onchocerca* nodules on iliac crests of an African
The adult filariae become encapsulated in fibrous material, which forms nodules in the subcutaneous tissues. They are found predominantly in the lower part of the body in Africa, whereas in South and Central America they are more commonly found on the head and upper trunk.

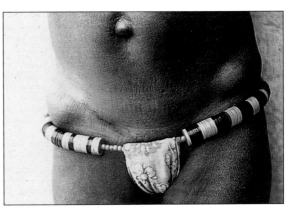

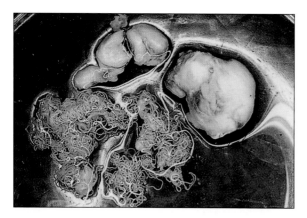

333 Macroscopic section of nodule
In this gross section of a nodule, the adult worms are seen entwined. (× 2.)

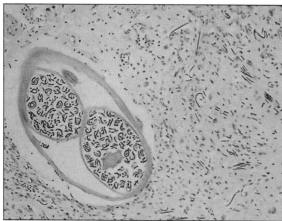

334 Transverse section of nodule
Section through an onchocercal nodule showing cross sections of a gravid female in a matrix of inflammatory cells and fibrinoid material, in which microfilariae are embedded. (*Phloxinetartrazine × 40.*)

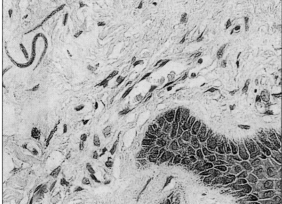

335 Microfilaria in skin biopsy
After discharge from the female uterus, the microfilariae migrate to the skin and the eye. (*H&E × 350.*)

336 Papular dermatitis in onchocerciasis
Early onchocerciasis is characterised by lesions in two main sites: the skin and the eye. This pruriginous condition, commonly called 'craw craw' in Africa, involves irregular, broad areas of the skin, where small papules form around the microfilariae.

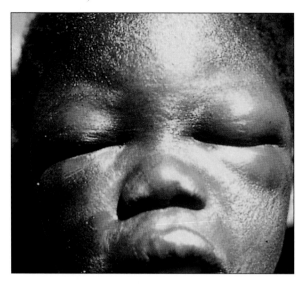

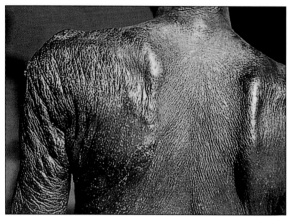

337 Mazzotti reaction in an African child
Treatment with even a single, very small dose of a micro-filaricide such as diethylcarbamazine can trigger a severe allergic reaction due to the rapid killing of skin-dwelling microfilariae. This was formerly used as a provocative diag-nostic test for onchocerciasis in individuals in whom micro-filariae could not be detected in skin snips. The reaction may also be positive in *Mansonella streptocerca* infections.

338 'Elephant' skin
Thickening and wrinkling of the skin give rise to the 'lizard' or 'elephant' skin appearance.

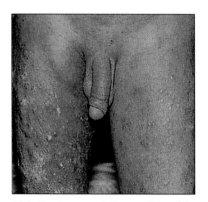

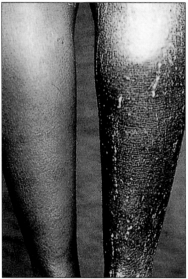

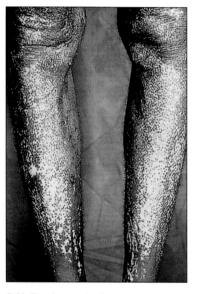

339 Onchocercal dermatitis with lichenification
This patient has swelling, lichenification and early hyperpigmentation of the right leg. In time, this will progress to the stage seen in **340**.

340 Advanced Sowda
This is a peculiar and quite common feature of onchocerciasis in Africa and Yemen. It is characterised by hyperpig-mentation (usually of one of the lower limbs), and it is often accompanied by inguinocrural lymphadenopathy.

341 Depigmentation
Pretibial atrophy and depigmentation in a patient with late (burnt-out) oncho-cerciasis. This condition is sometimes called 'leopard skin.'

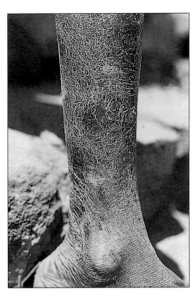

342 'Tissue paper' skin
In chronic infections, atrophy of the skin may occur, resulting in a 'tissue paper' appearance.

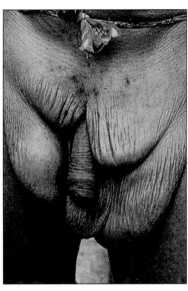

343 'Hanging groin'
Involvement of the inguinocrural glands can result in an appearance described as 'hanging groin.'

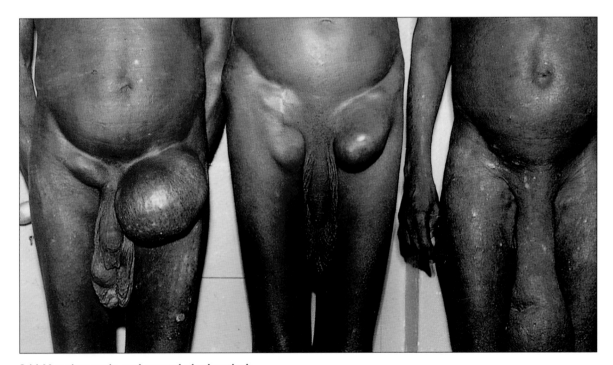

344 Hanging groin and scrotal elephantiasis
These three African patients show particularly severe anatomical changes due to onchocerciasis.

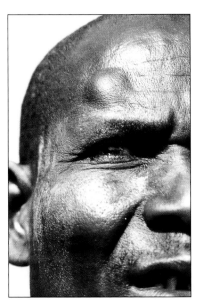

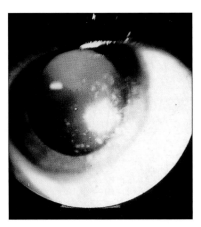

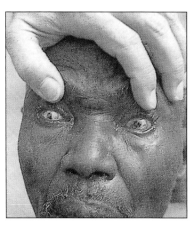

345 River blindness
From the female worm in the nodule of *Onchocerca volvulus* on the head of this blind African in Burkina Faso, large numbers of microfilariae will have penetrated the tissues of the eyes, eventually leading to blindness.

346 Early corneal involvement
The tissue reaction associated with dead microfilariae in the cornea gives rise to several 'snowflake-like' opacities, as seen in the figure. This punctate keratitis may clear with time.

347 Sclerosing keratitis
Heavy microfilarial infection of the cornea leads to the development of progressive, sclerosing keratitis, which commonly produces blindness, as seen in this African patient.

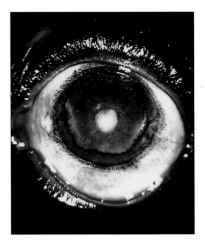

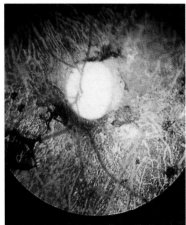

348 Cornea in sclerosing keratitis
Chemotherapy can now prevent such serious eye changes by destroying the microfilariae.

349 Optic atrophy
A variety of choroidoretinal lesions may follow damage by microfilariae to the anterior segments of the eye; optic atrophy may develop finally, as seen in this eye.

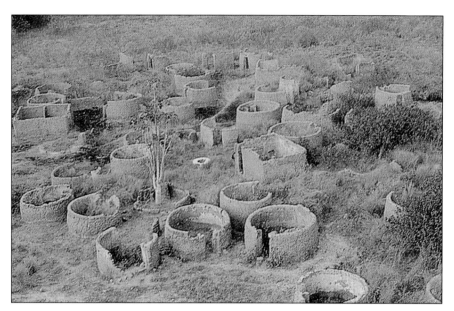

350 Abandoned village near the Volta River
High blindness rates in some areas have resulted in the depopulation of entire villages, as seen here. In the wake of the current eradication programme, it is to be hoped that this picture will become of historic interest only.

351 Helicopter spraying biological agent, BTI, over a breeding site of *Simulium damnosum* on the River Milo, Republic of Guinea
Fixed wing aircraft have also been used widely in the international Onchocerciasis Control Programme. Following the emergence of insecticide resistance to the organophosphate insecticide, temephos (Abate[R]), extensive use has also been made of the biological agent *Bacillus thuringiensis israelensis* H14 (BTI) to destroy the aquatic stages of *S. damnosum* in a 20-year campaign that has dramatically reduced the transmission of *Onchocerca volvulus* in much of the endemic area of West and Central Africa. However, the risk of reinvasion

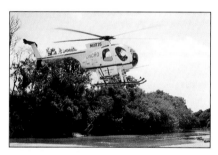

of infected areas by flies infected outside the controlled area continues to pose a serious threat.

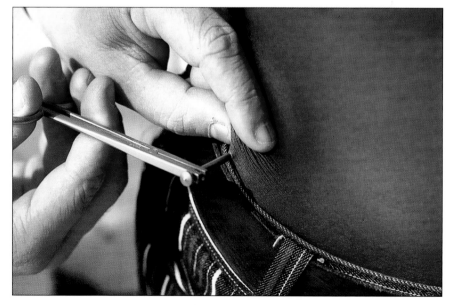

352 Skin-snip technique
A tiny piece of skin, often from the back of the shoulders, iliac regions or calf, is snipped off and placed in a drop of saline on a microscope slide under a coverslip, where it is left for several minutes at room temperature. The use of a scleral puncture as seen here permits the removal of a standard-sized sample to be taken for quantitative assessment of the microfilarial load. A simpler method is to raise the skin with a needle tip, then remove a piece of skin with a scalpel blade.

353 Living microfilariae of *Onchocerca volvulus*
After some time, actively moving microfilariae emerge from the skin into the surrounding saline where they can be counted. An enzyme-linked immunosorbent assay that is currently being evaluated uses a 'cocktail' of recombinant antigens as the basis of diagnosis and has shown some promise as a replacement for skin snips in diagnosis. However, the use of a non-radioactive polymerase chain reaction procedure on skin snips has proved more sensitive than visual examination and,

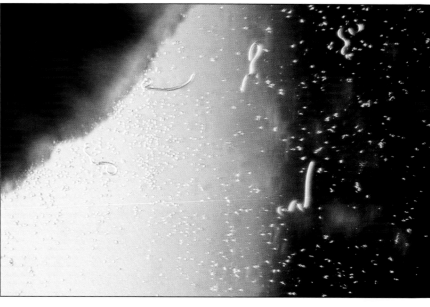

unlike serological tests, can distinguish between past and current infections. It is likely to gain in importance for the monitoring of the progress of control programmes rather than for individual diagnosis. (× 350.)

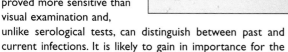

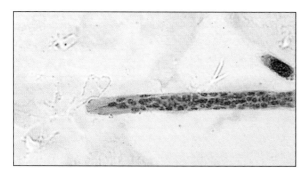

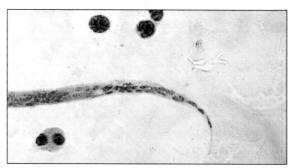

354 & 355 Microfilariae in skin snips
Onchocerca volvulus head (**354**, left) and tail (**355**, right) (× 930). (*c.f.* **301–307, 360** *and* **361**.)

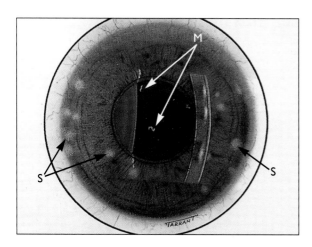

356 Slit-lamp examination of the eye Slit-lamp examination often reveals numerous microfilariae (M) in the anterior chamber of the eye. They are best sought in the inferior medial quadrant. This painting also shows numerous 'snowflake-like' opacities (S) in the cornea.

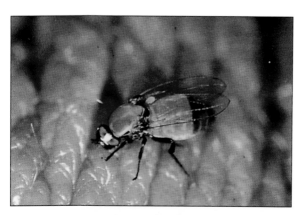

357 *Simulium ochraceum*
This simuliid fly and *S. metallicum* are two of the most important vectors of onchocerciasis in Central America. (× 12.)

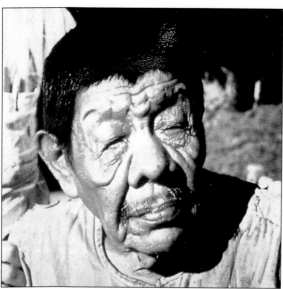

358 'Leonine facies' due to onchocerciasis in Guatemala
Estimates of the number of people infected in the New World are inaccurate but, for example, at least two million people inhabit the endemic areas of Venezuela. In Central America, onchocerciasis ('Erisipela de la costa') is characterised by an erythematous appearance of the face or upper trunk. It occurs in heavily infected young people, usually under 20 years of age. Purplish-tinged plaques or papules may be observed in Central America, usually in patients of an older age group. This condition, which is known as 'mal morado,' sometimes gives the leonine appearance seen here.

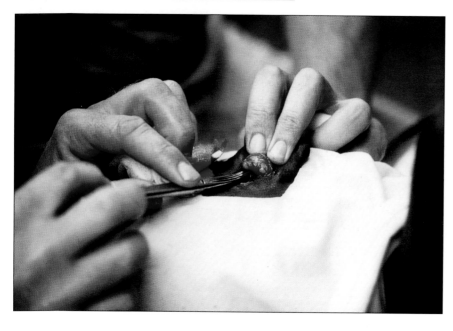

359 Nodulectomy
Serious eye changes can be prevented in some early cases by excising the nodules that contain the adult worms, thus preventing the continuing production of the microfilarae, which are the actual pathogenic agents in this disease. Nodulectomy has been widely employed in Central and South America. Control (by larviciding) in the New World has only been successful so far in Mexico and, to a lesser degree, in Guatemala.

OTHER FILARIASES

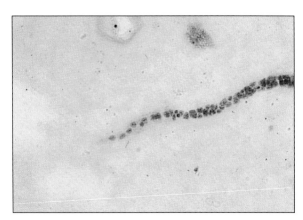 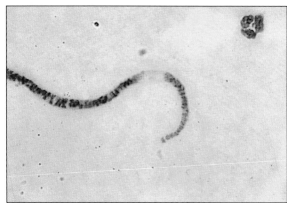

360 & 361 Microfilariae of *Mansonella streptocerca*
This skin-dwelling, unsheathed microfilaria must be distinguished from that of *Onchocerca volvulus* (**354** *and* **355**) in African patients. For this, a stained preparation should be examined (e.g. with haematoxylin). *M. streptocerca* produces few pathogenic effects; it is transmitted by *Culicoides grahami*, also infects chimpanzees, and is known only in Africa. Head (**360**, left), tail (**361**, right) (× 700). (*c.f.* **301–307, 354** *and* **355**.)

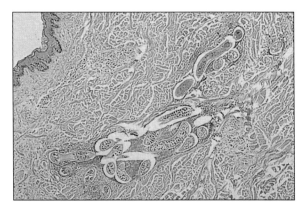

362 Adult female *Mansonella streptocerca* seen in a section of human skin
This low-power view shows the parasite within the dermis. Sections of microfilariae can be seen within the uterus (*H&E* × 100.) (AFIP No. 377582.)

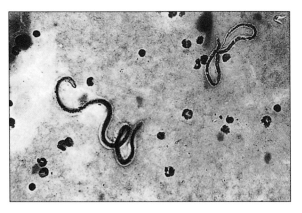

363 Microfilaria of *Mansonella ozzardi*
This unsheathed microfilaria (right) is found in the blood in parts of South America and the Caribbean. The microfilaria is readily distinguished from the larger and sheathed microfilaria of *Wuchereria bancrofti* (left), which also occurs in parts of South America. Vague symptoms of various types have been attributed to infection with the parasite, which is also transmitted by *Culicoides* spp. (× 340.)

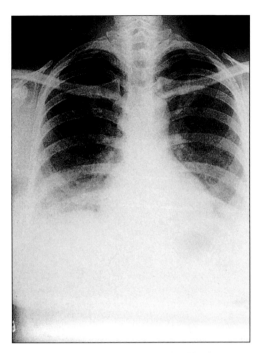 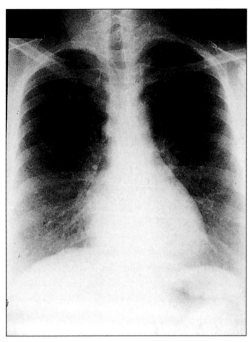

364 Tropical pulmonary eosinophilia (Löffler's syndrome)
This is a peculiar allergic reaction to filarial infections that may be of human or animal origin. It occurs principally in South Asia and affects Indians particularly. The condition is characterised by nocturnal cough and bronchospasm, with transient shadows in the lungs. Eosinophilia may be very marked. These radiographs are of the chest of a patient who returned from Sri Lanka with a severe wheeze and eosinophilia and who was found to have an extremely high antibody to filaria (no microfilaria were found on thick blood films). The condition responds well to specific filaricides. Left, before treatment; right, 10 days after treatment with diethylcarbamazine.

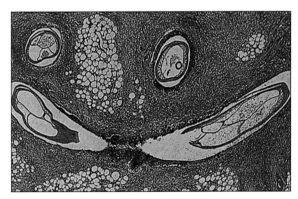 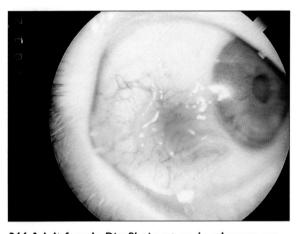

365 *Dirofilaria repens* in retrobulbar tissues
The adult of this filarial worm has been found in the eyelids and retrobulbar tissues of the eye of patients in Europe. *D. repens* is normally a parasite of dogs. (*H&E* × *10*.)

366 Adult female *Dirofilaria repens* in a human eye
The figure shows a mass situated under the bulbar conjunctiva of a 51-year-old Italian farmer. Excision and microscopic examination of the mass revealed an adult female of this nematode measuring 95 mm in length with a diameter of 0.45 mm. (By courtesy of Professor A E Bianco and Drs A Biglino and A Casabianca.)

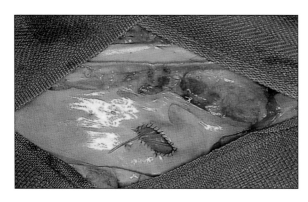

367 *Dirofilaria immitis* **in humans**
Several cases of infection with the common dog heartworm have been recorded in humans. This figure shows a 25 cm long, adult female *D. immitis* sited within the prosthetic portocaval shunt of a 32-year-old black woman in the southern USA who died of hepatic failure from chronic alcoholism. The nematode was first detected at post mortem examination.

OTHER ARTHROPOD-BORNE NEMATODES

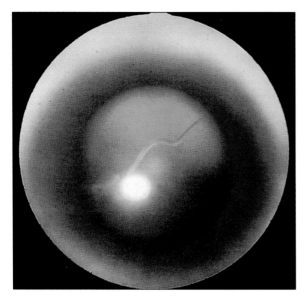

368 *Thelazia callipaeda* **in the human eye**
The adult worms of this spirurid nematode (see **Table 11**), which are 1–2 cm long, normally inhabit the lachrymal ducts and conjunctival sacs of dogs and rabbits. The females are viviparous and the first stage larvae in the lachrymal secretions may be picked up by eye-haunting flies such as those of the genera *Musca* and *Fannia*. The flies may then transfer the larvae to fresh hosts, including humans, in whom the worms develop to adults within 3–6 weeks. Seen here is an adult worm in the eye of a Malaysian man.

CHAPTER 2

Soil-mediated Helminthiases

Soil-transmitted helminthic infections are caused by two types of organisms: hookworms, which undergo a cycle of development in the soil (the larvae being infective) and a group of nematodes, which survive in the soil merely as eggs that have to be ingested for the cycle to continue.

The geographical distribution of the hookworms is limited by the requirements of the developing larvae for warmth and humidity. Generally speaking, the second type can occur not only in the tropics and subtropics but also in temperate regions. All of these helminthiases provide an index of the level of personal hygiene and sanitation in a community, because they depend for their dispersal, among other factors, on the indiscriminate deposition of faecal material on the ground and the use of untreated night soil as an agricultural fertiliser. In temperate regions, as in other areas, those infections that are spread directly (i.e. through the ingestion of eggs) are common in microenvironments that favour such spread (e.g. homes for mentally subnormal people, refugee camps, orphanages). The provision of adequate sewage disposal facilities virtually excludes these diseases.

Faecal contaminated soil in the neighbourhood of human habitations or on farmland is the source of hookworm infection for barefooted inhabitants. Conversely, the use of footwear greatly reduces the prevalence of *Necator americanus* infection but not necessarily that of *Ancylostoma duodenale* infection, which may also be acquired by the oral route (*see* **362**). Such people as rubber tappers in Malaya and farmers planting rice paddies commonly acquire infection from contaminated soil. Larvae of several animal hookworm species do not mature in humans, but the invasive larvae produce a transitory skin eruption as they migrate (cutaneous larva migrans). Visceral larva migrans may be due to infections with eggs of the dog or cat roundworm (*Toxocara canis, T. cati*). The larvae of these worms also do not mature in humans but may set up inflammatory reactions in the viscera (especially the liver) or the eye.

Generally speaking, the degree of harm done to the host is related to the worm burden in these helminthiases. Hookworm disease results when large numbers of adult worms are present and the loss of blood owing to the worms cannot be balanced because the host's diet is deficient in iron and other essential components. Moreover, multiple intestinal helminthic infection is the rule in many areas. Heavy infections with *Ascaris* may result in intestinal obstruction, particularly in children. Severe *Trichuris* infection of the large bowel can lead to anaemia and rectal prolapse in infants. The prevalence of human infection with the individual nematodes is indicated in **Table 11**.

369–383 The eggs of helminths

The morphology of helminth eggs that are detected in urine, faeces, sputum, etc., is usually sufficient to establish a diagnosis. Here, the eggs of species described in Chapters 2, 3 and 4 are shown at a single magnification for comparison. (*See* **Table 11** *for classification.* The eggs of the last three species are very difficult to distinguish.) *Schistosoma haematobium* (**369**), *S. mansoni* (**370**), *S. japonicum* (**371**), *Fasciola hepatica* (**372**), *Ascaris lumbricoides* (**373**), *Ascaris* (infertile) (**374**), *Paragonimus westermani* (**375**), *Diphyllobothrium latum* (**376**), hookworm (**377**), *Trichuris trichiura* (**378**), *Enterobius vermicularis* (**379**), *Vampirolepis nana* (**380**), *Hymenolepis diminuta* (**381**), *Taenia* (**382**), *Opisthorchis sinensis, Opisthorchis felineus, Heterophyes heterophyes* (**383**) (× 380). [Note: *V. nana* was formerly known as *Hymenolepis nana*.]

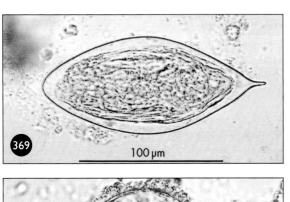

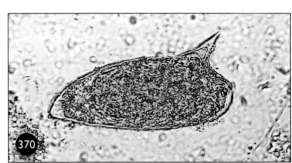

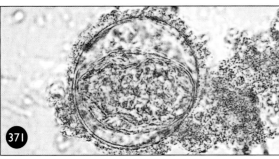

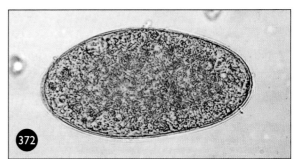

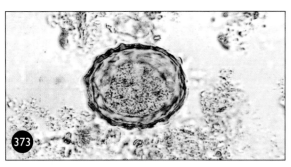

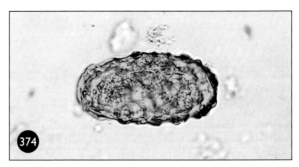

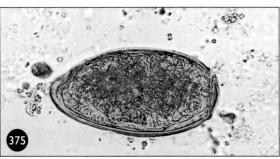

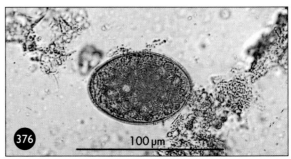

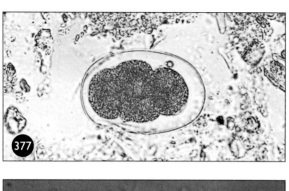

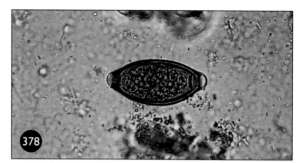

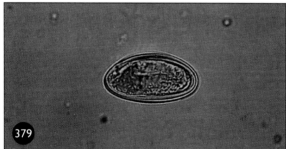

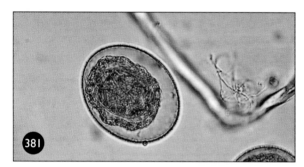

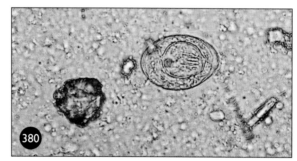

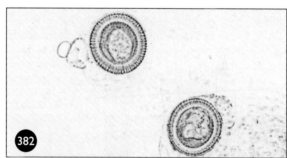

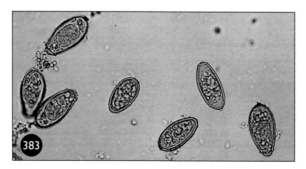

HOOKWORM INFECTIONS

ANCYLOSTOMA DUODENALE AND NECATOR AMERICANUS

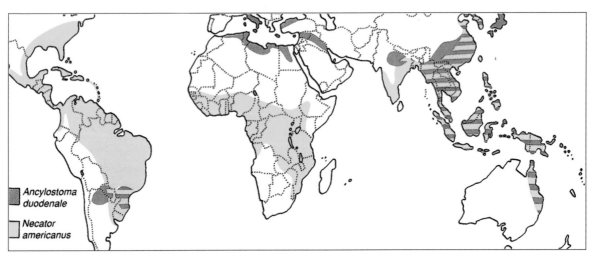

384 Distribution map of hookworm infection

The common hookworms of humans are *Ancylostoma duodenale* and *Necator americanus*. It is estimated that nearly a quarter of the world's population are infected with these species. One species usually predominates in any one locality; the map shows the approximate areas in which one or other species dominates. As the larvae can only develop in warm, moist soil, the distribution of the parasite is limited by climatic conditions.

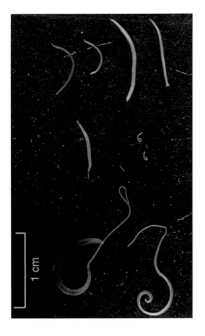

385 Comparative size of nematodes

First row	*Necator americanus* ♀ ♂	*Ancylostoma duodenale* ♀ ♂
Second row	*Enterobius vermicularis* ♀	*Trichinella spiralis* ♀ ♂
Third row	*Trichuris trichiura* ♀ ♂	

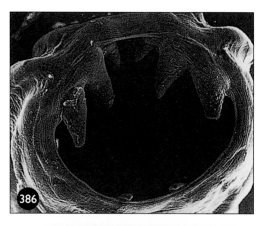

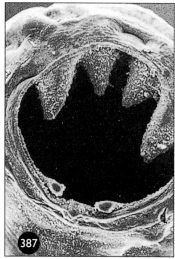

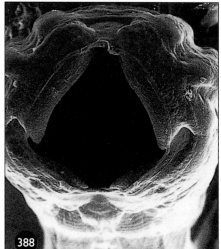

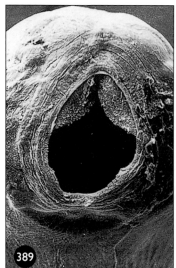

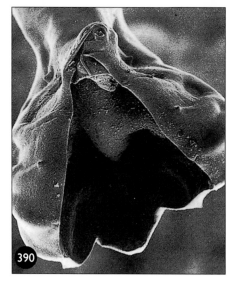

386–390 Identification of adult hookworms
Ancylostoma caninum (**386**, × *280*), *A. duodenale* (**387**, × *630*),
A. ceylanicum (**388**, × *670*), *N. americanus* (**389**, × *470*),
A. duodenale (**390**, × *470*). The different species may be distinguished by the characteristic morphology of the head capsule
(**386–389**) and male bursa (**390**), seen here in scanning
electromicrographs. The male bursae are distinguished by the
numbers and pattern of the 'rays.'

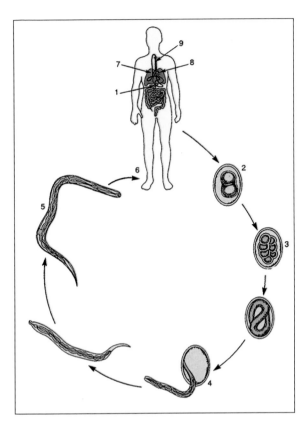

391 Life cycle of *Necator americanus* and *Ancylostoma duodenale*

Adults are attached to the walls of the jejunum (1) by the buccal capsule. Females lay large numbers of eggs, which are passed out with the faeces (2). The eggs mature through four-segment and eight-segment stages (3) to larvae that hatch in the soil (4). There they feed on bacteria and undergo two moults to produce filariform, infective larvae (5). These penetrate the skin of a new host (6), usually on the feet. They migrate into venules, entering the right heart (7) and lungs (8). Here they grow before penetrating from the capillaries into the alveoli. They enter the trachea (9) then the pharynx, are swallowed and pass into the small intestine (1) where they mature. *N. americanus* seems to enter the human body solely through the penetration of the skin by soil-dwelling, infective larvae. *A. duodenale*, on the other hand, is able to establish itself both percutaneously and via the ingestion of contaminated food and soil. It further differs from *N. americanus* in exhibiting the phenomenon of arrested development (i.e. the apparent ability to remain within the host at a larval stage for many months before finally reaching maturity). (*See also* **377** *and* **393–396**.)

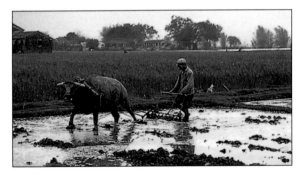

392 Ecology of geohelminth infection

In tropical and subtropical areas, wet soil (such as that found at the edges of rice fields, rubber plantations and the surroundings of villages in areas of high rainfall) supports the maturation of hookworm larvae from eggs deposited by indiscriminate defaecation; this limits their geographical distribution. In contrast, the well protected eggs of nematodes with a direct cycle of transmission (*Ascaris lumbricoides*, *Trichuris trichiura*) can survive in drier conditions even at freezing temperatures. (*See also* **485**.)

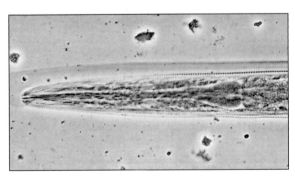

393 Filariform larva of hookworm

Eggs (**377**) passed in the faeces hatch into rhabditiform larvae in damp soil; they feed and undergo two moults to produce an infective, sheathed filariform larva. (× *350*.)

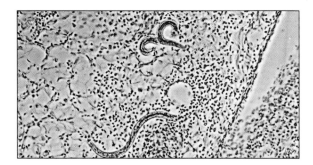

394 Larvae of hookworm in the lung of a dog
The infective larvae penetrate bare skin, usually of feet or legs, and, if they are in their correct host, enter the blood stream, to reach the lungs. The larvae then penetrate into the bronchioles, pass into the pharynx and are swallowed. They become attached to the small intestine and mature to adults. (× *100*.)

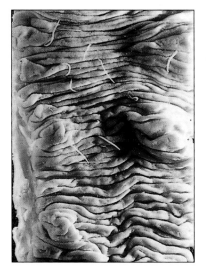

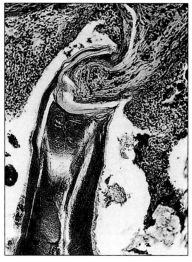

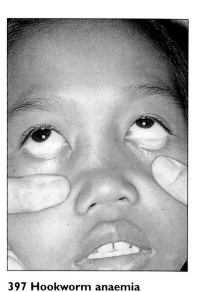

395 Adult hookworms *in situ*
The worms are about 1 cm long and characteristically curved. They are attached by their buccal capsules to the villi of the small intestine.

396 Section of adult *Ancylostoma duodenale in situ*
The hookworm feeds by sucking blood from the intestinal mucosa. It has been estimated that a single *A. duodenale* can withdraw as much as 0.2 ml a day, whereas *Necator americanus* withdraws 0.05 ml (× *17*.) (AFIP No. 33818.)

397 Hookworm anaemia
Severe anaemia is the classic feature of hookworm disease. This young Thai woman with a heavy load of *Necator americanus* had a haemoglobin concentration of 22 g/l.

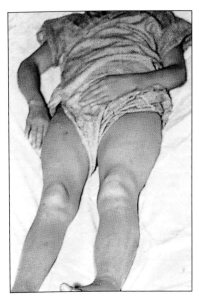

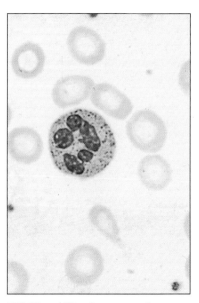

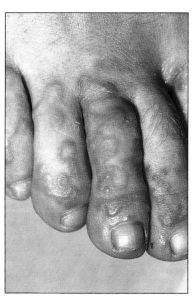

398 Clinical picture of gross hookworm disease

This results from a combination of a high hookworm load and low daily iron intake. The patients usually complain of lassitude and shortness of breath. Oedema and ascites, as seen in this young patient, also occur.

399 Blood film from a patient with hookworm anaemia

The typical anaemia resulting from severe hookworm infection is of the iron-deficiency type, with hypochromic, microcytic red cells and a low serum iron and low ferritin concentration. (× 1300.)

400 Cutaneous larva migrans ('creeping eruption') due to larvae of animal hookworms

Infective larvae of various species of animal hookworms (e.g. *Ancylostoma braziliense, A. caninum, A. ceylanicum*) often fail to penetrate the human dermis. They migrate through the epidermis leaving typical serpiginous tracks, known also as 'creeping eruption.' A severe infection is present on the toes of this patient who went for a beach holiday in the Bahamas. The patient was treated with a three-day course of albendazole.

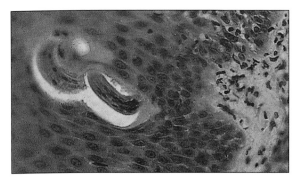

401 Larva of dog hookworm in the epidermis of a human foot

Portions of a larva are seen in longitudinal section. (*H&E × 400.*)

402 Adult *Ancylostoma caninum* in human ileum

In the humid north of Queensland, Australia, the larvae of this dog hookworm cause eosinophilic enteritis—a form of visceral larva migrans. The infection is probably acquired by the penetration of infective larvae from contaminated grass through the skin of the feet. Severe inflammatory lesions in the small intestine are associated with recurrent abdominal colic and sometimes diarrhoea, which is characterised by eosinophilia and is relieved by anthelminthic treatment. Resection of the severely inflamed segment of bowel shows oedema and eosinophilic inflammation of the wall. In the case seen here, the worm was situated in a nodule in the terminal ileum from where it could be removed under visual control through a fibre optic endoscope.

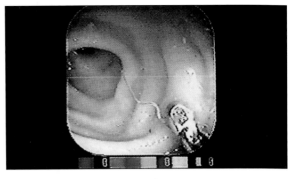

STRONGYLOIDIASIS

403 Distribution map of strongyloidiasis

Although mainly distributed in humid tropical and subtropical areas where its larvae can survive in the soil, *Strongyloides stercoralis* is also transmitted in some cooler areas (e.g. in warm and humid deep mines). It has also been reported to be spread on occasion from humans to humans by contamination with faeces containing infective rhabditiform larvae (e.g. in mental institutions and prisons). The map illustrates areas of high prevalence. There is an association between strongyloidiasis and human T-cell leukaemia virus-1 infection in the Caribbean and Japan.

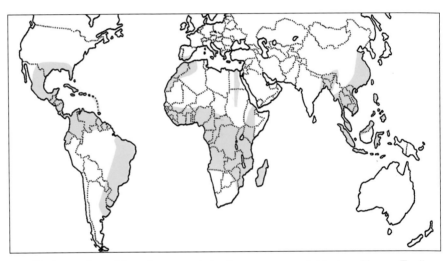

404 Life cycle of *Strongyloides stercoralis*

This tiny nematode has two generations: one free-living and the other parasitic. *I. The parasitic generation.* Males are rare and the females (1) are probably parthenogenetic, living in the mucosal glands of the small intestine. Eggs usually hatch in these glands into larvae, which are passed in the faeces (2). These rhabditiform larvae can develop into filariform larvae (3) in the ground, with the infective filariform larvae then penetrating the skin of a new host (4). The rest of the cycle in humans is as in hookworm infections. *II. Free-living generation.* Rhabditiform larvae (2) may develop into free-living males and females (5), which lay eggs (6) that hatch in the soil into rhabditiform (7), then infective filariform larvae (8). These too can penetrate the skin (4) and recommence a parasitic cycle in man. *III. Autoinfection.* Rhabditiform larvae (2) can mature into filariform larvae in the intestine; these can directly penetrate the perianal skin, causing autoinfection. *IV. Hyperinfection.* Rhabditiform larvae may penetrate the intestinal mucosa, causing massive autoinfection, usually in

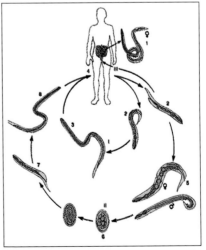

people with diminished immune responsiveness and in those treated with steroids (cycle not illustrated here).

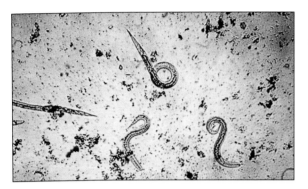

405 Rhabditiform larvae of *Strongyloides stercoralis* in faeces

The figure shows rhabditiform larvae, which are usually the only stage seen in faeces. Eggs, which are rarely seen, resemble those of hookworm but contain maturing larvae. Larvae of *S. stercoralis* can readily be distinguished (by their active, snake-like movements) from larvae of hookworms, which sometimes hatch in faecal specimens that have been left standing for some time ($\times$ 60). (*See also* **417**.)

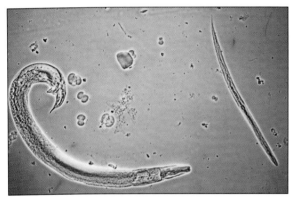

406 Adult male and free-living larva in soil ($\times$ 65.)

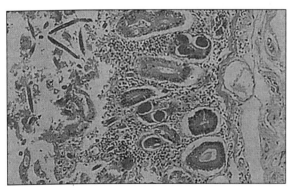

407 Sections of parasitic female and eggs embedded in jejunal mucosa

Free-living females (about 1 mm long) are smaller than the forms found in the intestine (up to 2.2 mm). Males are normally found only in the soil and are about 0.7 mm long. The parasitic females lying in the intestinal mucosa may reproduce parthenogenetically, with the eggs filtering through to the intestinal lumen or first hatching in the mucosa. ($\times$ 180.)

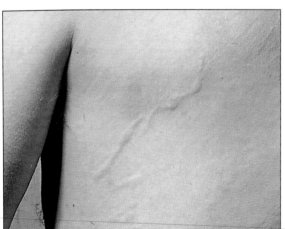

408 Migrating larvae of *Strongyloides stercoralis* in skin

Autoinfection can lead to severe 'creeping eruption,' which usually occurs on the back. This may occur many years (30 or more) after initial infection. Deep migration of the larvae may be associated with an 'eosinophilic lung' type of syndrome.

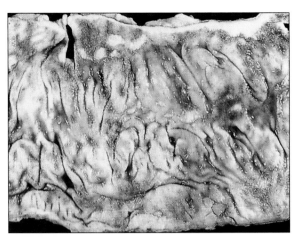

409 Appearance of colon at post mortem examination

The incidental administration of steroids and immuno-suppressive agents may greatly enhance infection with *Strongyloides stercoralis*, which may even be fatal, as in this case. Note the multiple ulcerations and thickening of the wall of the colon. There is also evidence that concurrent infection with human T-cell leukaemia virus-1 can be associated with an increased incidence of larvae in the faeces, possibly due to suppression of the normal IgE response to the helminths.

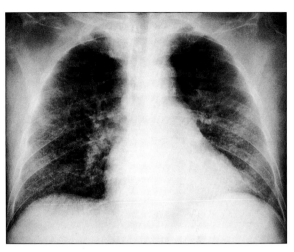

410 Haemorrhagic pneumonia in disseminated *Strongyloides stercoralis* infection

The chest radiograph shows bilateral, confluent, interstitial and alveolar infiltration.

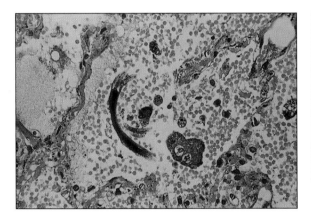

411 Section of lung from a patient with disseminated *Strongyloides stercoralis*

At post mortem examination the lungs of the patient whose chest radiograph is shown in **410** show haemorrhagic pneumonia with thickening of the alveolar walls, inflammatory infiltration with erythrocytes and eosinophils and sections of filariform larvae within an alveolus. In some cases eosinophils may be absent in this condition, which is fatal in 50 to 75% of all cases, even with intensive anthelminthic therapy. (*H&E* × *100.*)

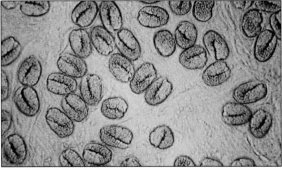

412 Eggs of *Strongyloides fülleborni* in faeces

Strongyloides fülleborni, a common intestinal nematode in African and Asian primates, is found in humans in several countries, including Zambia where 10% of human *Strongyloides* infections may be caused by this species. Massive infections with a subspecies of this nematode, *S. fülleborni kellyi*, cause an often fatal illness in infants in the west of Papua New Guinea, a country from which monkeys are absent. This condition, known as 'swollen belly sickness,' is characterised by respiratory distress, abdominal distension and generalised oedema. Very heavy egg loads, as seen here, occur in such cases. (× *300.*)

OTHER PHASMID NEMATODES OF HUMANS

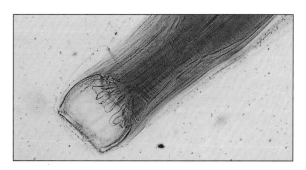

413 Head capsule of adult *Ternidens deminutus*
In some areas such as East Africa and Zimbabwe, infection commonly occurs with a hookworm-like parasite of monkeys, *T. deminutus*, which also infects monkeys in Asia. The adult worm, which is about 1 cm long, is found at any level in the small and large intestine. Normally infection is asymptomatic. ($\times$ *80*.)

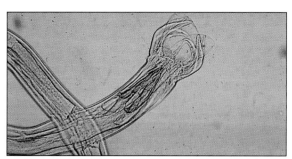

414 Eggs of *Ternidens deminutus* and hookworm compared
The eggs of *T. deminutus* (right) are usually mistaken for those of hookworm, but the adults passed accidentally during hookworm therapy are distinctive ($\times$ *125*). (See also **377**.)

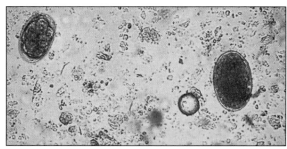

415 Adult male *Trichostrongylus*
Various species of *Trichostrongylus* inhabit the digestive tract of herbivores, burrowing into the mucosa (like hookworms) to obtain their nutrition. They have been encountered infrequently in humans, but in many different countries, although in one Iranian town they were said to be present in 70% of the population. They are readily distinguished from human hookworms by their smaller size and more slender shape. The male bursa is different in form from that of *Ancylostoma duodenale* (**390**). ($\times$ *100*.)

416 Adult female *Trichostrongylus*
The head of this tiny, very slender worm (about 0.5 cm long) lacks the distinct buccal cavity of the human hookworms (**386–389**). ($\times$ *50*.)

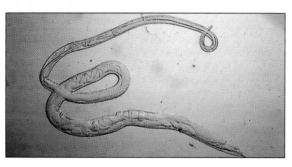

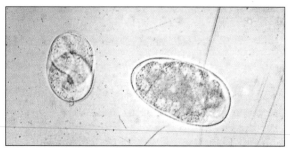

417 Eggs of *Trichostrongylus* and *Strongyloides stercoralis* in faeces
The hookworm-like egg of the *Trichostrongylus* (right) is much larger (about $80 \times 40 \mu$) than that of *S. stercoralis*, which contains an embryonic larva ready to hatch. ($\times$ *250*.)

INFECTION WITH *ASCARIS* AND RELATED NEMATODES

ASCARIASIS

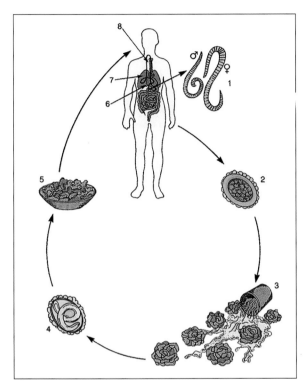

418 Life cycle of the roundworm *Ascaris lumbricoides*
Adult worms (1) live in the small intestine where they lay large numbers of eggs (2) that are passed out with the faeces. In the soil, they can readily contaminate vegetables, e.g., when night soil (3) is used as fertiliser. The larvae develop inside the eggs (4), which are swallowed when they are present in uncooked food (5). The eggs enter the jejunum (6) where the larvae hatch, penetrate the mucosa and are carried through the hepatic circulation to the heart and lungs (7). There they grow, moulting twice before escaping from the capillaries into the alveoli. They again enter the stomach via the trachea and oesophagus (8) and thence pass to the small intestine where they grow to adulthood. (*See also* **373** *and* **374**.)

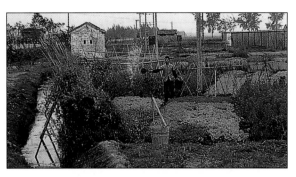

419 Ecology of infection with *Ascaris* and *Trichuris*
The use of fresh night soil to fertilise green-leaf vegetables, which are then eaten without adequate washing is a sure way to maintain the transmission of these roundworms. Their prevalence in a community is a good indicator of the standards of personal hygiene and sanitation. As their eggs can survive even in a cold climate, their distribution is global.

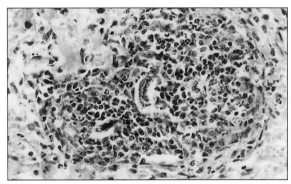

420 *Ascaris lumbricoides* larvae migrating in lung
The figure shows a section of a larva in the interstitial tissue of the lung. This stage is associated with eosinophilia; pneumonitis may accompany heavy infestations. ($\times 110$.)

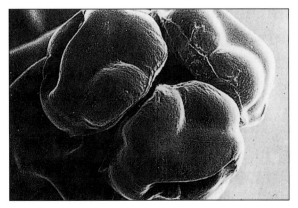

421 Head of adult
This scanning electron micrograph shows the typical head structures of *Ascaris lumbricoides*. ($\times 110$.)

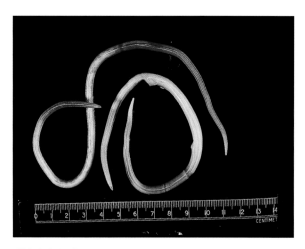

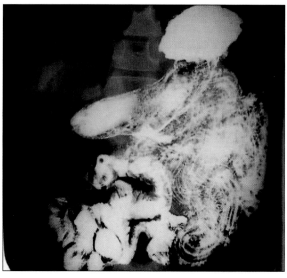

422 Adult *Ascaris lumbricoides*
After returning to the gut, the larvae mature into adult roundworms in the small intestine. The adult males are about 15–30 cm long and females 20–35 cm. The adults, if sufficient in number, can cause bowel obstruction (see **424**), and individual worms can migrate up the bile duct causing obstructive jaundice (see **425**).

423 *Ascaris lumbricoides* seen in radiograph
The adults may be seen (often incidentally) as filling defects on a barium meal.

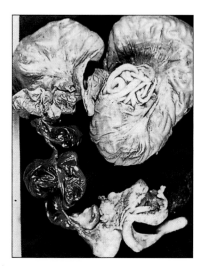

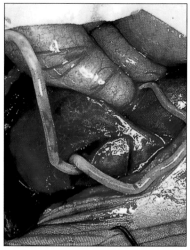

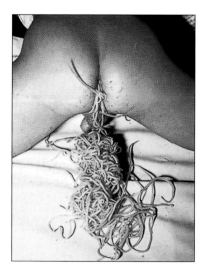

424 Obstruction due to roundworms
Heavy infections, especially in children, may lead to intestinal obstruction. Volvulus is an additional complication in this intestine from a 2-year-old child.

425 Adult roundworms migrating in liver
The adult worms have a marked tendency to penetrate any available hole in their vicinity and may escape through abdominal fistulae following operation. They may also lead to biliary obstruction and occupy the appendix.

426 Massive *Ascaris* infection in a child
A large bolus of roundworms expelled following anthelminthic treatment.

TOXOCARIASIS

Visceral larva migrans results from accidental infection of humans with eggs of the ascarid roundworm of the dog, *Toxocara canis*, and cat, *T. cati*. The life cycle in the animal host is the same as that of *Ascaris*, but the invasive larvae in humans become arrested in various tissues, where they are gradually phagocytosed; in the process, they induce marked eosinophilia and local tissue reaction, most commonly involving the liver and eye sites. Other helminths that can cause visceral larva migrans include *Ancylostoma caninum*, producing eosinophilic enteritis (see **402**), and *Baylisascaris procyonis* (see **Table 11, 432**), a parasite of the raccoon in North America, which can cause damage to the central nervous system and eye.

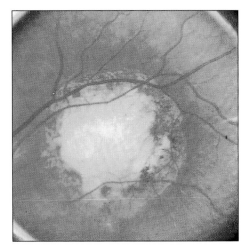

428 Larva of *Toxocara* in the human eye
The penetrating larva has become encysted, leading to the formation of a large granuloma, seen here at the posterior pole of the fundus. The granuloma resembles a retinoblastoma and may lead to blindness. Unless a correct diagnosis is made, the eye may mistakenly be enucleated.

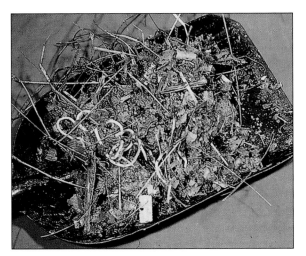

427 Adult *Toxocara canis*
The worms seen here were from a puppy following anthelminthic therapy. The adults are about 10 cm long and similar in general appearance to *Ascaris lumbricoides*. Uncontrolled contamination of soil by dogs and cats is common everywhere. Like those of *Ascaris*, the eggs of *T. canis* and *T. cati* can survive even in a cold climate.

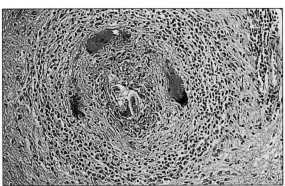

429 Larvae of *Toxocara canis* in the human brain
The larva is seen in the centre of the granuloma formed by mononuclear cells, eosinophils and multinucleated giant cells. (H&E × 120.)

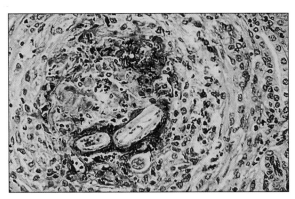

430 Migrating larvae in the human kidney
In this section, a larva is seen in the kidney surrounded by an inflammatory exudate and fibroblasts. (H&E × 300.)

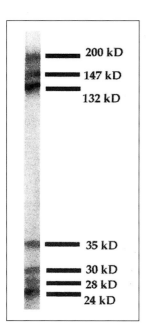

431 Serological diagnosis
The diagnosis is supported by a positive serological response to specific *Toxocara* antigens such as the excretory/secretory antigens produced by culturing second stage larvae. In this figure of a positive Western blot result, the top three bands at 200, 147 and 132 kD represent cross reactions that can occur with other nematodes such as *Strongyloides stercoralis*, *Enterobius vermicularis* and even the cestode, *Taenia saginata*. A specific response is shown by the presence of the bands at 35, 30, 28 and 24 kD.

BAYLISASCARIS PROCYONIS

432 Cross section of a larva of *Baylisascaris procyonis* from a child with neural larva migrans
The parasite was discovered in a brain biopsy from a teenage boy with a history of pica living in California. The adult nematode is found in the small intestine of the majority of peridomestic raccoons in the western USA (80% or more in some areas), and the larva is an increasingly reported cause of visceral larva migrans. Infection is acquired when eggs on contaminated soil (raccoon 'latrines') are accidentally ingested. The larvae, 1.5 to 2 mm long,

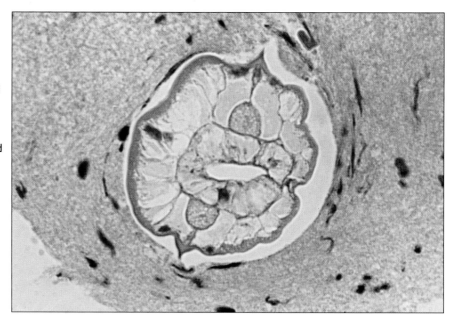

hatch in the stomach and migrate through the tissues but do not develop fully, except in their natural host in which they produce typical, ascarid adults from 14 to 18 cm long. In accidental hosts such as humans, from 5 to 7% of larvae are believed to migrate to the eye and central nervous system, where they can cause extensive lesions. (*H&E × 1440.*)

TRICHURIASIS

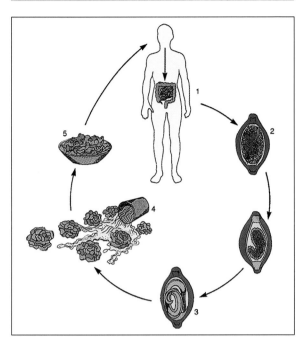

433 Life cycle of the whipworm, *Trichuris trichiura*
Adults inhabit the caecum (1) and sometimes the colon and rectum, where they are attached to the mucosa. Eggs passed with the faeces (2) mature in the soil to larvae (3), which remain in the eggs. Eggs can readily contaminate vegetables (e.g. when night soil is used as fertiliser (4) or when sanitary habits are otherwise primitive), and are then swallowed in uncooked food (5). The eggs hatch in the small intestine, and the developing larvae pass directly to their attachment sites in the large intestine. Females commence egg laying after about three months. (*See also* **378** *and* **385**.)

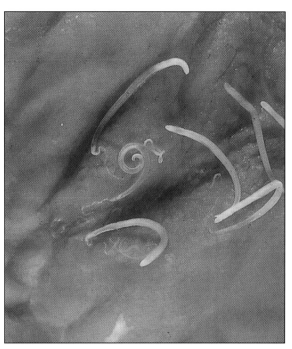

434 Adult female and male morphology
Three to 10 days after the eggs are ingested, the young worms pass down to the caecum where the whip-like anterior portion becomes entwined in the mucosa. The adult worms are about 3–5 cm long, with the females being slightly larger than the males, which are coiled. The adult worms (one male and several females) are seen in this figure of the caecal mucosa (× 2.) (AFIP No. 69–3583.)

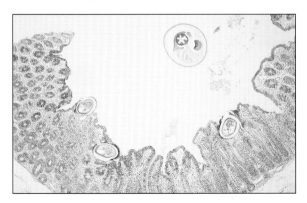

435 Cross section of *Trichuris trichiura* associated with caecal tissue
The section shows a cross section of an adult worm free in the lumen and sections of the slender anterior end apparently inserted in the mucosa. (*H&E* × 13.)

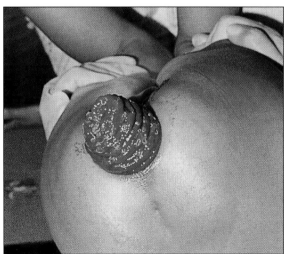

436 Rectal prolapse
Heavy infections may cause rectal prolapse following chronic bloody diarrhoea with abdominal pain in infants and children, especially if they are undernourished.

CHAPTER 3

Snail-mediated Helminthiases

With the exception of the angiostrongyliases (*see* **Chapter 4**), which are nematode infections transmitted accidentally to humans in the course of their complex life cycles in rodents and other mammals, the important group of snail-transmitted helminthiases are all caused by trematodes (flukes), which undergo a complicated cycle involving various species of land or aquatic snails.

Six hundred million people are exposed to schistosomiasis and over 200 million are estimated to be infected. The three common species, *Schistosoma mansoni, S. haematobium* and *S. japonicum*, cause a heavy morbidity and contribute in certain areas to the high mortality rate found among adolescents and young adults. Infection with these parasites is a major cause of cancer in the endemic countries. In the case of *S. haematobium* infection, for example, it has been estimated that its prevention would reduce the global rate of bladder carcinoma by 5000 to 10 000 cases annually. Since infection occurs by penetration of the skin by water-dwelling infective stages (cercariae), transmission tends to increase in parallel with the extension of land utilisation by irrigation. Hence, schistosomiasis is a positive obstacle to agricultural and economic development in many parts of the developing world.

Apart from schistosomiasis due to *S. haematobium* and *S. mansoni*, for which humans are the main reservoir of infection, *S. japonicum* has an important animal reservoir, whereas the other snail-mediated helminthiases are zoonoses. Like many zoonoses, they are relatively uncommon, with notable, highly localised exceptions. Despite the availability of excellent molluscicides and anti-schistosomal drugs, remarkably little overall success has met attempts to control the schistosomiases in many endemic countries up to the present time, although important progress has been made in reducing the morbidity and mortality they cause. Some progress has been made towards the development of anti-schistosomal vaccines, but none is available for human use at present.

The public health importance of food-borne, intestinal, liver-fluke and lung-fluke infections has, until very recently, been grossly underestimated; indeed, our knowledge of the epidemiology of some species is still limited. It is, however, now realised that at least 40 million people are infected with liver-dwelling and lung-dwelling trematodes. These flukes have a somewhat more complicated life cycle than the schistosomes, in that the cercariae develop a resting stage (the metacercaria) which, in turn, must be ingested for infection to occur. As the metacercariae are found usually on various water plants, on fish or on crustaceans, infection with these worms tends to be localised to areas in which particular local eating habits bring humans and the metacercaria together. Thus, clonorchiasis and opisthorchiasis are restricted to regions where raw fish is commonly ingested (notably in parts of Southeast Asia and the former

USSR), fasciolopsiasis to regions where, for example, water caltrops and water chestnuts are eaten uncooked, and paragonimiasis to regions where the appropriate crustaceans form part of humans' diet in one culinary delicacy or another. Most of these flukes are primarily parasites of animals other than humans (e.g. *Fasciola hepatica* is essentially a parasite of sheep that infects humans following the ingestion of watercress or other aquatic plants from contaminated, wet pastures). In certain villages in Northeast Thailand, for example, *Fasciolopis buski* has been found to infect nearly 100% of the population and *Opisthorchis viverrini* 90%, even though they are zoonoses. An indication of the numbers of human infections with these trematodes is given in **Table 12**.

The diagnosis of snail-mediated helminthiases rests mainly on the demonstration of the parasites (e.g. as eggs in urine or faeces) or on medical imaging techniques of adults within various tissues. Serological procedures and skin testing are of value in some types of infection.

Table 12 Digenetic trematodes of medical importance and their prevalence[1]

Superorder	Order	Superfamily	Genus and species	Estimated cases	No.
ANEPITHELIOCYSTIDA	STRIGEATOIDEA	Schistosomatoidea	*Schistosoma mansoni*	57 million	1
			S. haematobium	78 million	2
			S. japonicum	69 million	3
			S. intercalatum	thousands	4
			S. mattheei	thousands	5
			S. mekongi	thousands	6
	ECHINOSTOMIDA	Paramphistomatoidea	*Gastrodiscoides hominis*	rare[2]	7
			Watsonius watsoni	rare	8
		Echinostomatoidea	*Fasciola hepatica*	} 2.4 million	9
			F. gigantica		10
			Fasciolopsis buski	0.2 million	11
			Echinostoma hortense	thousands	
			E. ilocanum	thousands[3]	12
			Echinochasmus lilliputanus	thousands	
EPITHELIOCYSTIDA	PLAGIOCHIIDA	Plagiorchioidea	*Dicrocoelium dendriticum*	rare	13
			Nanophyetus salmincola	rare	14
			Paragonimus westermani	21 million[4]	15
			P. africanus	rare	16
			P. uterobilateralis	thousands	17
			P. mexicanus	} > 2 million	
			P. ecuadoriensis		
	OPISTHORCHIIDA	Opisthorchioidea	*Opisthorchis felineus*	> 1 million	18
			O. viverrini	10 million	19
			Clonorchis sinensis[5]	7 million	20
			Heterophyes heterophyes	thousands	21
			Metagonimus yokogawai	0.5 million	22

Note: The numbers in the right-hand column refer to **Table 13** in which are indicated the molluscs that serve as intermediate hosts for these trematodes. Some species referred to as rare may occur in high prevalence in certain foci where local food habits make the intake of the infective stages more common. The list in this table is by no means inclusive. At least 70 species of intestinal trematodes have been recorded in humans.

[1] See Footnote to [1] **Table 11**. Numerous other species rare in man are listed in WHO (1995) *T.R.S.* 849.
[2] Said to be common in Assam where a prevalence of over 40% was found in certain foci.
[3] Prevalence rates average 5% in northern Luzon (Philippines).
[4] See other data in **Table 14**. The estimate of 21 million includes all *Paragonimus* species of humans.
[5] Now referred to as *Opisthorchis sinensis* by some authors.

SCHISTOSOMIASIS

437 Life cycle of *Schistosoma mansoni*

The schistosomes provide a classic example of the life cycle of trematodes. The three common parasites of humans, *Schistosoma haematobium*, *S. japonicum* and *S. mansoni*, have a similar life cycle. Eggs (1) that are passed in urine (*S. haematobium*) or faeces (*S. japonicum* and *S. mansoni*), hatch in aggregations of water such as ponds, lake edges, streams and canals. From the eggs, miracidia (2) hatch into the water where they penetrate into suitable snails. In the snails, they develop two generations of sporocysts (3A, 3B), the second of which produces fork-tailed cercariae (4). These cercariae penetrate the skin (5) when a new host comes into contact with contaminated water. Once through the skin, the cercariae shed their tails and become schistosomulae, which migrate through the tissues until they reach the portal venous system of the liver. Here, males and females (6) copulate before settling down in pairs in the venous system of the liver. From there *S. haematobium* migrates usually to the venous plexus of the bladder, and other species (including the geographically localised *S. intercalatum* and *S. mekongi*) to the rectum (7), where eggs are laid. The eggs penetrate the bladder or rectum from where they reach the exterior. Eggs laid by worms in the liver itself lead to local fibrotic changes and cirrhosis. (*See also* **369–371, 440–442, 444–452, 456, 466** *and* **491–494**.)

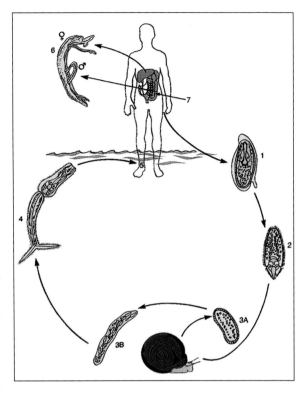

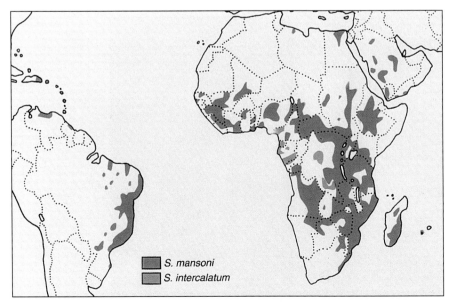

438 Distribution map of *Schistosoma mansoni* and *S. intercalatum*

The distribution of schistosomiasis is regulated by both the presence of susceptible snail intermediate hosts and human sanitary habits. *S. mansoni* occurs in Africa, the Middle East, some Caribbean islands and parts of South America. It was introduced from the Old World into the New World, where potentially susceptible species of *Biomphalaria* were already present. (Adapted from WHO *Map No. 92720*.)

S. mansoni
S. intercalatum

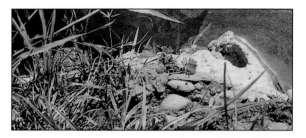

439 Ecology of intestinal schistosomiasis
Human faeces deposited at the edge of a pond in which snail hosts of *Schistosoma mansoni* were breeding. Eggs enter the water to hatch and perpetuate the cycle of transmission.

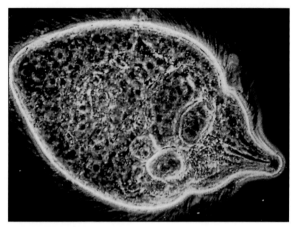

440 Hatched miracidium of *Schistosoma mansoni*
The three common species of schistosomes infecting humans have easily recognisable eggs, although those of *S. haematobium* may be confused with those of *S. intercalatum* (**491**). Miracidia can often be seen inside mature eggs. As many eggs deposited in the tissues in old infections may be non-viable, the detection of miracidia ('miracidia hatching test') in urine or stool specimens diluted in water can give a valuable indication of the activity of an infection. (× *600*.)

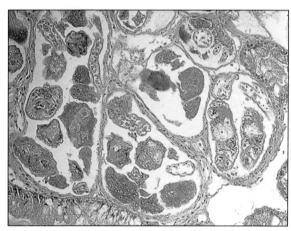

441 Section of 'mother' sporocyst in the hepatopancreas of a snail
The cycle in the snail is of variable duration, depending on the species of parasite and host and on the environmental conditions, but it is usually only one month. Cercaria develop in the second generation ('daughter') sporocysts. The figure shows several coils of the sporocyst in the hepatopancreas and sections of cercaria. (*Acetic carbol fuchsin* × *130*.)

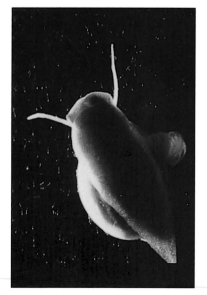

442 A snail 'shedding' living bifurcate cercaria of *Schistosoma mansoni*
Once snails start to 'shed' cercariae, they continue to do so during daylight hours for up to as many as 200 days. A heavily infected snail may shed 1500 to 2000 cercariae a day. (× *4.4*.)

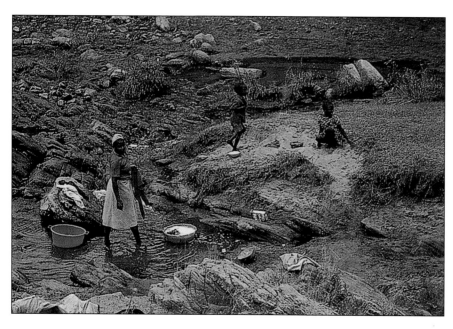

443 Site of human infection with *Schistosoma mansoni* These women and their children became infected by cercariae while washing clothes in contaminated water. The provision of a piped water supply to the village drastically reduced the amount of transmission.

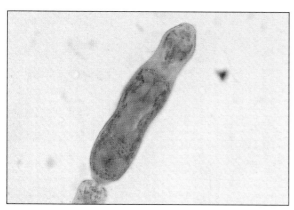

444 Head of cercaria
The apical and ventral suckers of the future schistosomule are clearly seen in this preparation. (*Mayer's haemalum × 310.*)

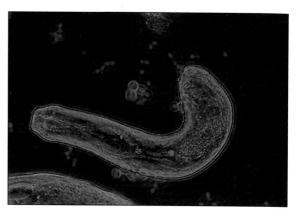

445 Schistosomule of *Schistosoma mansoni*
(*Phase contrast × 350.*)

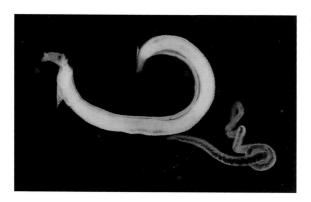

446 Living male and female *Schistosoma mansoni*
The slender female (right) is normally seen within the gynaecophoral groove of the male (left). (× 14.)

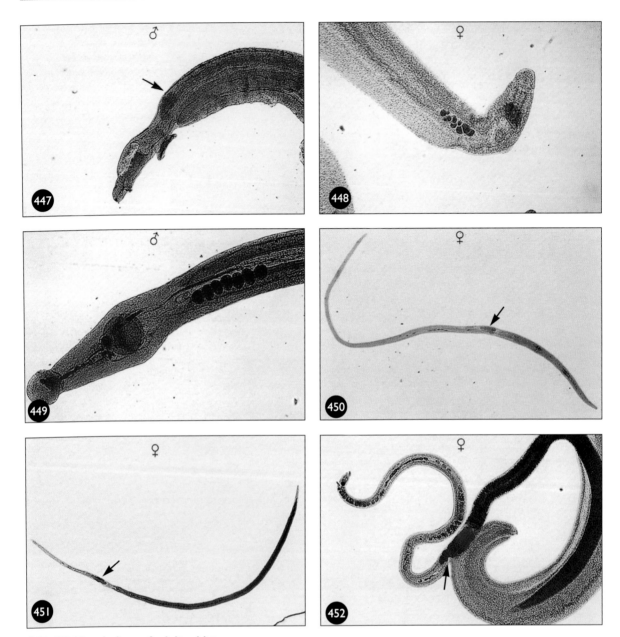

447–452 Morphology of adult schistosomes
Mature males and females live in copulating pairs. The common species are recognised by the characters shown in the figures. Testes of males: *Schistosoma haematobium* (**447**); *S. mansoni* (**448**); *S. japonicum* (**449**). Ovaries of females: *S. haematobium* (**450**); *S. mansoni* (**451**); *S. japonicum* (**452**). (× 25.)

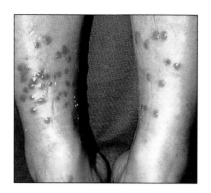

453 Dermatitis from avian cercariae in a Japanese patient

Penetration of the skin by cercariae may give rise to an itchy rash known as 'cercarial dermatitis.' This is occasionally seen in countries free of human schistosomiasis due to invasion by the cercariae of avian schistosomes, which are otherwise non-pathogenic to humans.

SCHISTOSOMA MANSONI

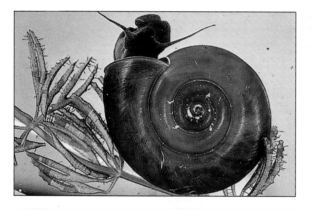

454 Intermediate host of *Schistosoma mansoni*

The snail intermediate hosts of *S. mansoni* are various species of *Biomphalaria* ($\times$ 4.) (*See also* **Table 13**.)

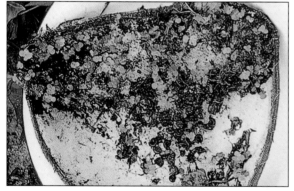

455 Sampling snail populations

A scoopful of *Biomphalaria sudanica*, a host for *Schistosoma mansoni* in Lake Victoria.

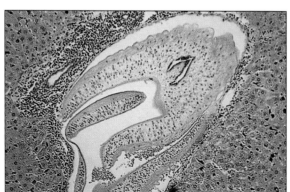

456 Adult *Schistosoma mansoni* in portal tract

Male and female schistosomes lodge *in copula* in the portal tract, mesenteric or vesical plexuses. The figure shows a cross section of a male and female *S. mansoni* in a branch of the portal vein. (*H&E* $\times$ *44*.)

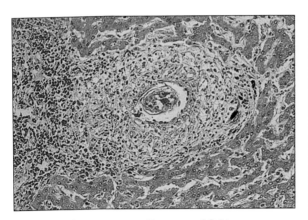

457 Granuloma surrounding egg of *Schistosoma mansoni* in liver

Eggs (**370**) may lodge ectopically in any tissues, where they cause characteristic granulomas. It has been suggested that toxic substances associated with the ova trigger the fibrotic process. In histological sections, the ova are seen in the portal and periportal regions. All types of reaction may be present from acute eosinophilic cellular infiltration (as seen here) to the dense collagenous deposition that leads to periportal fibrosis (*See also* **469**). (*H&E* × 90.)

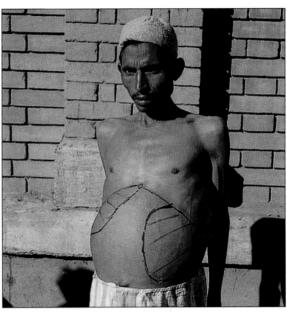

459 Egyptian splenomegaly

The combination of enlarged, irregularly fibrosed liver and greatly enlarged spleen is commonly called 'Egyptian hepatosplenomegaly.'

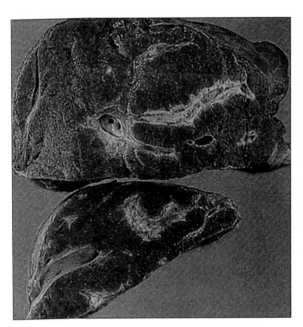

458 Periportal fibrosis of the liver

Periportal fibrosis ('pipestem fibrosis') is the classic pathological hepatic lesion. The white areas, which may be round, ova, or stellate, are due to the terminal fibrotic reaction originally caused by the presence of the ova in and around the portal venous radicles. (*See also* **487**.)

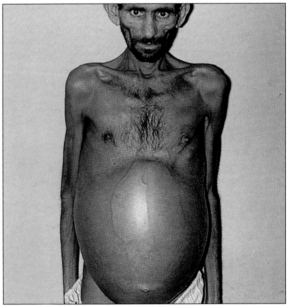

460 Ascites secondary to chronic portal hypertension in a Brazilian

The classic, clinical feature of chronic *Schistosoma mansoni* infection is portal hypertension. The opening up of a secondary, circulatory shunt leads to the development of varices in the oesophageal and gastric veins, ascites and gross splenomegaly.

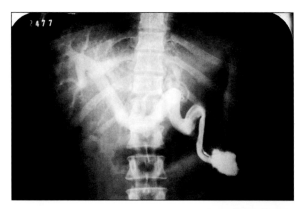

461 Angiogram showing portal hypertension caused by *Schistosoma mansoni*
This radiograph was taken before surgery in this Brazilian man.

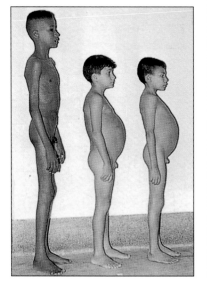

462 Growth retardation by chronic infection with *Schistosoma mansoni*
A combination of undernutrition and chronic infection with *S. mansoni*, especially around the time of puberty, can lead to significant retardation of growth. The boys seen here in the northeast of Brazil are (left to right) 14, 13 and 12 years old. The two on the right with hepatomegaly have schistosomiasis. Similar changes are seen in children infected with *S. japonicum*.

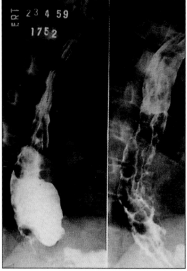

463 Radiograph of oesophageal varices
Oesophageal varices such as those shown in this gastrografin swallow can rupture, leading to a fatal haematemesis.

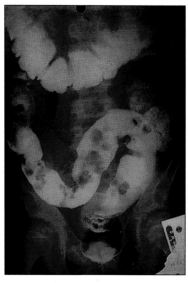

464 Barium enema of colonic polyposis
Diarrhoea is a common complaint in the early stages of *Schistosoma mansoni* infection. Extensive polyposis of the colon sometimes occurs. These lesions are reversible with antischistosomal drug therapy.

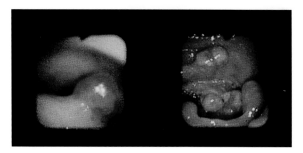

465 Sigmoidoscopic view of colonic polyps
Two views of polyps in the descending colon.

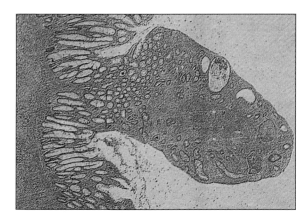

466 Biopsy specimen showing *Schistosoma mansoni* eggs in a colonic polyp

Diagnosis is usually confirmed by demonstrating eggs of *S. mansoni* in the stool. The Kato–Katz technique is one of the simplest quantitative prodecures to evaluate egg loads in faeces. However, intestinal biopsy through a proctoscope or sigmoidoscope is also an effective means of finding eggs and establishing a definitive diagnosis of *S. mansoni* infection. It may also give positive results in patients with *S. haematobium* or *S. japonicum* (*See also note on 'miracidia hatching test'*, **440**). (*H&E* × *25.*)

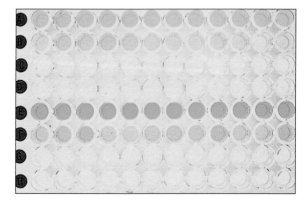

467 Enzyme-linked immumosorbent assay

This, one of the most sensitive tests currently available for the detection of antischistosomal IgG, IgM or IgE, is probably of most value for the screening of expatriates for recently acquired infection with any of the species of *Schistosoma* and to distinguish acute from chronic infections. In this example of an IgG ELISA, alkaline phosphatase-p-nitrophenyl phosphate was used as indicator in rows A–D and horseradish peroxidase in rows E–H, with different sera in each of the rows. A and E show a strong positive reaction, B and F a weak positive reaction and C and G a negative reaction; D and H are the buffer controls. Detection of circulating antigen with monoclonal antibodies is now shown to be more specific and sensitive both for diagnosis and for the confirmation of cure after intervention. Skin tests, which are relatively unreliable, have now been abandoned.

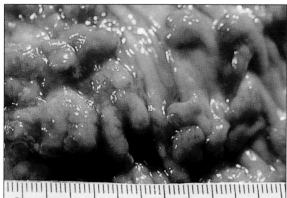

468 Polyposis of colon at post mortem examination

Massive polyposis of the colon with fatal intestinal haemorrhage seen at post mortem examination in an Egyptian farmer.

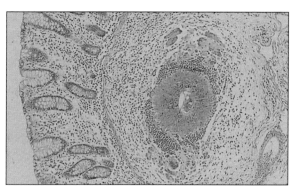

469 Hoeppli reaction

The fibrotic granuloma around this dead ovum in the colon is known as a Hoeppli reaction. (*H&E* × *70.*)

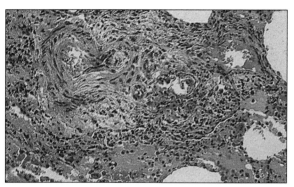

470 Ectopic infection—*Schistosoma mansoni* infection of lung

Typical eggs may appear in the sputum when the lungs are affected. Such ectopic lesions usually contain large numbers of ova in necrotic material surrounded by eosinophils, and multinucleated giant cells. They may also involve the central nervous system. (*H&E* × *100.*)

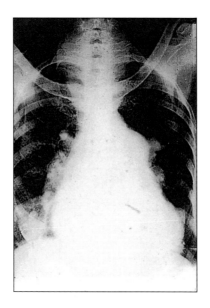

471 Radiograph of 'cor pulmonale' due to schistosomiasis
Eggs that reach the lungs by metastatic-blood spread lead to periarteritis. This is followed by fibrosis of the pulmonary arterioles with pulmonary hypertension and, finally, enlargement of the right heart (i.e. cor pulmonale).

SCHISTOSOMA HAEMATOBIUM

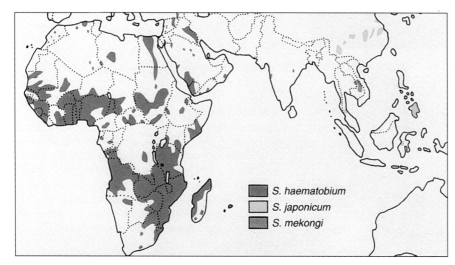

S. haematobium
S. japonicum
S. mekongi

472 Distribution map of *Schistosoma haematobium*, *S. japonicum* and *S. mekongi*
S. haematobium is found in Africa and the Middle East; *S. japonicum* is endemic in the Far East, Southeast Asia and the Philippines; *S. mekongi* is limited to parts of Laos, Kampuchea and South Thailand, bordering the lower Mekong River basin. (Adapted from WHO *Map No. 92721*.)

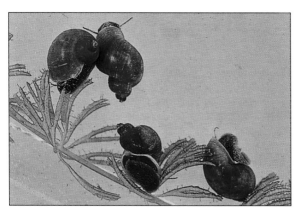

473 Intermediate hosts of *Schistosoma haematobium*
The intermediate hosts of *S. haematobium* are species of *Bulinus* (× 3.5). (See also **Table 13**.)

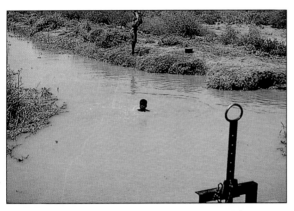

474 Ecology of *Schistosoma haematobium* infection
Increased land use through the development of irrigation projects (as in Egypt, the Sudan and Kenya), may result in an increasing incidence of *S. haematobium* transmission through *Bulinus* snails breeding in the irrigation canals, which are favourite swimming places for children. In the village near this canal, 62% of children from 2–6 years were infected.

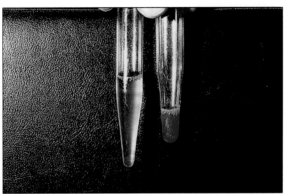

475 Haematuria
Often best seen at the end of urination, haematuria is a characteristic early clinical feature of infection with this parasite. Typical, terminal spined eggs of *Schistosoma haematobium* (see **321**) may be found in the centrifuge deposit. (*See also note on 'miracidial hatching test,'* **440**.)

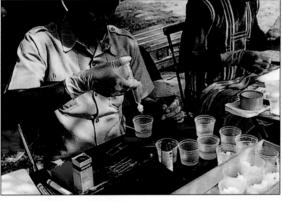

476 Village survey for urinary schistosomiasis
A simple and effective technique to detect eggs in urine is to pass samples through a nylon-mesh filter attached to a 10 ml syringe. The filter is removed and examined under the microscope using a × 10 objective, and the eggs collected on it are counted. A simple dipstick test for protein and blood is a useful supplementary method of assessing the prevalence of those passing eggs and may even replace microscopy. This procedure, which saves labour, time and money, facilitates the delivery of treatment programmes in communities for which such intervention might otherwise be delayed (or not provided at all) and is valuable for assessing the effectiveness of such programmes.

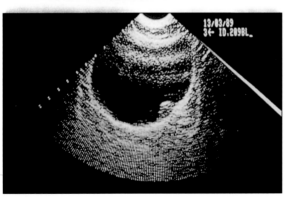

477 Ultrasonic probe of bladder in early infection
A large polyp can be seen in this ultrasonic probe of a bladder early in infection with *Schistosoma haematobium*. Unlike radiography, ultrasonography with portable equipment can readily be used in a simple peripheral medical centre or even under field conditions by specially trained personnel. It is an invaluable procedure for assessing morbidity in individuals or in community surveys (e.g. to evaluate the progress of control campaigns).

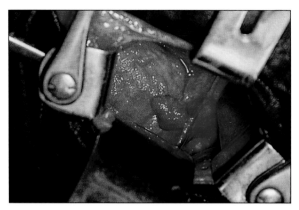

478 Nodules due to *Schistosoma haematobium*
The appearance of a nodular lesion in the vesical wall as seen at open operation is well shown here.

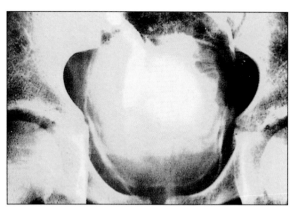

479 Radiograph of bladder with calcification
Widespread fibrosis and eventually calcification of the bladder wall result in this 'foetal head' appearance.

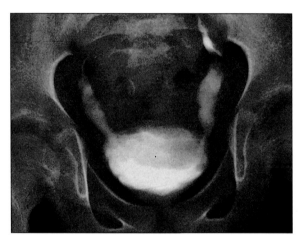

480 Intravenous urogram of dilated ureters
Gross tortuosity and dilation of the ureters result from stenosis of the ureteric orifices, possibly due to calcification.

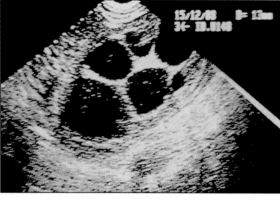

481 Ultrasonogram showing severe hydronephrosis
Unilateral and bilateral hydronephrosis due to vesical and ureteric destructive lesions are not uncommon in infection with *Schistosoma haematobium*. Hydronephrosis due to *S. haematobium* infection in children is often reversible with adequate antischistosomal drug therapy. The non-invasive technique of ultrasonography has largely replaced urography in the investigation of severe urinary tract lesions due to *S. haematobium* in a hospital environment.

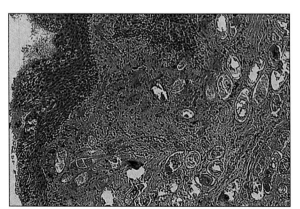

482 Eggs in section of bladder
Schistosome ova laid by female worms in the vesical plexus are retained in the vesical tissues and later become calcified. (*H&E × 50.*)

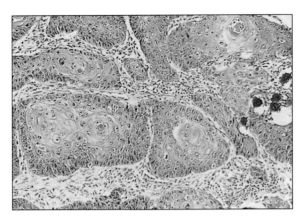

483 Squamous cell carcinoma of the bladder
In areas where *Schistosoma haematobium* infection is intense, the incidence of bladder cancer is high. Squamous cell carcinoma is the type most commonly found, and ova of *S. haematobium* are often present in such tumours. Adenocarcinoma also occurs. (*H&E* × 90.)

SCHISTOSOMA JAPONICUM AND *S. MEKONGI*

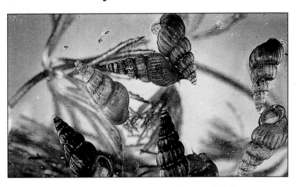

484 *Oncomelania*, intermediate host of *Schistosoma japonicum*
Various species of the amphibious genus *Oncomelania* serve as intermediate hosts for *S. japonicum*. In the lower Mekong River basin, a river-dwelling snail, *Tricula aperta*, is the intermediate host for *S. mekongi*—a trematode closely related to *S. japonicum* (× 3). (*See also* **Table 13**.)

485 Ecology of *Schistosoma japonicum* and *S. mekongi*
These infections are zoonoses. *S. japonicum* is found in a wide variety of vertebrate hosts, including domestic animals and bovines. Human infection often occurs in farm workers (e.g. when planting rice in contaminated paddy fields, as seen here) (*see also* **392**). In contrast, *S. mekongi* is associated more with rivers; it is likely to increase as irrigation works in the lower Mekong River basin are extended. In some Kampuchean 'floating villages,' up to 47% of sampled villagers have been found infected with this parasite.

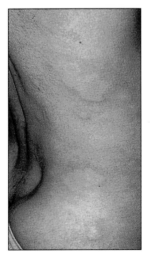

486 'Katayama fever'
The acute phase of moderate or heavy infection with schistosomes may present as a febrile reaction with hypereosinophilia that can last for several days or weeks. 'Katayama fever,' which is commonest in infection with *Schistosoma japonicum*, less common with *S. mansoni* and rarely seen with *S. haematobium*, appears with the onset of oviposition. It results from the formation and circulation of antigen–antibody immune complexes, which provoke a type of serum sickness and may be complicated by glomerulonephritis. Massive giant urticaria occurred in this man soon after infection with *S. mansoni*.

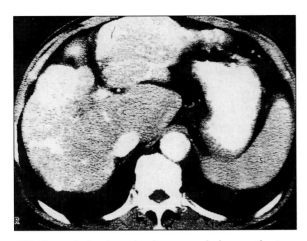

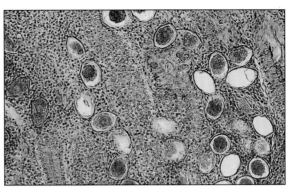

489 Eggs of *Schistosoma japonicum* in wall of colon
The adult worms do not invade the vesical plexus, but usually inhabit the mesenteric plexus. The diagnosis of *S. japonicum* infection can usually be made by finding typical eggs in the faeces. However, it is more common for eggs of *S. japonicum* to be deposited in ectopic sites than those of other schistosome species. (*H&E* × *150.*)

487 Liver cirrhosis and splenomegaly in a patient with *Schistosoma japonicum*
Severe hepatic fibrosis and massive splenomegaly occur in *S. japonicum* infection (in the same manner as in *S. mansoni*—see **459** and **460**), often with ascites. In this computed tomogram of a 58-year-old Japanese man, the presence of fibrosis around the portal tracts is seen as light-coloured lines in the liver. *S. mekongi* may also produce severe changes like these.

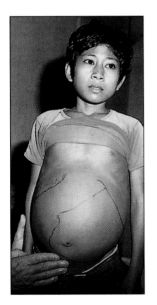

488 Philippino boy with gross splenomegaly
Advanced lesions due to *Schistosoma japonicum* may also be seen in children and adolescents.

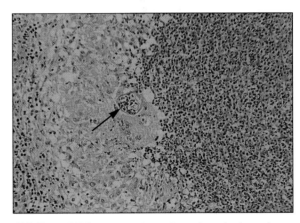

490 Ova of *Schistosoma japonicum* in spinal cord
Schistosomal lesions in the spinal cord or brain may contain large numbers of ova in necrotic material, often surrounded by eosinophils. Patients with cerebral schistosomiasis usually present with epileptiform attacks. This post mortem specimen from a 24-year-old Japanese male shows marked cellular reaction, including a multinucleated giant cell around a dead ovum (arrow) in the spinal cord. (*H&E* × *200.*)

SCHISTOSOMES FOUND UNCOMMONLY IN HUMANS

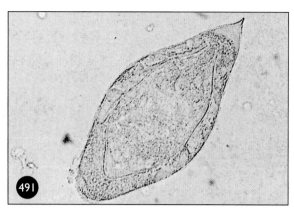

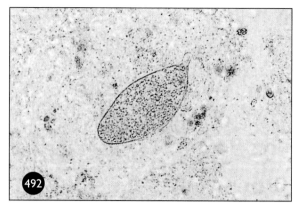

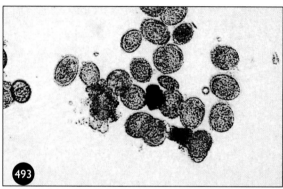

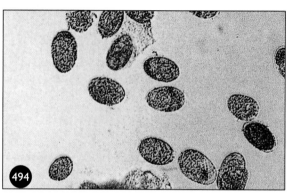

491–494 Eggs of unusual schistosomes seen in humans
The eggs of *Schistosoma intercalatum* (**491**) are similar to those of *S. haematobium* but are found only in the faeces. *S. mattheei* (**492**), which occurs in sheep and cattle, has been found in humans on rare occasions (× 290). *S. mekongi* (**493**) is easily mistaken for *S. japonicum*, which is shown here for comparison (**494**). (× 140.)

INTESTINAL FLUKES

(See **Tables 12** *and* **13**.)
Zoonotic intestinal infections have been recorded in humans with at least 70 species of trematodes, most of which are acquired by eating raw or inadequately cooked fish that contains encysted metacercariae. In other species, the metacercariae are eaten with raw amphibians, aquatic arthropods, molluscs or plants.

Most infections are symptomless and are revealed only during surveys or when the hosts are given drugs to expel the more important trematodes such as *Fasciolopsis buski*. Although many species are minute, and hence often over-looked, their prevalence in endemic foci may be high. For example, *Echinostoma hortense* acquired from raw loach occurs in up to 22% of people in some villages of southern Korea, whereas *Echinochasmus lilliputanus* was found in a similar proportion of some villages in parts of China. *Nanophyetus salmincola*, acquired by eating raw salmon or trout, is endemic in Khabarovsk territory (Russia), where up to 60% of local ethnic minorities may be infected in some villages.

The eggs of the minute intestinal trematodes are virtually indistinguishable by normal microscopy of stool specimens. **Table 13** includes only those species to which reference is most commonly made and is by no means all inclusive.

495–502 Snail intermediate hosts of trematode infections of humans
Several the molluscs listed in **Table 13** are shown here: *Oncomelania nosophora* (× 7.7) (**495**); *Thiara granifera* (× 2.0) (**496**); *Biomphalaria glabrata* (× 4.1) (**497**); *Biomphalaria sudanica* (× 1.7) (**498**); *Bulinus (Bulinus) senegalensis* (× 4.8) (**499**); *Bulinus (Physopsis) globosus* (× 2.5) (**500**); *Segmentina* sp. (× 5) (**501**); *Lymnaea truncatula* (× 5) (**502**).

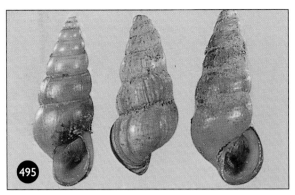

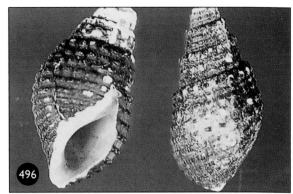

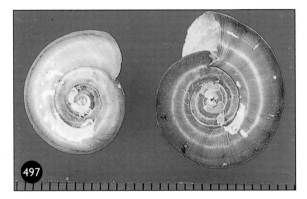

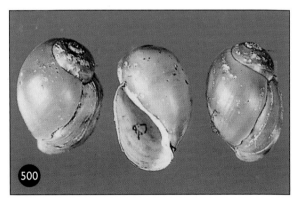

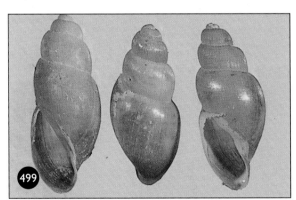

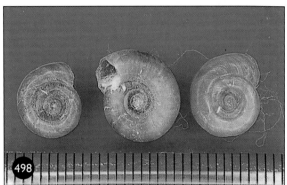

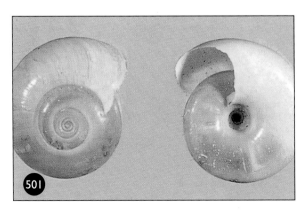

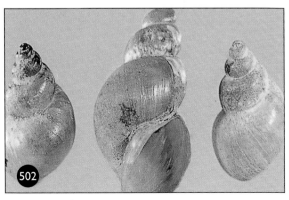

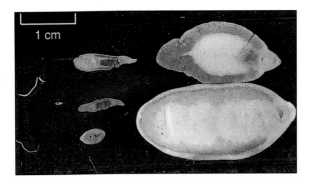

503 Comparative sizes of flukes
From left to right: first column—*Schistosoma mansoni* ♂ and ♀; second column—*Heterophyes heterophyes*; third column—*Opisthorchis felineus, O. sinensis, Paragonimus westermani*; fourth column—*Fasciola hepatica* and *F. buski.*

Table 13 Snails and other molluscs of medical importance (class Gastropoda). (The relation of the genera to the helminths that infect them is indicated by reference to the numbers in **Table 12.** The most important helminths are indicated in bold type.)

Subclass	Order	Family	Genera and species	Helminths
STREPTONEURA	PROSOBRANCHIATA (fresh water)	Bithyniidae	*Bithynia* spp.	**18, 19, 20**
			Parafossularis spp.	**20**
		Pamatiopsidae	*Oncomelania* spp.	**3**
			Tricula aperta	**6**
		Thiaridae	*Thiara granifera*	**15, 22**
		Pleuroceridae	*Semisulcospira libertina*	**15, 22**
		Pilidae	*Pila conica*	12
	(brackish and sea water)	Patamididae	*Cerithidia cingulata*	21
			Pirenella conica	21
EUTHYNEURA	PULMONATA BASOMATOPHORA (fresh water)	Planorbidae	*Biomphalaria* spp.	**1**
			Bulinus (Bulinus) spp.	**2**
			Bulinus (Physopsis) spp.	**2, 4, 5**
			Segmentina hemisphaerula	12
			S. trochoideus	11
			Hippeutis cantori	11
			H. umbilicalis	13
			Gyraulus convexiusculus	12
			G. prashadi	12
			? *Indoplanorbis exustus*	7
		Ancylidae	*Ferrissia tenuis*	**2**
		Lymnaeidae	*Fossaria* spp.	**9, 10**
			Lymnaea spp.	**9, 10**
			Stagnicola bulimoides	9
			Pseudosuccinia columella	**9, 10**
	STYLOMMATOPHORA (land snails)	Helicidae	*Helicella candidula*	13
		Enidae	*Zebrina detrita*	13
		Cionellidae	*Cionella lubrica*	13
			Achatina fulica	⎫
			Bradybaena similaris	⎬ 1,2
			Subulina octona	⎭
	SYSTELLOMMATOPHORA	Veronicellidae	*Veronica leydigi*	

[1] *Parastrongylus contonensis.* The land planarian *Geoplana septemlineata* has also been found infected with this nematode. *Achatina fulica* may be kept in non-endemic areas as a 'pet'; care is needed to ensure that infected snails are not imported.

[2] *P. costaricensis* is acquired from the slug *Vaginulus plebeius.*

FASCIOLOPSIASIS

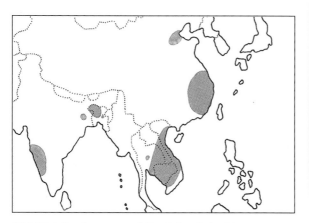

504 Distribution map of *Fasciolopsis buski*
F. buski is limited to areas of the Far East and Kalimantan (Indonesia). In certain foci (e.g. in northeast Thailand), almost the entire population of some villages may be infected.

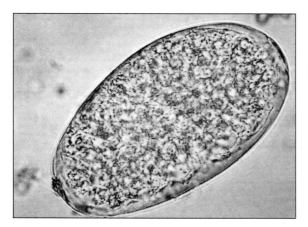

505 Egg of *Fasciolopsis buski* Miracidia, hatching from eggs passed in the faeces after shedding their ciliated coats, invade snails of various genera, including *Segmentina* and *Hippeutis*. The reproductive cycle in the snail differs from that of the schistosomes. After development through the sporocysts and two generations of rediae (see **514**), cercariae emerge into the water. They then encyst on aquatic plants such as the water caltrop (**508**) and water chestnut (**525**). (× 240.)

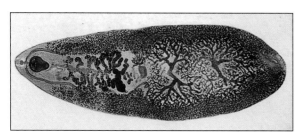

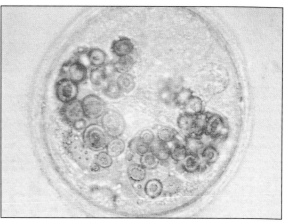

506 Metacercaria of *Fasciolopsis buski*
The metacercaria of *F. buski*, with its cyst wall. (× 220.)

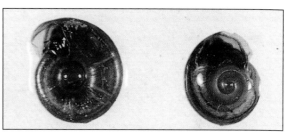

507 *Segmentina hemisphaerula*
This snail and a number of species of *Hippeutis* are the first intermediate hosts of *Fasciolopsis buski*. (× 2.7.)

508 The water caltrop
'Plantations' of water caltrop are harvested in endemic areas. The characteristic fruits of this plant are commonly eaten raw, and the meta-cercariae are thus swallowed. Water chestnuts (**525**) also often serve as a source of infection to children, who peel the raw plants with their teeth, thus ingesting the attached metacercariae.

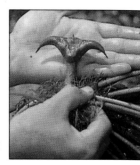

509 Adult *Fasciolopsis buski*
The adult *F. buski* is the largest parasitic trematode of humans and may reach 7.5 cm in length. Larvae mature in about three months, when the adults attach to the mucosa of the duodenum and jejunum. They can produce local trauma or, in heavy infections, obstruction, together with toxic effects that may be due to absorption of their meta-bolic products and subsequent sensitisation of the host. The pig is the main animal reservoir of infection for humans.

UNCOMMON SPECIES

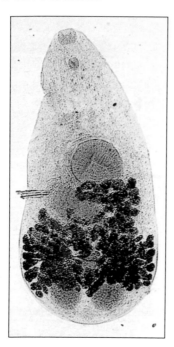

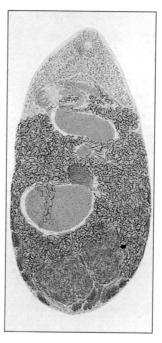

510 Adult *Heterophyes heterophyes*
This is a widely distributed (from Egypt to the Philippines) tiny trematode, one of the large family Heterophyidae, with a typical life cycle in brackish water snails (e.g. *Pirenella*) (see **Table 13**). Up to 1% of villagers in some foci in the northern Nile Delta are infected, and rates as high as 24% have been recorded in foci in Khuzestan; elsewhere, it is usually rare. The cercariae encyst on fish such as the mullet and infect humans when improperly cooked fish is eaten. The adult trematode shown here lives in the middle part of the small intestine. The eggs (see **383**) are very similar to those of *Clonorchis* and *Metagonimus*. (× 45.)

511 Adult *Metagonimus yokagawai*
This is the most common heterophyid fluke of the Far East, but it is also found in the Mediterranean basin. The life cycle is similar to that of *Heterophyes*, and the eggs of the two genera can be differentiated only with difficulty. The adult worm shown here is also very small (1.4 × 0.6 mm) and lives in the upper and middle jejunum. Several genera of snails, including *Semisulcospira* (see **Table 13**), are the first intermediate hosts for the species. The prevalence rate in the Korean Republic averages 4.8%, with rates over 20% in several foci there and in the eastern provinces of the former USSR. The cercariae encyst on various species of freshwater fish. (× 45.)

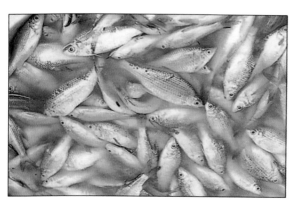

512 Cyprinoid fish in an Eastern market
The mullet and other fish living in fresh or brackish waters are common intermediate hosts for *Heterophyes heterophyes* and *Metagonimus yokagawai*. The metacercariae are attached under the scales or in the skin.

LIVER AND LUNG FLUKE INFECTIONS

Over 100 species of snails have been implicated as hosts of the four commonest liver flukes (*see* **Table 12**), whereas 150 species of freshwater fish, 60 species of crustacea and 20 species of plants are involved in the cycles of these and other trematode species, which infect 40 million people.

Opisthorchiasis (excluding that caused by *Opisthorchis sinensis*, of which there are seven million cases), formerly believed to be most prevalent in Southeast Asia, is now admitted to be extremely common in parts of the former USSR, affecting about 1.2 million, with almost 100% infection rates in some foci, especially of western Siberia. Altogether, at least 10 million people have opisthorciasis. As many as 10% of those infected may develop cholangiocarcinoma. A high proportion (up to 20%) of Southeast Asian immigrants to Europe or North America have been found infected with *Opisthorchis* (or *Clonorchis*). Moreover, it is now estimated also that the lungs of about 21 million individuals are infected with various species of *Paragonimus*, which is often mistaken (and thus wrongly treated) for pulmonary tuberculosis. In part of northeastern India, for example, 60% of patients receiving such therapy were found to have pulmonary flukes, whereas in Ecuador, where at least two million are infected, 13% in one clinic had paragonimiasis, not tuberculosis.

OPISTHORCHIS SINENSIS*

*(Previously called *Clonorchis sinensis*. The infection is still commonly referred to as clonorchiasisis.)

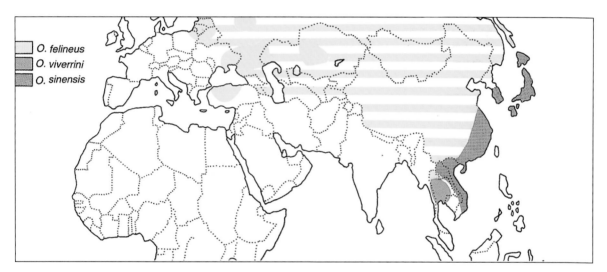

513 Distribution map of *Opisthorchis* species in humans
Parasitic food-borne trematodes of this genus are very widely distributed in the Old World. *O. sinensis* is also known as the Chinese or oriental liver fluke; it is found in humans and also in other fish-eating mammals in the areas shown. *O. felineus* is now known to have a much wider distribution, whereas that of *O. viverinni* is localised in parts of Thailand and neighbouring countries.

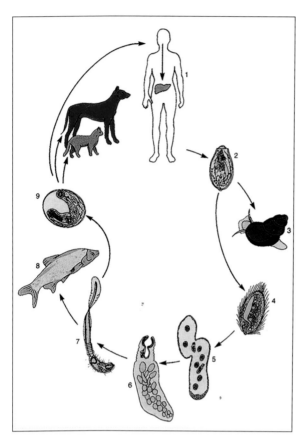

514 Life cycle of *Opisthorchis sinensis*
The adult flukes living in the biliary tree of the liver (1) produce operculated eggs (2), which are passed in the faeces. When ingested by the snail host (3), miracidia (4) hatch from the eggs to produce sporocysts (5) in which develop a single generation of daughter cells (rediae) (6). Within these develop lophocercous (i.e. single-tailed) cercariae (7), which leave the snails to enter various freshwater fish (8) in which they encyst to form metacercariae (9). When the fish is eaten by a carnivore, the young trematodes emerge and eventually pass up the common bile duct, finally reaching the smaller branches of the biliary tree where they mature. (*See also* **383**.)

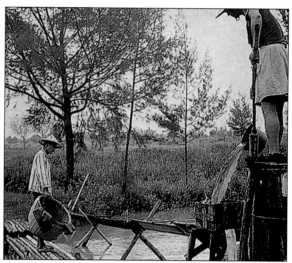

515 Ecology of *Opisthorchis sinensis* infection
Latrines used to be built over the edges of fishponds into which faecal material containing helminth eggs would drop. This provided an ideal way of infecting cultivated fish and perpetuating the cycle of transmission. Although this practice has been greatly reduced, it is still common practice to pour fresh night soil into fishponds, as seen here.

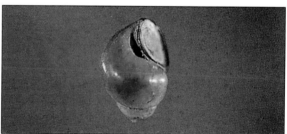

516 Intermediate host of *Opisthorchis*
Bithynia funiculata is one of the species of this genus in which *O. sinensis* will develop. Other molluscan genera (*see* **Table 13**) can serve as intermediate hosts. (× 3.2.)

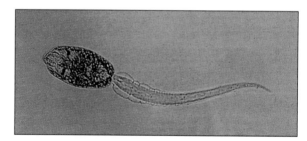

517 Cercaria of *Opisthorchis sinensis*
The lophocercous cercariae escape from the snail to encyst under the scales of various species of freshwater cyprinoid fish. (× 62.)

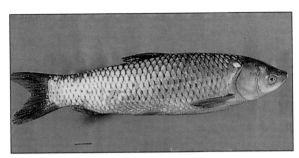

518 *Ctenopharyngodon idellus*
This fish is a common host for metacercariae of *Opisthorchis sinensis*.

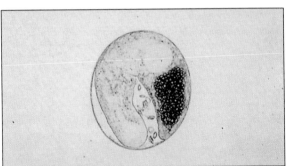

519 Metacercaria in fish
Humans are infested by eating raw or incompletely cooked fish, a common delicacy among many Chinese. Metacercariae are thus ingested and excyst in the duodenum. (× 160.)

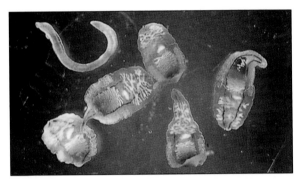

520 Living adult *Opisthorchis sinensis*
The young worms migrate up the common bile duct to the liver. At maturity they may reach 2 cm in length. (× 2.5.)

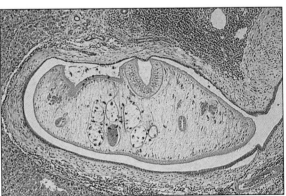

521 Section of *Opisthorchis sinensis* in bile duct
Direct mechanical damage and possibly toxic effects of the adult worms lead to fibrotic changes in the bile ducts. (× 25.)

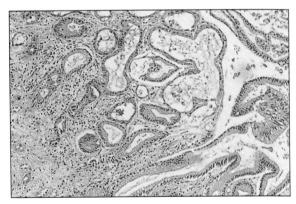

522 Cholangiocarcinoma of the liver
Severe chronic infection with *Opisthorchis sinensis* may lead to marked pericholangitic fibrosis and finally multifocal cholangiocarcinoma of the liver. In this case, metastases were widely distributed throughout the body. (*H&E* × 80.)

OPISTHORCHIS FELINEUS AND O. VIVERRINI

The distribution of *Opisthorchis felineus* and *O. viverrini* is shown in **513**. *O. felineus* is common in domestic cats, dogs and some other animals in eastern and southeastern Europe, as well as many parts of the former USSR. In the Far East it is largely replaced by *O. viverrini*, which occurs mainly in northeast Thailand, where it infects up to 90% of the population in some villages. Cats, as well as humans, serve as reservoirs of infection. The life cycles are similar to that of *O. sinensis*, with snails of the genus *Bithynia* serving as intermediate hosts (*see also* **516**).

523 Ecology of *Opisthorchis viverrini*
Humans are infected by ingesting the metacercariae in cyprinoid fish. The figure shows a typical village fishpond in northeast Thailand. Both the snail and fish populations of the ponds increase during the rainy season.

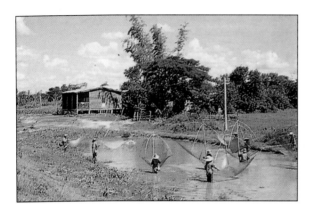

524 Metacercaria in fish
Most infection is from uncooked fish. In northeast Thailand, the fish sauce 'koipla' is the most important source. (× *230*.)

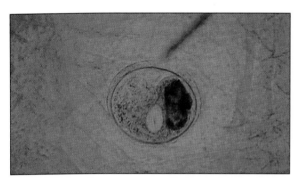

525 *Cyprinus carpio*, host for metacercariae of *Opisthorchis felineus*
These freshwater fish are often infected in the Far East and are a common source of infection in northeast Thailand. This shopper's basket also contains water chestnuts on which metacercariae of *Fasciolopsis buski* may encyst (*see* **506**).

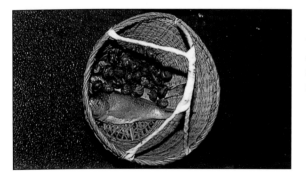

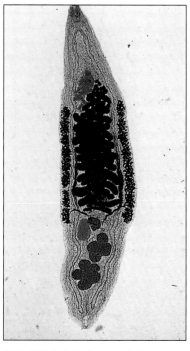
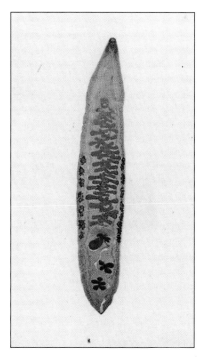
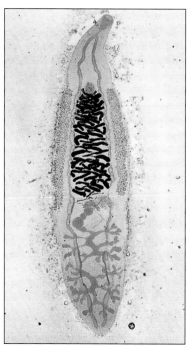

526–528 Adult flukes of *Opisthorchis felineus*, *O. viverrini* and *O. sinensis*
The adults of *O. felineus* (**526**, left) and *O. viverrini* (**527**, centre), which are similar to those of *O. sinensis* (**528**, right), live in the bile ducts and produce similar pathological changes. They can be distinguished by such structural details as the numbers, positions and shapes of the testes in the posterior parts of the worms (the lower thirds in these figures). (× 7.7.)

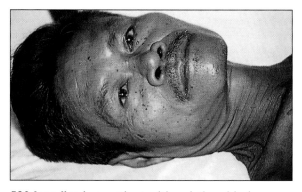

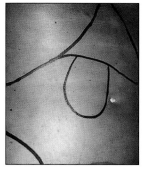

530 Gross enlargement of the gall bladder in opisthorchiasis
This figure shows the grossly enlarged gall bladder of the patient seen in **529**.

529 Jaundice in a patient with opisthorchiasis
This adult Thai man was heavily infected with *Opisthorchis viverrini*.

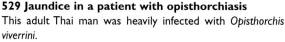

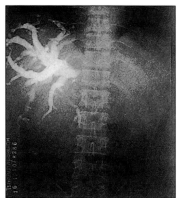

531 Cholangiogram of patient with opisthorchiasis
This radiograph shows dilation of the main bile ducts and disorganisation of the biliary tree.

DICROCOELIUM DENDRITICUM

532 Life cycle of *Dicrocoelium dendriticum*

The only trematode of medical importance in which the life cycle involves insects is a cosmopolitan parasite normally found in the biliary tract of sheep. It has evolved a bizarre method to ensure its transmission. (1) Eggs passed by infected sheep are eaten by various species of land snails in the intestine from which miracidia hatch. (2) The miracidia form several generations of sporocysts and finally tailed cercariae, which accumulate near the snails' surface. (3) This leads to their ejection by the molluscs in small balls of slime, each of which may contain several hundred cercariae. (4) The slime balls are eaten by ants, the second intermediate hosts, in the body cavities of which most of the parasites encyst as metacercariae. However, a few encyst in the suboesophageal ganglion. (5) Their presence causes the ants to behave in a remarkable fashion, climbing to the tips of vegetation where they remain overnight, ready to be ingested by grazing animals in the cooler hours. The next day when the temperature increases, they descend to the shelter of the cooler microclimate provided near the soil. (6) Once taken up by the herbivore (or, accidentally, by humans), the para-

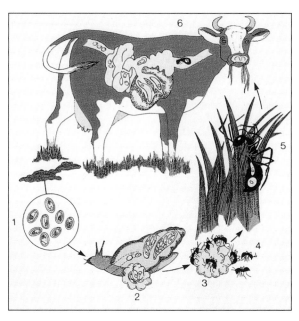

sites excyst in the duodenum from where they migrate to their definitive sites in the smaller bile ducts.

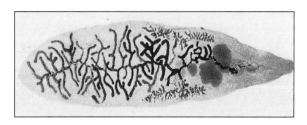

533 Adult *Dicrocoelium dendriticum*

Maturation of the flukes takes between six and seven weeks, and individual animals may harbour as many as 50 000 adult flukes. The adult, which grows up to 1.5 cm long, lives in the biliary tract, especially the small bile ducts. The eggs are similar to those of the *Opisthorcis* group (see **383**). Infection in humans, understandably, is rare. In West Africa, zoonotic infection with *Dicrocoelium hospes* has been reported, with species of *Dorylus* and *Crematogaster* serving as secondary hosts. ($\times$ *4.5*.)

FASCIOLA HEPATICA AND F. GIGANTICA

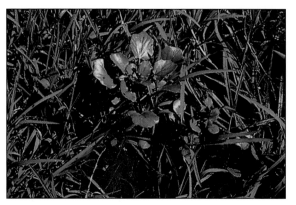

534 Watercress, a source of infection of fascioliasis

Infection with *Fasciola hepatica* is cosmopolitan in herbivores that graze in wet pasturage where the intermediate hosts—snails of the genus *Lymnaea*—are found. About two million people are believed to be infected with *Fasciola* acquired from metacercaria-infected aquatic plants. In temperate climates, humans are most often infected by eating wild watercress on which metacercariae have encysted. It grows commonly in swampy pasture by small streams. *F. gigantica*, the common liver fluke of cattle in the Middle East, much of Africa and Asia, occasionally infects humans.

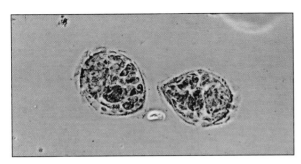

535 Miracidia of *Fasciola hepatica*
Motile miracidia hatch from eggs passed in faeces and infect snails of the genus *Lymnaea*. (× 225.)

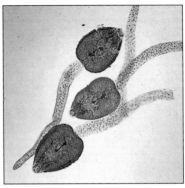

538 Cercariae of *Fasciola hepatica*
The cercariae, which have unforked tails, encyst on aquatic vegetation to form metacercariae. (× 85.)

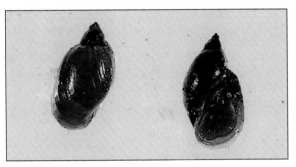

536 *Lymnaea swinhoei*
This snail is a host for *Fasciola hepatica* in parts of China. In Europe the usual intermediate host is *L. truncatula* (see **502**). (× 7.)

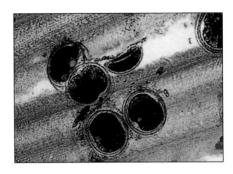

539 Metacercariae on grass
These are found on grass or other moist herbage such as watercress (**534**). When the metacercariae are ingested, the cycle recommences. (× 75.)

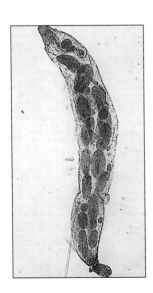

537 Redia from intermediate host
Rediae develop in the hepatopancreas, with the formation of cercariae. (× 30.)

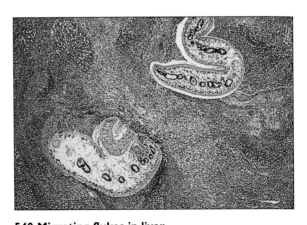

540 Migrating flukes in liver
After being swallowed, the metacercariae pass through the intestinal wall and penetrate the liver capsule to enter the liver parenchyma. The figure shows a sheep liver with migrating, immature flukes. (*H&E* × 20.)

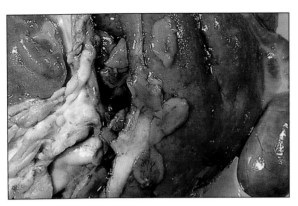

541 Adult flukes in bile ducts of a sheep liver
The adult flukes penetrate into the bile ducts where they cause damage to the biliary tract. Eggs (see **372**) are passed with the bile into the faeces.

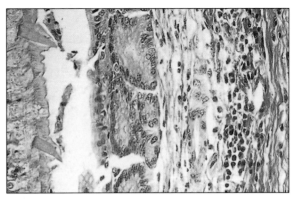

542 Adult *Fasciola hepatica* in section of liver
The surface spines of the adult fluke produce mechanical damage to the biliary epithelium. (*H&E × 350.*)

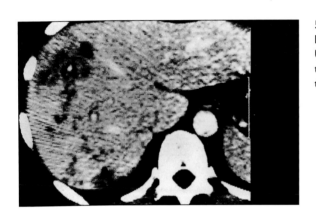

543 Computed tomogram of *Fasciola hepatica* in human liver
Using contrast, cystic filling defects suggestive of this trematode infection can be visualised. They usually disappear after therapy.

PARAGONIMIASIS

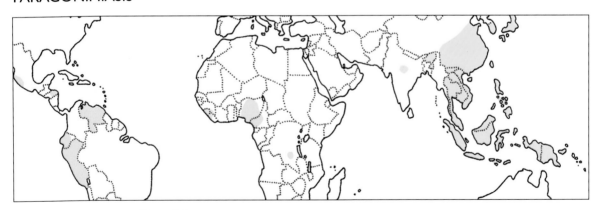

544 Distribution map of lung flukes
Paragonimiasis, affecting over 20 million people worldwide, is caused by numerous species of lung flukes (see **Table 14**). *Paragonimus westermani* is the commonest parasite responsible for human infection in the Far East, where it is has a wide range of mammalian reservoirs. Human infections with *P. heterotremus* are well known in Thailand and with *P. pulmonalis* in the Far East. *P. africanus* and *P. uterobilateralis* have a focal distribution in humans in West Africa. *P. mexicanus* and other species commonly produce human infection in parts of Central and South America. The so-called 'lung flukes' have the further distinction of becoming localised at times in the brain where they may give rise to major neurological symptoms.

Table 14 Species of *Paragonimus* recorded in humans

Species	Geographical area	Natural final hosts[1]
ASIA and PACIFIC		
Paragonimus westermani westermani	China, Thailand, Malaysia, Sri Lanka	dog, wild canids, cat, wild felids, civets, mongooses, macaques
P. westermani japonicus	Japan	mainly raccoon dog, fox
P. westermani filipinus	Philippines, Taiwan	dog, cat, rat
P. westermani ichunensis	Northern China, former USSR	dog, cat, tiger, raccoon dog, wolf
P. pulmonalis	China, Taiwan, Korea, Japan	dog, cat, tiger, wild boar
P. miyazakii	Japan	dog, cat, weasel, sable, wild boar, raccoon dog, badger
P. heterotremus (= P. tuanshanensis)	China, Laos, Thailand	dog, cat, leopard, rat, bandicoot
P. skrjabini (= P. szechuanensis)	China	cat, dog, ? weasel, masked palm civet
P. hueitungensis	China	
P. ohirai	Japan	rodents, insectivores, dog, raccoon dog, badger, pig, wild boar, weasel
P. iloktsuenensis	Taiwan, Japan	dog, weasel, rodents, insectivores
P. sadoensis	Japan	weasel, cat
AFRICA		
P. africanus	Cameroon, Zaire, Nigeria, Ghana	dog, civet, mongoose, drill, potto
P. uterobilateralis	Cameroon, Nigeria, Guinea, Ivory Coast, Liberia	dog, civet, mongoose, rat, shrew
NORTH and SOUTH AMERICA		
P. mexicanus	Mexico, Guatemala, Costa Rica, Panama, Peru, Ecuador	opossum, wild felids, canids, coati, raccoon, skunk
P. caliensis	Panama, Colombia, Peru	opossum
P. peruvianus	Peru	opossum, cat
P. ecuadoriensis	Ecuador	coati

[1] In addition to humans. Other species occur only in domestic or wild animals.

545 Life cycle of *Paragonimus pulmonalis*

This may be taken as a typical example of the genus. (1) Humans, the definitive hosts, are infected when they eat the flesh of crustacea containing living metacercariae. The metacercariae hatch in the duodenum, and the young flukes penetrate the gut wall, the mesentery and the diaphragm to the pleural cavity. Within 2–3 weeks, the worms, which are hermaphroditic, penetrate beneath the lung capsule where they meet and cross fertilise. Adult trematodes (2) become partly encapsulated in the parenchymal tissue, where they lay eggs (3) that pass into the alveoli and are coughed up or swallowed. Eggs that reach water hatch into miracidia (4), which penetrate snails of an appropriate species. These are the first intermediate hosts. In the snails (5) they form sporocysts from which develop two generations of daughter cells (rediae), which give rise in about three months to very short-tailed (microcercous) cercariae (6); after emerging into the water the cercariae seek their crustacean (secondary intermediate) host (7) into which they penetrate to encyst in the gills or muscles as metacercariae (8). *P. pulmonalis* can also be acquired by eating uncooked flesh of the wild boar (9), which serves as a paratenic host of this species (i.e., a supernumerary intermediate host). Domestic cats (10) and dogs can also serve as definitive hosts for numerous species of *Paragonimus* in the Far

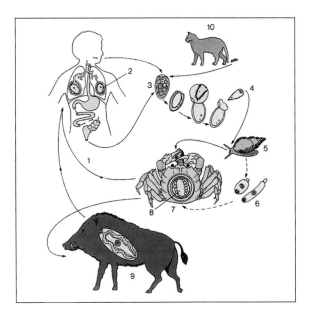

East and in West Africa. Like *P. westermani*, *P. heterotremus* may invade the brain and subcutaneous tissues but often only causes a type of larva migrans in humans.

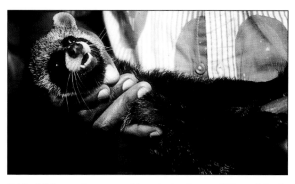

546 African civet cat, *Civettictis civetta* (Viverridae)
This carnivore is a primary reservoir host for both *Paragonimus africanus* and *P. uterobilateralis* in West Africa. The West African long-nosed mongoose, *Crossarchus obscurus*, is also an important host for *P. uterobilateralis* in Liberia as well as being infected by *P. africanus* in countries further east. The palm civet, *Paradoxurus hermaphroditus* (Viverridae), is one of the feral reservoir hosts of *Paragonimus* in Thailand and other Far East countries.

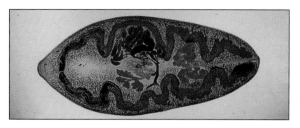

547 Adult *Paragonimus westermani*
The adult fluke lives normally in the lungs. Preserved specimens, as seen here, become flattened and distorted during preparation (× 5.2). It is rather lemon shaped and about 1 cm long when alive (see **553**).

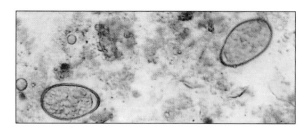

548 Eggs in human sputum
Eggs are passed in the sputum or swallowed to be passed later in the faeces. The miracidia hatching from the eggs penetrate snails of various genera, including *Semisulcospira* and *Thiara* (see **Table 13**). After the usual cycle of development in the snail, microcercous cercariae emerge and encyst inside freshwater crayfish and crabs. Various crab-eating carnivores thus become the natural reservoirs of *Paragonimus* species. (See *also* **375**.) (× 150.)

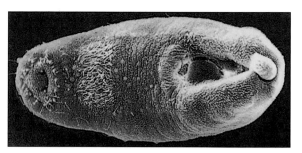

549 Microcercous cercaria of *Paragonimus pulmonalis*
Ventral view of the cercaria of this species, which is widely distributed in Korea, China (including Taiwan) and Japan, where the infection is acquired from crabs or crayfish. (*SEM* × 510.)

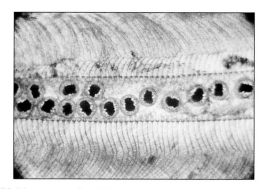

550 Metacercaria of *Paragonimus pulmonalis* along a gill bar of the crab *Eriocheir japonicus*
Compare with the smaller metacercaria of *Opisthorchis sinensis* (**519**). (× 7.)

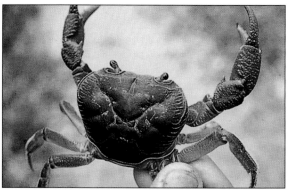

551 *Ranguna smithiana*, a host of lung fluke
Crabs are commonly eaten raw or in the form of an uncooked paste, with which the metacercariae are ingested. This species is a host of *Paragonimus westermani* and *P. heterotremus* in Thailand.

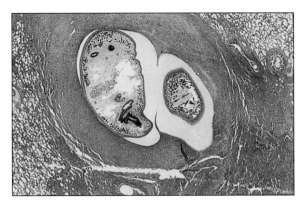

552 Section of lung
The figure shows a section of lung containing encapsulated, adult *Paragonimus westermani*. (*H&E × 20.*)

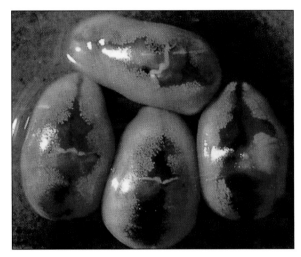

553 Living adult *Paragonimus westermani*
Compare the appearance with that of the prepared specimen in **547**, which is the condition figured in most textbooks. (× 4.3.)

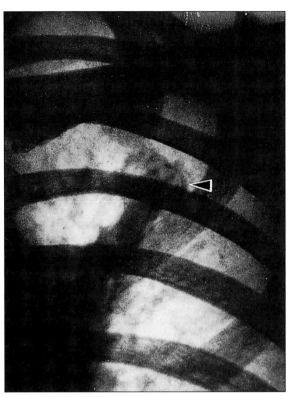

554 Chest radiograph
Human infection is manifested by cough, haemoptysis and other signs and symptoms, which are commonly confused with those of tuberculosis. Typical shadows caused by the encysted adult trematodes may be seen on this radiograph of a seven-year-old Japanese girl who was infected with *Paragonimus pulmonalis* after eating the flesh of the crab, *Eriocheir japonicus*. Note the ring shadow in the left lobe. There were also nodes in the hilar area. Numerous eggs were present in her brown-coloured sputum.

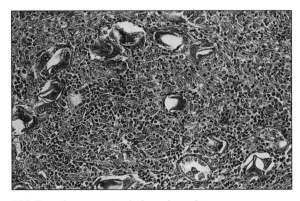

555 Eggs in mesenteric lymph node
In this section, several disintegrating eggs of *Paragonimus westermani* are seen in a granuloma containing numerous eosinophils in a mesenteric node. (*H&E × 100.*)

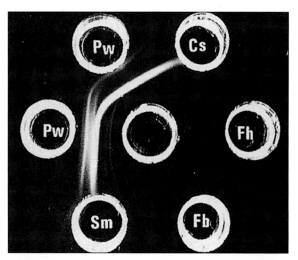

556 Gel diffusion test for paragonimiasis
The reaction of antigen derived from adult worms with serum antibodies can be a useful diagnostic aid. More sensitive tests now include a dot-enzyme-linked immunosorbent assay, based on a specific monoclonal antibody, which detects *Paragonimus* antigens in the serum.

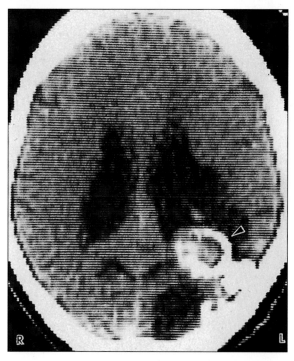

557 Cyst of *Paragonimus* in the brain
This 59-year-old woman, who lived in China as a teenager, presented with a history of epileptic convulsions once or twice a year for over 40 years. They followed an initial pulmonary infection, which was probably acquired when she was about 16 years of age. Computed tomography revealed a large, calcified mass caused by encystation of an adult fluke, probably *Paragonimus westermani*, in the left occipital region. The peripheral brain tissue was shrunken and the left lateral ventricle dilated.

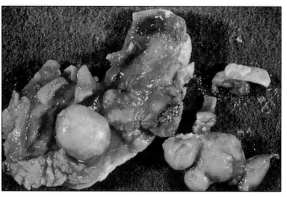

558 *Paragonimus* cyst extracted from brain
A cyst of *Paragonimus westermani* found at autopsy in the brain of a 21-year-old Japanese girl. Unlike the patient in **557**, such individuals usually present with epilepsy occurring for the first time in adult life.

CHAPTER 4

Infections Acquired through the Gastrointestinal Tract

Many of the important pathogens that gain entry through the gastrointestinal tract are cosmopolitan in their distribution. They include viruses, bacteria, protozoa, helminths and endoparasitic arthropods. The first three of these can be directly infectious for humans when they are passed in the faeces but, in the case of helminths, the eggs may become infectious only after maturation in the soil (e.g. *Ascaris lumbricoides*) or after passing through an intermediate host (e.g. *Taenia saginata*)★. Some of the pathogens pass from the intestinal tract to cause systemic infection and may localise in other organs (e.g. poliomyelitis, acute viral hepatitis (*see* **Table 15**), trichinosis). Localised infection of the gastrointestinal tract itself with pathogenic viruses or bacteria (*see* **Table 16**) accounts for a high proportion of deaths in infants and young children in developing countries, where the standards of hygiene and nutrition are often already at very low levels.

The most important pattern of transmission is the passage of infective material from human faeces into the mouth of a new host, which is known as 'faeco–oral' transmission. This occurs mostly through inapparent faecal contamination of food, water and hands, the three main points of contact with the mouth. Some of the pathogens

that infect through the mouth are not excreted in the faeces (e.g. guineaworm infection is acquired by drinking contaminated water, but the larvae escape through the skin). On the other hand, although the ova of *Necator americanus* are passed in the faeces, the route of human infection is by direct penetration of the skin by the larvae after a period of incubation of the egg in the soil.

A number of the infections that are acquired through the gastrointestinal tract, such as cholera and typhoid, characteristically occur in epidemic form. The spread of cholera, for example, is facilitated by the potentiating combination of a symptomless carrier state with both widescale local and international travel. It was feared that the pandemic of the El Tor biotype would soon be replaced by the more virulent 0:139 serovar, which has recently appeared in Southeast Asia although, so far, this has not been realised. Even the protozoal pathogen, *Cryptosporidium parvum*, may cause severe, waterborne epidemics, as has occurred recently in the USA and elsewhere. Other infections may be more localised, affecting people from the same household or institution (e.g. amoebiasis or enterobiasis); hospitals housing the mentally subnormal are particularly vulnerable to such conditions.

The importance of some of the rare, protozoal infections such as the Microsporidia is only being appreciated now that they are appearing as concomitant infections in people with depressed immune responsiveness (e.g. in AIDS).

★ Helminthiases acquired from the soil are included in Chapter 2 and those requiring a snail intermediate host in Chapter 3. A number of the latter are also acquired via the oral route.

VIRAL INFECTIONS

POLIOMYELITIS

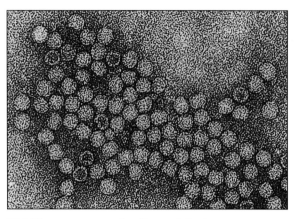

559 Ultrastructure of poliomyelitis virus
Spherical particles measuring 25 nm in diameter are apparent in this electron micrograph; both 'full' and 'empty' particles are shown. Once considered to be mainly a disease of the industrialised world, poliomyelitis, thanks to effective vaccination, is now mainly a problem in the developing countries throughout which it was, until very recently, widespread. (× *126 000.*)

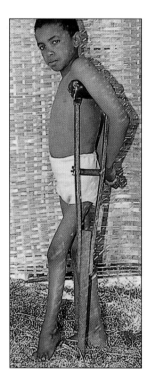

560 Ethiopian boy with paralysis of left leg
Today, young indigenous children in the developing countries are predominantly affected, along with non-immunised expatriates of all ages. A global campaign to eliminate the disease in developing countries has made spectacular progress in recent years. In India alone, for example, 200 000 cases were reported in 1989. By 1993, only 8000 new cases were reported globally to the WHO, and 141 countries were apparently free of the disease.

ACUTE VIRAL HEPATITIS

Acute viral hepatitis and its sequelae are a major problem, particularly in the tropics and subtropics, although the viruses are cosmopolitan. The viruses so far identified are reviewed in **Table 15**.

Hepatitis A (HAV) and HEV, formerly called HNANB(E), are transmitted by the faeco–oral route. HBV (hepatitis B virus), HCV, HDV and HFV are transmitted by parenteral infection; they are dealt with in Chapter 9 (see **1021–1027**). Yellow fever is highlighted in Chapter 1 (**18–21**). Hepatitis may also be associated with cytomegalovirus, Epstein–Barr virus and filoviruses (see **Table 25**). HAV is commonly acquired from contaminated food, with shellfish being a notorious source of infection. It can occur in epidemic fashion and may affect more than 90% of the adult population in some developing countries. It does not usually have serious consequences. HEV may be the commonest agent of acute viral hepatitis in developing countries and can result in serious disease in pregnant women.

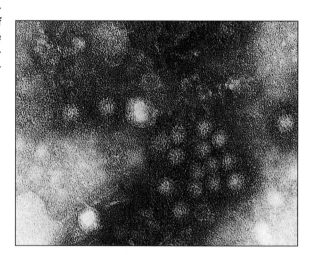

561 Ultrastructure of hepatitis A virus
The electron micrograph of this enterovirus shows the (27 nm in diameter) particles that were found in faecal extracts from an adult volunteer during the acute phase of hepatitis A infection after inoculation with serum. The particles are heavily coated with antibody present in convalescent serum. The incubation period is between two and four weeks and the infection, which may be with or without jaundice, is often mild. The virus causing hepatitis E is a calicivirus with a longer incubation period. Although usually producing a mild illness, the infection can be particularly dangerous during pregnancy when it may cause a high mortality. (× *220 000.*)

Table 15 Hepatitis viruses[1]

Name	Type or genus	RNA/DNA	Transmission mode	Course of infection	Notes
HBV	hepadnavirus (similar to retroviruses)	DNA	via blood and blood products, usually by inoculation; perinatal infection from mother	incubation 1–3 months, then immune-mediated acute hepatitis	high proportion become chronic carriers; chronic active infection leads to cirrhosis, hepatocellular carcinoma (i.e. oncogenic)
HCV = HNANB(P)	togavirus	RNA	as HBV plus other modes (90–95% of transfusion induced HNANB)	incubation 2 months; hepatitis less severe than HBV infection	may give chronic carrier state with same sequelae as HBV
HDV (delta)	'defective virus'	RNA	transfusion, heterosexual transmission	incubation 2–12 weeks; requires HBs antigen; ('piggy-back virus'); superinfection may give fulminating hepatitis	commonest in Africa and South America—probable cause of Labrea fever
HAV	heparnivirus ('enterovirus 72')	RNA	faeco–oral route; water, shellfish etc.	incubation 2–4 weeks; often mild infection with or without jaundice	can give epidemic spread, > 90% of adults infected in developing countries
HEV = HNANB(E)	calicivirus	RNA	faeco–oral route; mainly water	incubation 6–8 weeks; mild except in pregnancy	mortality up to 20% in pregnancy
HFV	not known	?	accounts for 5–10% of HNANB(P) infections	little known	little known
Yellow fever	togavirus	RNA	vector-borne	incubation period 3–6 days; usually severe hepatitis, high mortality rate	see 18–21

[1]Hepatitis may also be associated with infection by cytomegalovirus, Epstein–Barr virus and filoviruses (*see* **Table 25**).

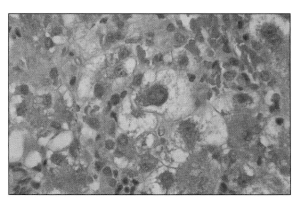

562 Section of liver in acute viral hepatitis
The changes seen here are found in both hepatitis A and hepatitis B infection. Marked swelling of the hepatocytes (which have indistinct or lysed membranes) and loss of cytoplasmic contents cause this 'ballooning degeneration.' (× *800*.) (AFIP No. 71–1396; *see also* **1025**.)

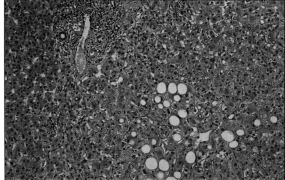

563 Acute spotty hepatitis
This liver in mild viral hepatitis (which was caused by hepatitis E or hepatitis C) shows macrovesicular fat in the centrilobular area and diffuse microvesicular fat with infiltration of inflammatory cells in the portal triad (*H&E* × 60). (*See also* **1025**.)

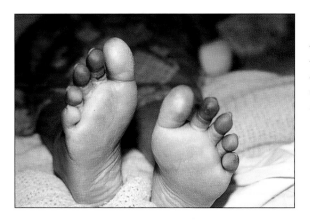

564 Peripheral vasculitis in a patient with hepatitis C
Hepatitis C is produced by a positive single-stranded RNA virus of the Flaviviridae family. It a common viral infection of the liver and can occasionally present with systemic features of a vasculitis, as demonstrated here, with severe involvement of the terminal digits of the foot due to an immune-related, essential, mixed cryoglobulinaemia.

ACUTE VIRAL GASTROENTERITIS

Acute viral gastroenteritis is a major cause of morbidity and mortality, especially in infants and young children in the developing countries, where it is the leading cause of death in those under four years of age. It has been estimated that over 500 million children are infected and that 5–10 million die yearly from infectious gastroenteritis.

565 Infant with viral gastroenteritis
Among the viruses that have been identified as responsible for acute gastroenteritis in children are a variety of rotaviruses, adenoviruses, astroviruses and caliciviruses including Norwalk and Norwalk-like virus (see **Table 16**). Infection results in severe dehydration, which calls for energetic oral replacement therapy, with glucose and electrolytes or parenteral rehydration in the most severe cases. Malnourished infants are at

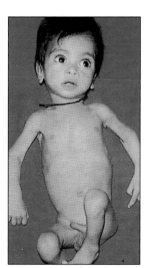
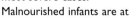

particular risk. Note here the flaccidity and other signs of dehydration in this infant.

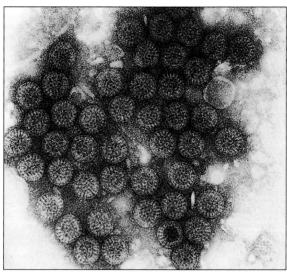

566 Rotavirus causing viral gastroenteritis
Rotaviruses, of which at least seven groups and two subgroups can infect humans, are responsible for about 20% of all diarrhoeal infections in developing countries. This electron micrograph shows particles approximately 75 nm in diameter that were found in faeces. They have a characteristic, wheel-like appearance. (*EM × 125 000.*)

Table 16 Major viral and bacterial pathogens causing acute diarrhoea[1]

Pathogen	Pathogenesis	Notes
VIRUSES		
Rotaviruses (Rotaviridae)	Destroy tips of microvilli; new cells absorb less water, salts and sugars.	Global. Cause 140 million cases and 1 million deaths yearly. Major cause in developing countries.
Adenoviruses (Adenoviridae)	Less severe but more prolonged than above. Types 40, 41 main pathogens.	Second most important agents in developing countries.
Astroviruses (Astroviridae)	Mild gastroenteritis, may occur in outbreaks.	Mainly children < 7 years.
Caliciviruses (Caliciviridae)	Mild gastroenteritis, may occur in outbreaks.	Older children.
Norwalk and Norwalk-like viruses (Caliciviridae)	Mild gastroenteritis, may occur in outbreaks.	Older children and adults.
BACTERIA		
Salmonella species (except *S. typhi*, *S. paratyphi*)	Invade lamina propria of ileocaecal region; prostaglandins released, trigger cyclic AMP; active fluid secretion.	Were commonest in Western World; mainly zoonotic
Escherichia coli —enterotoxigenic	Pilli bind bacteria to mucosal cells, secrete exotoxins; these increase cyclic GMP, causing fluid secretion.	Major cause in children in developing countries and of 'Turista'
—enteropathogenic	Adhere to enterocytes, destroy microvilli.	Babies and infants in developing countries
Helicobacter pylori	Stomach is normal site, invades mucosa.	High prevalance in adults in developing world associated with gastric adenocarcinoma
Vibrio cholera	Biotypes of serovar 0:1 vary in virulence factors and toxin production; toxin activates cyclic AMP, blocks absorption of salt, increases fluid secretion.	El Tor replaced classic biotype but virulent serovar 0:129 now spreading.
Shigella species	Enteropathogenic, causing ulcers in distal ileum and colon.	Major cause in young people in developing countries.

[1]Excluding typhoid and paratyphoid, which cause systemic infection. *See also* Protozoal Infections, p. 172.

BACTERIAL INFECTIONS

SALMONELLOSIS—TYPHOID (ENTERIC) FEVERS

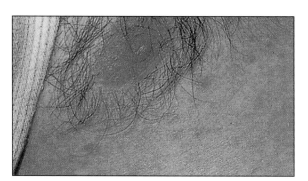

567 Rose spots

Species of *Salmonella* cause only a small proportion of the diarrhoeal infections (about 2.5%) in developing countries. The most important member of this genus is *Salmonella typhi*, the cause of typhoid (enteric fever). The classic rose spots of typhoid (1 to 3 mm in diameter) may appear irregularly, usually on the abdominal wall, lower thorax and back of the trunk.

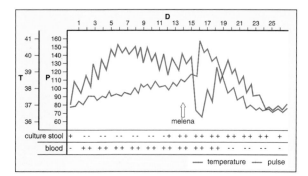

568 Temperature chart

The fever, which often rises in a stepwise fashion, is high and accompanied by confusion and severe prostration ('typhoid state'). There is often a dissociation between pulse and temperature (Faget's sign) and an accompanying leucopenia. The tongue is frequently coated (in contrast to kala-azar, when it is usually clean—see **222**). [D—day of illness; T—temperature (°C); P—pulse rate.]

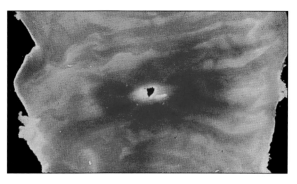

569 Ulceration of Peyer's patches

Intestinal haemorrhage and perforation are the two most serious complications of typhoid fever. They are due to ulceration of Peyer's patches.

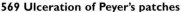

570 Temperature chart in salmonellosis associated with *Schistosoma mansoni* infection

An association exists between fever occurring in chronic *Salmonella typhi* infection and concomitant *S. mansoni* infection. In such cases, clearance of the helminth infection is needed before the *Salmonella* organisms can be eliminated. [D—day of illness; T—temperature (°C).]

'NON-SPECIFIC' ACUTE INFECTIOUS DIARRHOEA

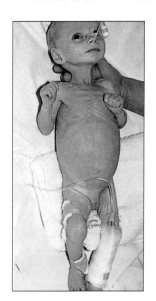

571 Dehydration due to gastroenteritis

Severe dehydration due to diarrhoea and vomiting is the salient diagnostic feature of acute infectious diarrhoea of bacterial origin. As in the treatment of viral gastroenteritis, oral rehydration with a solution containing salts and glucose and intravenous fluid replacement have revolutionised the treatment of 'non-specific' diarrhoeal diseases of bacterial origin.

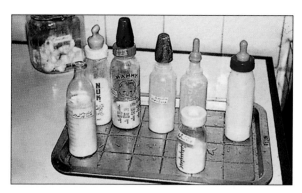

572 Sources of infantile infectious diarrhoea

Gastroenteritis due to a variety of bacteria, as well as to viruses (see **565** *and* **566**), is one of the major causes of childhood mortality in the tropics. The substitution of the milk bottle for breast feeding is increasing, rather than decreasing, the problem. Mismanagement of artificial feeding is a serious cause, due to contamination of feeds with pathogenic organisms.

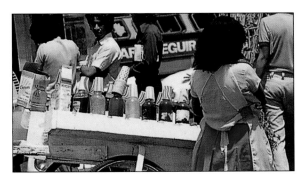

573 Origin of 'Turista'
Dirty food containers contaminated with pathogenic bacteria are another common cause of non-specific gastroenteritis (often called 'Turista'), especially in travellers.

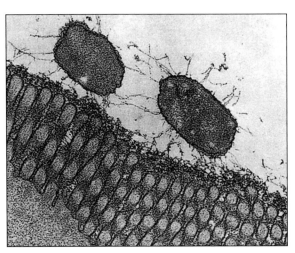

575 Enterotoxigenic *Escherichia coli*
These organisms are a major source of diarrhoea in the tropics and subtropics, accounting for about 15% of all cases; enteropathogenic *E. coli* causes about 2.5% of all cases. The bacteria are seen here adhering via pili to the brush border of human intestinal mucosa, which remains intact. (*EM* × *16 000.*)

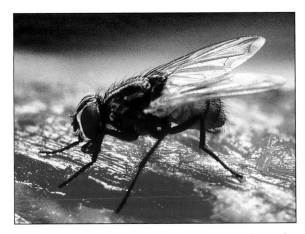

574 Female *Musca domestica*, the common housefly, feeding on raw meat
As with cockroaches, flies are indiscriminate feeders. The insects lower their mouthparts onto the food, which is sucked up directly if already liquid or semi-liquid. If settled on solid organic matter, the flies first cut off tiny pieces with their prestomal teeth then regurgitate saliva or their crop contents onto them before sucking the food up into the crop. This procedure provides adequate opportunity to contaminate food or drinks with previously ingested pathogens. (× *7.5.*)

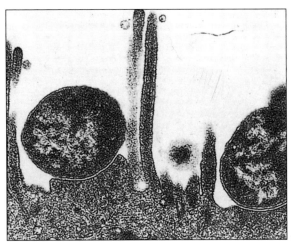

576 Enteropathogenic *Escherichia coli*
The bacteria are closely adherent to the microvilli, which undergo localised destruction. (*EM* × *16 000.*)

CHOLERA

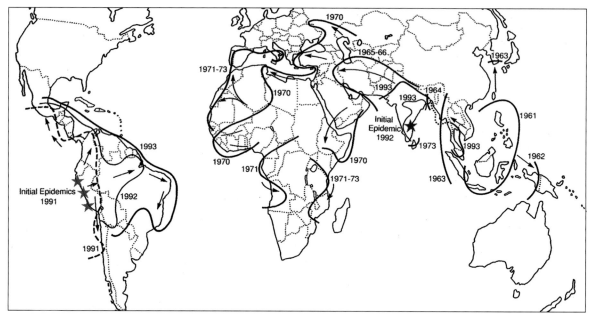

577 Pandemic spread of *Vibrio cholerae*

Cholera, which is one of the major causes of severe acute infective diarrhoea, is not restricted to the tropics or subtropics but occurs mainly in such areas because of its association with contaminated drinking water. *V. cholerae* exists in numerous serovars of which serovar 0:1 is the most important. This has been divided into two toxigenic biotypes of which the classic one (which carried a high mortality) occurred worldwide but has since all but disappeared in countries where clean water supplies became available. It was replaced in most areas from about 1960 onwards when the less virulent El Tor biotype appeared and spread in epidemic fashion. The map illustrates the progressive waves of the extension from its original focus in Indonesia in what has been called the 'seventh pandemic.' Between 1961 and 1990, cholera El Tor spread throughout Asia and Africa; the infection only reached the Americas in 1991 (*red stars*). An explosive epidemic commenced in early 1991 in Peru and spread rapidly across Latin America; within two years, over 73 000 cases with over 6300 deaths had occurred in 21 countries. The rapid spread of the recently discovered 0:139 serovar from its epicentre (*blue star*) to neighbouring countries of Southeast Asia in 1992 and 1993 is also indicated on this map.

578 An ancient epicentre of cholera

Mass assemblies of pilgrims for religious activities such as that seen here on the River Ganges are an important source of epidemic cholera, as well as other water-borne infections. Symptomless carriers, who may represent 75% of those infected with the El Tor serovar, are very important in the epidemiology of this disease as they may transport the organisms over long distances and from country to country. In October 1992, a hitherto unknown toxigenic serovar, now designated 0:139, was identified in epidemics of a cholera-like illness in Madras, India and in Bangladesh. This new organism which, unlike El Tor in that region, affected mainly adults, carried a high mortality. Within six months it had affected over 100 000 cases, among whom there were nearly 1500 deaths. This type of cholera, which spread rapidly in the Far East where it replaced El Tor (*see* **577**), was believed by some authorities to be the beginning of the 'eighth pandemic'; cases have been identified in international travellers as far away as England and the USA. The classic toxigenic 0:1

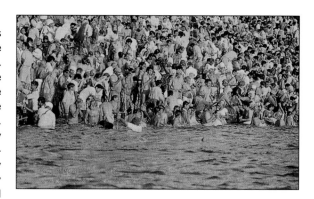

serovar of *Vibrio cholerae* is now limited to small areas in Bangladesh. Immunity to 0:1 strains does not protect against 0:139 which may, in a few individuals, invade the blood stream and give rise to bacteraemia. 0:139, which was the dominant cholera pathogen in the Calcutta area in 1992–93 and 1996–97, is now known to possess wide clonal diversity.

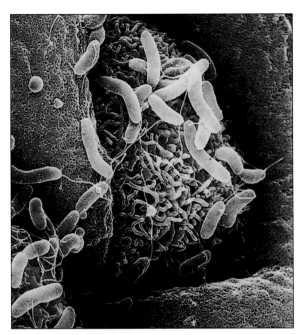

579 Cholera vibrios

Vibrios are very sensitive to an acid environment, and relatively few survive in individuals with normal gastric acidity. Stored cooked rice, milk and milk products with a high pH that become contaminated make excellent media for the multiplication of the organisms. Those vibrios that pass the stomach enter the small intestine and adhere to its luminal cells. This scanning electron micrograph shows *Vibrio cholerae* adhering to mucous cells of human ileum. The vibrios produce a mucinase that may help them to penetrate the mucus. ($\times$ *11 000*.)

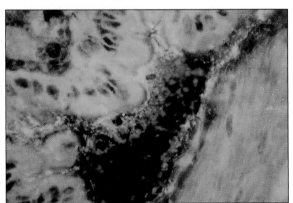

580 *Vibrio cholerae* in the jejunal lumen

The vibrios, stained green with a fluorescein-labelled antibody, can be seen here to lie entirely within the bowel lumen; they do not penetrate the intestinal mucosal cells. All pathogenic strains produce an enterotoxin that enters enterocytes via a surface receptor. Within the cells it accelerates the production of adenylcyclase, which leads to the overproduction of cyclic AMP. The accumulation of cAMP both inhibits the absorption and stimulates the excretion of sodium chloride, as well as the secretion of bicarbonate. The effect of this is to cause a massive loss of water and electrolytes—it is this that gives rise to the profuse, watery diarrhoea ($\times$ *300*.) (AFIP No. 75–3993.)

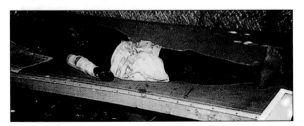

581 A 'cholera cot'

The disease is characterised by severe vomiting as well as the diarrhoea ('rice-water stools'). Ten per cent of the patient's body weight can be lost in a few hours. Nursing of patients in a 'cholera cot' facilitates their handling. A rapid assessment of the volume of fluid loss can be made by collecting the watery stools in a graduated bucket placed under the large central hole in the waterproof sheet on which the patient lies. This patient's severe dehydration necessitated intravenous fluid and electrolyte replacement as the first stage of treatment.

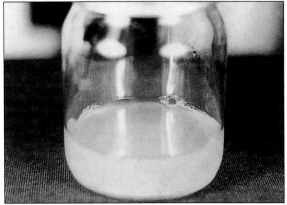

582 'Rice-water stool' of cholera

The fluid stool is free of blood and has an inoffensive, slightly fishy odour.

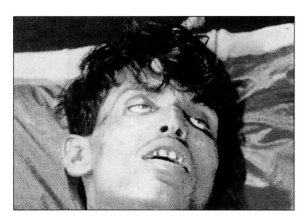

583 'Choleraic facies'

The massive fluid loss results in severe dehydration, which is the primary cause of death. Rapid rehydration with isotonic salts and glucose is life saving. This man shows the typical 'choleraic facies' with deeply sunken cheeks and eyes; he recovered completely with rehydration. Even for severely dehydrated patients, oral replacement therapy with simple salt–glucose solution may be adequate provided they are not vomiting.

584 Use of plastic water container in cholera control

The vast majority of cholera infections are acquired from faecally contaminated drinking water. This often occurs within households where open water containers are in use. The distribution of cheap, closed, plastic containers for boiled water, with a tap (such as that seen here being used by a girl in a rural Bolivian house), proved to be a major factor in limiting the spread of cholera in the recent epidemic in Latin America.

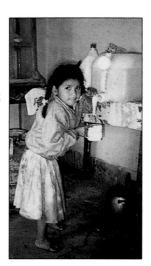

585 Seafood as a source of cholera infection

Raw or improperly cooked seafood (e.g. shellfish and crabs) has been incriminated as a source of infection with El Tor cholera. Infections arose in the USA in 1991 in individuals who ate crabs such as these that were imported by travellers from Ecuador. Endemic cholera is also known to exist in some coastal areas of North America, China and a few other countries, where the vibrios have been identified in brackish coastal waters. *Cyclops* water fleas have been shown to harbour the organisms, which produce a chitinase that may permit them to attach to the hosts. The water fleas are consumed by larger arthropods such as crabs and crayfish. These, and various molluscs such as oysters, may form part of the natural cycle of some strains of *Vibrio cholerae*, which could account in part for the transcontinental spread of the vibrios, probably in ships' ballast tanks.

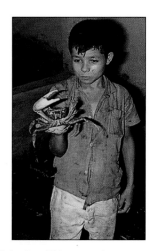

HELICOBACTER PYLORI

586 *Helicobacter pylori*

This microaerophilic, Gram-negative bacterium with a complex terminal flagellum occurs on the mucosa of the stomach and duodenum of up to 80% of adults living in developing countries, where the incidence increases with decreasing socioeconomic status and poor nutrition. The prevalence is much lower in the Western World. *H. pylori* is associated with peptic ulceration and is the probable cause of the high rate of gastric adenocarcinoma in developing countries. (× 11 000.)

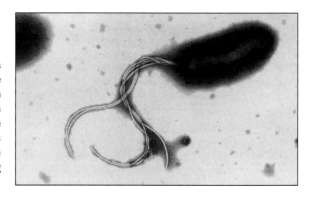

SHIGELLOSIS

587 Shigellosis affecting the sigmoid colon
Like *Vibrio cholerae*, the bacteria causing shigellosis produce an enterotoxin. Transmission is mainly faeco–oral and is associated with poor hygienic conditions. Not surprisingly, shigellosis is most prevalent in the poorer, developing countries. Four species are responsible for most human infection; *Shigella dysenteriae, S. flexneri, S. sonnei* and *S. boydii*. They affect initially the distal small intestine, causing painful cramps, fever and bloody diarrhoea. Once in the colon they multiply in the lamina propria and destroy the overlying mucosa. The figure shows a sigmoidoscopic view of colonic mucosa from a fatal case of *S. dysenteriae* infection.

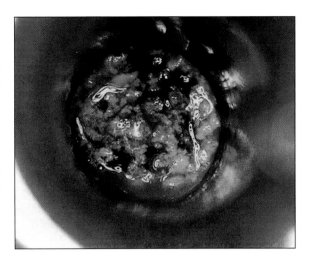

ENTERITIS NECROTICANS ('PIGBEL')

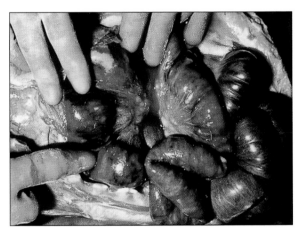

588 Enteritis necrotica seen at operation
'Pigbel' is a segmental disease of the intestine (usually the ileum), most commonly seen in the highlands of Papua New Guinea; it is caused by infection with a widely distributed soil organism, *Clostridium welchii* (= *C. perfringens*) type C. A carrier state clearly exists, as the organisms can be found in the faeces of 70% of highland villagers, although human to human transmission does not seem to occur. The infection is acquired by eating improperly cooked, infected pig meat, usually at ceremonial feasts, in an area where the diet is usually very low in protein (consisting mainly of baked sweet potatoes). Vaccination with *C. welchii* type C β toxoid gives protection lasting a few years.

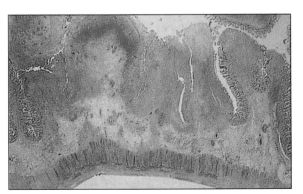

589 Necrosis of small intestine in 'Pigbel'
The main lesion is patchy necrosis of the small intestine, starting in the mucosa and extending through to the serosal wall, as seen here. Resection of the infected segment is indicated. (*H&E* × 150.)

BRUCELLOSIS

Goats, sheep, cows, pigs and camels are the common animal reservoirs of infection with *Brucella abortus, B. melitensis* and *B. suis.* Infection is commonly acquired by drinking unpasteurised milk or milk products. Brucellosis is an important cause of morbidity in the Middle East, especially for many desert-dwelling pastoralists.

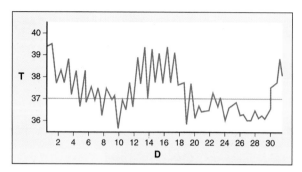

590 Temperature chart
Common initial symptoms of brucellosis are fever, which may be intermittent or undulant (as illustrated here). Moderate leucopenia with a relative lymphocytosis and hepatosplenomegaly are often encountered. In some areas, the fever is atypical. A persistent raised IgM is suggestive of brucellosis, but a high *Brucella*-agglutination titre or positive blood culture will confirm the diagnosis. [D—day of illness; T—temperature (°C).]

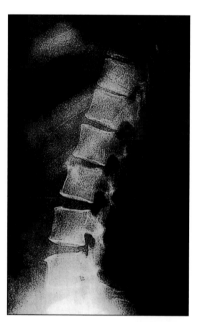

591 Radiograph of *Brucella* spondylitis
The earliest symptom of this condition is pain localised to the affected region of the spine (commonly the lumbar spine). Radiologically, narrowing of the disc spaces, erosion of the vertebral margins, collapse of the vertebrae and, characteristically, the development of proliferative changes with unison of osteophytes are seen. Although such arthritic changes are common manifestations of chronic brucellosis, the infection may also present protean neurological signs, sometimes suggestive of disseminated sclerosis. Acute meningoencephalitis with fatigue, demyelinating neuropathy and spastic paraplegia are usually forms of presentation of neurobrucellosis.

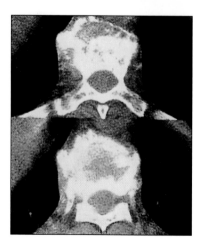

592 Computed tomogram of *Brucella* spondylitis
This CT scan illustrates typical degenerative changes in the vertebrae associated with spondylitis in a Kuwaiti patient with chronic brucellosis.

MELIOIDOSIS

593 Left upper pneumonia due to melioidosis

This disease, which occurs mainly in Southeast Asia and northern Australia, is due to infection with *Burkholderia* (formerly *Pseudomonas*) *pseudomallei* (Whitmore's bacillus). Diabetes mellitus and chronic renal disease are common predisposing factors. The route of infection is uncertain, but it may be water borne or air borne, or may be acquired by contamination of wounds with soil. Inapparent infections are probably widespread as surveys, for example in Thailand, have shown that 30–50% of those examined have been seropositive but asymptomatic. The disease may present as acute septicaemia followed by multiple organ abscess formation, or may be subacute from the start. Septicaemic melioidosis carries a 40% mortality rate. Chronic infections in children may present as a parotid abscess. This is the radiograph of a Thai patient showing consolidation and cavitation of the left upper zone. The diagnosis is indicated by a positive haemaglutination test or IgG-based enzyme-linked

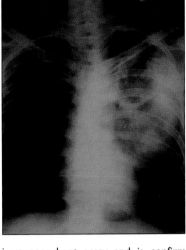

immunosorbent assay and is confirmed by culturing the organism from different body fluids on a selective medium such as Ashdown's.

594 Parotid abscess caused by *Burkholderia pseudomallei*

The parotid gland is a common site for localised melioidosis in children, with other common sites being the skin and soft tissues, liver, spleen and lymph nodes. This Thai boy shows a suppurating left parotid abscess. (© D. A. Warrell.)

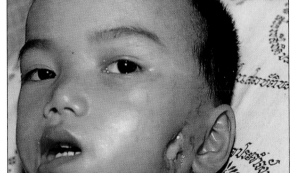

LEPTOSPIROSIS
(See **Table 4**.)

595 *Leptospira interrogans*

Leptospirosis is a zoonotic infection with one of a variety of organisms of the *Leptospira interrogans* species complex. The spirochaetes are readily seen in silver-stained preparations, especially with a phase contrast microscope. The disease is usually acquired from either contact with infected animals or, more commonly, from water contaminated with animal urine. The commonest source of human infection is from rats or mice (serotype *L. icterohaemorrhagiae*), and occasionally from dogs (serotype *L. canicola*). The disease is global in distribution but more common in tropical areas. (× 1050.)

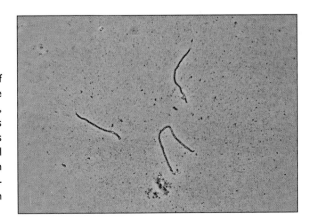

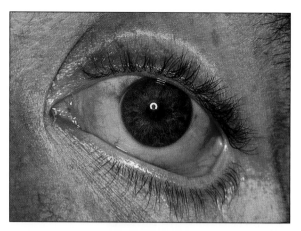

596 Subconjunctival haemorrhages in leptospirosis
The infection can follow one of three courses. Asymptomatic or atypical infection occurs in probably 90% of cases and, in some tropical areas, leptospirosis may account for up to 15% of all patients with undiagnosed pyrexia. Although this form can be mild, the infection may develop into a generalised septic form within one to two weeks. This is characterised by fever, myalgia and often subconjunctical haemorrhages. The photograph shown here was of a patient in the second week following the onset of symptoms. The most dangerous form due to *L. icterohaemorrhagiae* (Weil's disease) may be very severe and can involve several organs, with jaundice, renal failure, haemorrhage and vascular collapse.

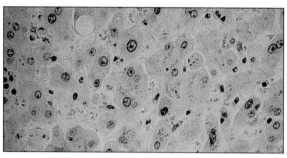

597 Hepatic changes in leptospirosis
In severe cases—even where hepatic dysfunction and jaundice are present—hepatocellular necrosis is unusual, but large amounts of bilirubin can be seen in the hepatocytes. After specific chemotherapy, the liver function usually returns to normal. (*H&E × 200.*)

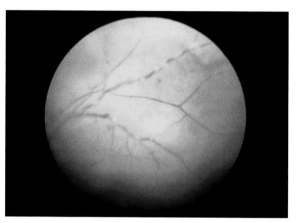

598 Uveitis in leptospirosis
During the recovery phase of leptospirosis, iridocyclitis or uveitis (as seen here) may be associated with the immunological response, often several weeks or months after the initial infection. This photograph of the fundus was taken three months after the patient developed acute, systemic leptospirosis.

PROTOZOAL INFECTIONS

(*See* **Table 17.**)

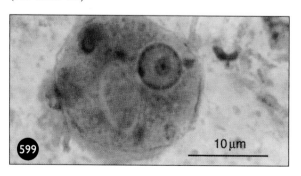

10 µm

599

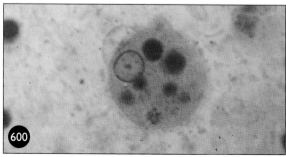

600

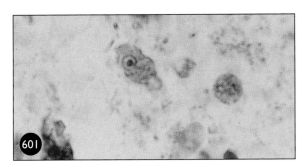

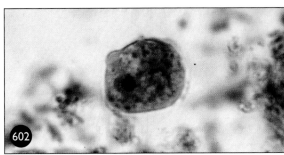

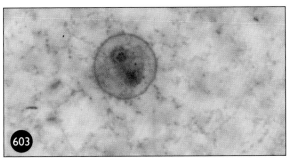

599–603 Trophozoites of intestinal protozoa
Entamoeba coli (**599**), *E. histolytica* or *E. dispar* (**600**),
Endolimax nana (**601**), *Iodamoeba bütschlii* (**602**),
Dientamoeba fragilis (**603**). *E. histolytica* cannot be distin-
guished morphologically from *E. dispar*. (**599 *and* 600**
trichrome stain; **601–603** *haematoxylin*). (× *1500*.)

Table 17 Protozoa (phyla Ciliophora and Sarcomastigophora, subphylum Sarcodina) of medical importance

Phylum	Subphylum etc.	Order	Genus and species
APICOMPLEXA (see **Table 5**)			
CILIOPHORA	RHABDOPHORA	Vestibuliferida	*Balantidium coli*
SARCOMASTIGOPHORA	MASTIGOPHORA (see **Tables 7, 8, 9** and **18** SARCODINA Superclass RHIZOPODEA		
		Amoebida	*Entamoeba coli*
			E. histolytica[1]
			E. dispar[1]
			E. gingivalis
			Endolimax nana
			Iodamoeba bütschlii
			Acanthamoeba culbertsoni[2]
			A. polyphaga[2]
			A. castellani[2]
			A. hatchetti[2]
			Blastocystis hominis[3]
		Schizopyrenida	*Naegleria fowleri*[2]
		Leptomyxida	*Balamuthia mandrillaris*[2]

[1] *E. histolytica* causing human amoebiasis, is clearly distinguishable by isoenzyme and genomic characters from *E. dispar*, which is non-pathogenic in humans.
[2] Pathogenic 'free-living' species. The other amoebae are obligatory parasites.
[3] This anaerobic, gut-dwelling protozoan has recently been ascribed to the order Amoebida.

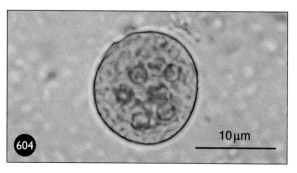

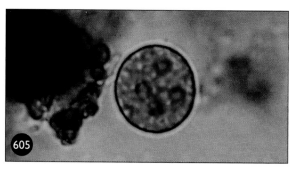

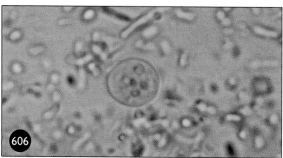

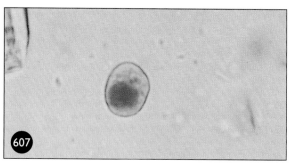

604–607 Cysts of intestinal protozoa
Entamoeba coli (**604**), *E. histolytica* or *E. dispar* (**605**), *E. nana* (**606**), *Iodamoeba bütschlii* (**607**). *E. histolytica* cannot be distinguished morphologically from *E. dispar.* (*Iodine* × 1500.)

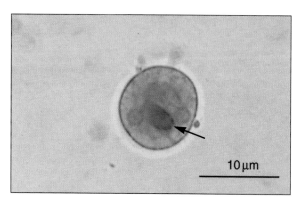

608 Chromatoid bodies in *Entamoeba histolytica* and *E. dispar*
These characteristic structures (arrow) are readily demonstrated with Sargeaunt's stain. (× 1500.)

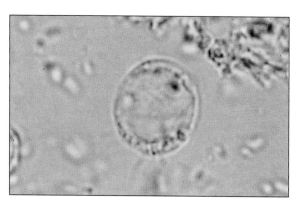

609 *Blastocystis hominis*
This common faecal organism, which was formerly believed to be a commensal fungus, has recently been shown to be an anaerobic protist, one of a very heterogeneous group of organisms that includes such widely divergent organisms as brown algae (kelp) and diatoms. Molecular and immunological analysis suggests that several species may be present in the human gut. *B. hominis* may be associated with acute enteritis in some immunocompromised individuals. (*Iodine* × 1500.)

AMOEBIASIS

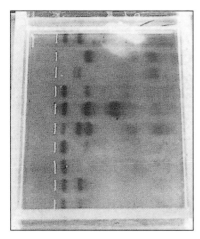

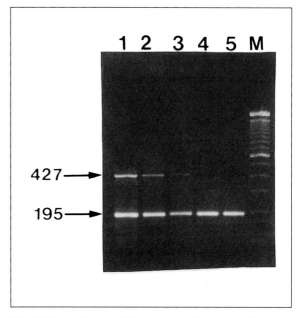

610 '*Entamoeba histolytica*' zymodemes

Amoebiasis caused by invasive *E. histolytica* is acquired from the ingestion of infective cysts in food or drinks contaminated by faeces (often from food handlers), or possibly transported by insects such as flies and cockroaches. By enzyme electrophoresis, a number of zymodemes of this parasite were distinguished in trophozoites cultured from cysts in human faeces. Only a few zymodemes were found to be associated with pathogenicity, the remainder seeming to be harmless commensals. DNA characterisation and other research has confirmed that there are two genetically distinct, but morphologically indistinguishable, species: *E. histolytica*, which is pathogenic but varies in its virulence, and *E. dispar*, which is non-pathogenic. A recently developed enzyme-linked immunosorbent assay based on *E. histolytica*-specific monoclonal antibodies now permits the two parasites to be distinguished in faecal or other specimens.

611 Differentiation of *Entamoeba histolytica* from *E. dispar* by polymerase chain reaction

The most sensitive method for the identification of these parasites in faeces is the polymerase chain reaction. In this figure the band at 195 base pairs in lanes 1 to 5 shows the presence of 1000 trophozoites of *E. dispar* that were seeded into a 50 mg sample of faeces. The band at 427 base pairs in lanes 1 to 5 was produced by 1250, 250, 50, 10 and 2 trophozoites of *E. histolytica* added to aliquots of the faecal sample. Lane M indicates the molecular weight standards.

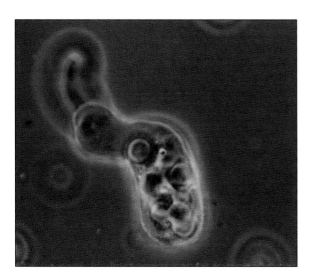

612 Living *Entamoeba histolytica*

Relatively rapidly moving trophozoites of *E. histolytica* containing ingested erythrocytes may be found in a freshly passed specimen. They are clear evidence of infection with a true *E. histolytica* unlike the presence of cysts alone. (*E. dispar*, unlike *E. histolytica*, does not ingest red cells or invade the intestinal tissue). In amoebic dysentery the stool is loose, containing mucus and blood mixed with faecal material. This is distinct from bacterial dysentery in which there is a cellular exudate. The commonest sites for localisation of *E. histolytica* in the intestine are the caecum and descending colon. Secondary sites, which are reached by haematogenous invasion or direct spread, are the liver, brain, lung and skin. (*Phase contrast* × *1200*.)

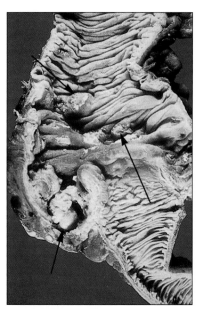

613 Postoperative specimen of the terminal ileum and caecum in a patient with perforation due to amoebiasis
The figure shows numerous distinct ulcers (*arrowed*) in a patient who developed an acute abdomen requiring surgery after returning from India with an acute diarrheoal illness. Stool microscopy was negative for amoebae but histology demonstrated the characteristic, erythrocyte-ingesting trophozoites of *Entamoeba histolytica*. In fulminating infections, the destruction of all layers of the intestinal wall is extensive and ulcerations may be confluent. Such lesions are often seen in pregnancy and the puerperium.

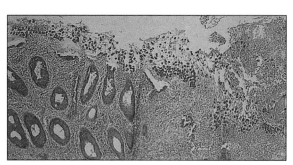

614 Amoebic typhlitis
Computed tomography of the lower abdomen in a patient presenting with abdominal pain and diarrhoea showed massive oedema of the ascending colon after the patient returned from a holiday in Thailand. A rectal swab showed the presence of the characteristic trophozoite forms of *Entamoeba histolytica*. The patient was managed conservatively with parenteral metronidazole and recovered well.

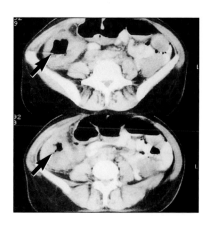

615 Section of colon wall as seen in a biopsy specimen
Typical 'flask-shaped' ulcers are seen in the intestinal wall, which is invaded by *Entamoeba histolytica* trophozoites. The intervening mucosa is usually normal. In this low-power view, large numbers of trophozoites can be seen both on the surface of, and invading, the mucosa. (*PAS × 30.*)

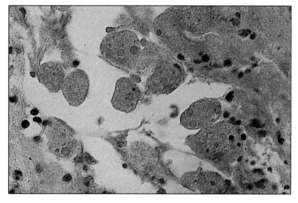

616 *Entamoeba histolytica* in mucosa of the colon
Numerous trophozoites with ingested erythrocytes are visible in this high-power view. (*PAS × 180.*)

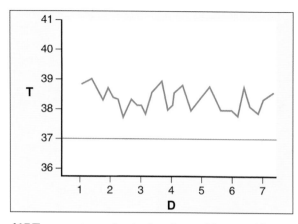

617 Temperature chart of patient with amoebic liver abscess
The triad of swinging temperature, profuse sweats and neutrophil leucocytosis is indicative of liver abscess, especially when associated with pain in the right hypochondrium and a raised hemidiaphragm. [D—day of illness; T—temperature (°C).]

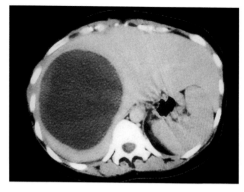

619 Amoebic liver abscess
An amoebic abscess of the liver is usually single and the volume of the contents of the lesion can vary from 500 to 1500 ml. The diagnosis is greatly facilitated by visualisation of the abscess on a computed tomogram. A massive abscess is seen here in the right lobe of the liver. Such lesions are usually associated with pain in the right upper quadrant and fever.

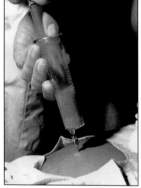

620 Aspiration of liver abscess
Aspiration of large abscesses is sometimes needed as an adjunct to specific chemotherapy for successful treatment, especially when the abscess is very large or close to the surface of the liver with the risk of rupture. The pus is said to be 'chocolate-coloured'; some have likened it to 'anchovy sauce.'

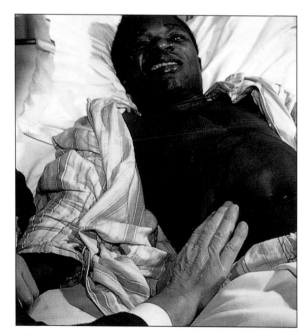

618 African patient with amoebic liver abscess
Palpation of the right hypochondrium in this patient with an enlarged, tender liver, has obviously elicited severe pain, as reflected in his face.

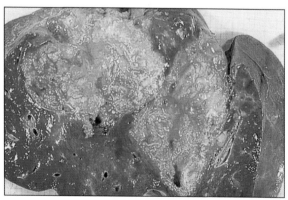

621 Macroscopic appearance of liver abscess at post mortem examination
The shaggy, irregular periphery consists of stroma and layers of compressed liver parenchyma.

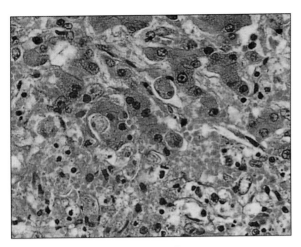

622 Section of amoebic liver abscess
Trophozoites, some containing ingested red blood cells, are seen in the tissues at the edge of the abscess and may be found in the pus if it is examined immediately after aspiration. (*H&E × 150.*)

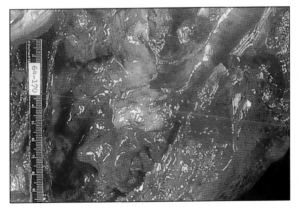

623 Amoebic abscess of lung
Extraintestinal infections occur commonly in the liver, but any site of the body may be affected. The lung and the pericardium are sometimes affected by rupture of a hepatic abscess through the diaphragm. Typical amoebic pus may be coughed up in the sputum.

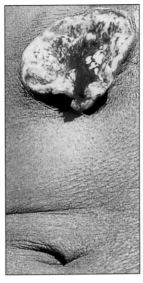

624 Amoebiasis of the skin
Amoebic infection of the skin may arise by direct spread from a primary abscess. This patient was erroneously operated on for a perforated duodenal ulcer and no antiamoebic drugs were given. Sloughing of the skin occurred and amoebae were recovered from the skin lesion.

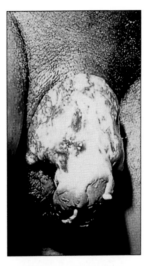

625 Amoebic balanitis
Amoebic infection of the genital organs can result from sexual intercourse. Although cysts are exceptionally common in homosexual males, the majority are attributable to non-pathogenic *Entamoeba dispar.*

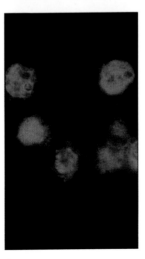

626 Fluorescent antibody staining of *Entamoeba histolytica*
The fluorescent antibody test, which is the most sensitive immunodiagnostic test available for invasive forms of amoebiasis, has proved a valuable adjunct to direct microscopical diagnosis. Fluorescence of cultured *E. histolytica* exposed to serum from a patient with hepatic involvement is seen in this figure. (× *780.*)

GIARDIASIS

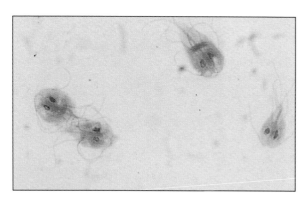 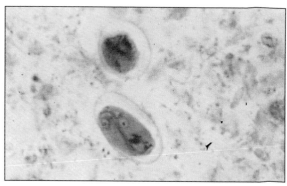

627 & 628 *Giardia lamblia* trophozoites and cysts
Giardiasis is probably the commonest, globally distributed, water-borne protozoal infection. It has been estimated, for example, that two million new infections may be acquired in the USA each year from contaminated water. The flagellated trophozoites (**627**, left) attach by their suckers to the surface of the duodenal or jejunal mucosa. The ovoid cysts in faeces (**628**, right) have a very distinctive structure. They are able to survive standard chlorination procedures, and filtration is required to ensure their exclusion from the drinking water supply. (**627** *Giemsa* × *1000*; **628** *trichrome* × *1230*.)

Table 18 The protozoa (class Zoomastigophorea) of medical importance

Phylum/Subphylum	Class	Order	Genus and species
SARCOMASTIGOPHORA *SARCODINA* (see **Table 17**)			
MASTIGOPHORA	ZOOMASTIGOPHOREA (no vector)		
		Retortamonadida Diplomonadida Trichomonadida	*Chilomastix mesnili* *Giardia lamblia* *Trichomonas vaginalis* *T. hominis* *Dientamoeba fragilis*[1]
	(invertebrate vector)	Kinetoplastida	*Leishmania* spp. (see **Tables 8** and **9**) *Trypanosoma* spp. (see **Table 7**)

[1]This parasite is now considered to be a flagellate and not an amoeba.

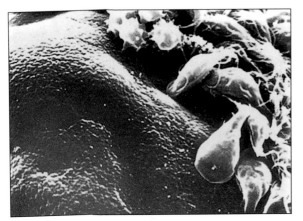

629 Scanning electron micrograph of *Giardia lamblia* in jejunal biopsy

The trophozoites are attached to the surface of the jejunal epithelium by sucker-like organelles, which leave pit marks when they detach. Their ability to produce at least 12 variable surface proteins assists the trophozoites to evade host antibodies. Infection may therefore become chronic. (× 1000.)

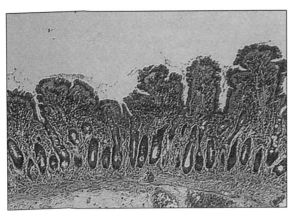

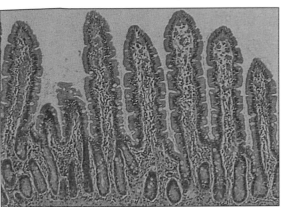

630 & 631 Jejunal epithelium

Severe infection with *Giardia lamblia* can result in partial villous atrophy of the duodenum or jejunum, with resulting flattening of the villi (**630**, top) compared with the normal pattern (**631**, bottom). Although the organism is commensal in many individuals, it is considered particularly pathogenic in children in the New World and is a common cause of diarrhoea and a malabsorption syndrome characterised by steatorrhoea in travellers. Although in severe infections the trophozoites or cysts can usually be found in the faeces, they may be very sparse in chronic infections. The trophozoites can sometimes be obtained via a duodenal aspirate, but serological methods have also been developed. An enzyme-linked immunosorbent assay (ELISA) to detect IgM in serum provides evidence of current infection. A polyclonal antigen-capture ELISA can be used to demonstrate submicroscopic infections in faeces, and an IgA-based ELISA will detect specific antibodies in saliva. (*H&E* × *40*.)

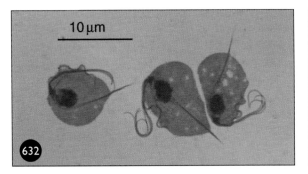

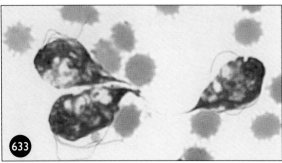

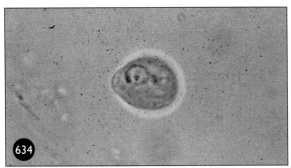

632–634 Other parasitic flagellates
Trichomonas vaginalis trophozoite as seen in culture (**632**) (see also **822**), *Chilomastix mesnili* trophozoite (**633**) and cyst (**634**). *C. mesnili* is non-pathogenic. (Trophozoites *Giemsa*, cyst *eosin* × 1800.)

COCCIDIAL INFECTIONS
(See **Table 5**.)

Most of the coccidial infections in humans are zoonoses. In immunocompetent individuals they usually produce mild, self-limiting infection. However, toxoplasmosis in pregnancy poses a serious danger for the foetus, whereas most, if not all, of the parasites are able to cause serious pathological changes in immunocompromised people—notably those with HIV infection of whom, for example, as many as 10% may pass oocysts of *Cryptosporidium parvum* (see **641–643**).

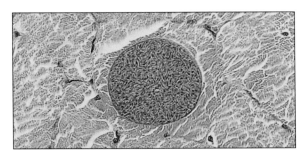

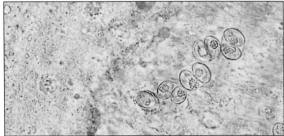

635 Section of sarcocyst in human muscle
In the muscles of the intermediate host, *Sarcocystis* forms fusiform cysts containing large numbers of bradyzoites. Although it is rarely diagnosed in life, this condition may be common in humans, who harbour the sarcocysts of a number of different species, none of which has so far been identified. '*Sarcocystis lindemanni*' is no longer considered to be a valid species but is thought to represent accidental zoonotic infection with a variety of species of this genus. (*H&E* × 375.)

636 *Sarcocystis hominis*-like oocysts in intestinal epithelium
This coccidian parasite is common in humans and is acquired from the consumption of raw or inadequately cooked beef in which the sarcocyst stage occurs. In this case, humans are the definitive host. Sporulated oocysts or single sporocysts are passed in the faeces. *S. suihominis* is acquired from pork. (*Phase contrast* × 400.)

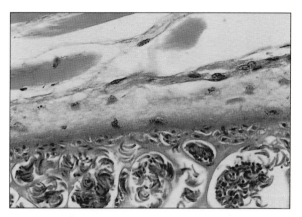

637 Sarcocystis hominis
The individual bradyzoites are seen within a large, fusiform sarcocyst in bovine muscle. (*H&E × 400.*)

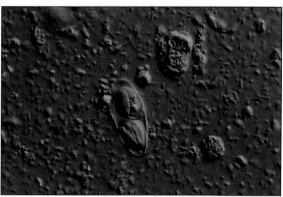

638 *Isospora belli* oocysts
Unsporulated oocysts of this species are passed in the faeces, but they sporulate on storage to form eight sporozoites (of which five can be seen in this figure). The infection may be associated with diarrhoea, due to development of the parasite in the intestinal epithelium, or may be symptomless. Coccidian oocysts stain dark red with a modified Ziehl–Neelsen stain. (*Nomarksi optics × 450.*)

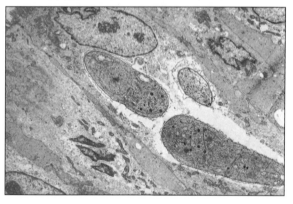

639 *Isospora belli* in a mucosal cell of the ileum of a patient with AIDS
The intracellular position of an immature oocyst containing sections of three sporozoites is clearly seen in this electron microscope image. In such immunocompromised individuals extraintestinal tissue cysts may also be located in lymphatic tissues such as those in liver, spleen and lymph nodes. (× 2200.)

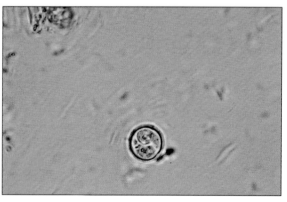

640 Sporulated oocyst of *Cyclospora cayetanensis*
This eimeriid parasite, which was first described in Peru in children with mild diarrhoea, has now been identified in countries as disparate as Mexico and the USA, the UK, Haiti, Nepal and Australia. Schizogony occurs within epithelial cells of the small intestine. When allowed to sporulate, for example in dichromate solution at 25–30°C for one or two weeks, *C. cayetanensis* produces two sporocysts, each with two sporozoites. Mixed infections with *Cryptosporidium* are common, and the two infections were formerly confused, especially because both may be associated with mild but chronic diarrhoea. Both are probably acquired from oocyst-contaminated water. A zoonotic reservoir of *C. cayetanensis* has not yet been identified. (*Saline × 900.*)

641 Oocysts of *Cryptosporidium parvum* and *C. cayetanensis* compared

C. parvum is enzootic in young calves. It is usually passed to humans in water containing oocysts, which survive normal chlorination and filtration. It causes outbreaks of self-limiting, mild diarrhoea in infants and small children (e.g. in day-care centres), but can also affect older people. Surveys have demonstrated a high level of seropositivity in normal, asymptomatic adults—over 50% in one outbreak. In 1993 over 400 000 people had diarrhoea when lake water near Milwaukee became contaminated after heavy rains. The use of the Ziehl–Neelsen stain on faecal smears or concentrates (made by sugar flotation) is a valuable technique both to detect the oocysts and particularly to reveal the existence of mixed infections. Both parasites stain red with Ziehl–Neelsen stain. However, *C. cayetanensis* typically takes up variable amounts of the stain and the oocysts are larger (8–10 μm, compared with 4–6 μm). The irregular staining

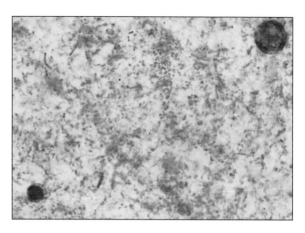

helps to distinguish *C. cayetanensis* from the same-sized oocysts of *Toxoplasma gondii*, which are, of course, not found in human faeces (*Ziehl–Neelsen × 850*.)

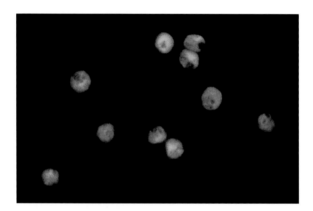

642 Auramine stain for oocysts of *Cryptosporidium parvum*

Fluorescent staining of oocysts with auramine is a useful technique for detecting these tiny objects in faecal or other specimens. They can be detected in about 5% of young children with diarrhoea but do not persist if the child is immunologically normal. (× 670.)

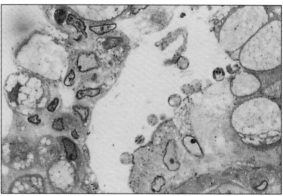

643 *Cryptosporidium parvum* on the surface of human jejunum

The presence of *C. parvum* on the surface of intestinal mucosa causes mild diarrhoea in normal subjects but in immunocompromised individuals can give rise to profuse and intractable, chronic diarrhoea. (*H&E × 750*.)

644 Differentiation of genotypes of *Cryptosporidium parvum* by polymerase chain reaction (PCR)

Genotyping by the PCR-restriction fragment linked poly-morphism (RFLP) technique of isolates from human and animal faeces has revealed at least eight genotypes. Genotype 1, which has only been found in humans, was responsible for a third of a sample of over 1400 faecal samples in the UK in 1998 and 1999. Two thirds were of genotype 2, which is found in a broad host range, whereas rare infections were caused by genotype 3. In this figure the *TRAP-C2* gene has been amplified followed by RFLP analysis using two restriction enzymes, *Hae*III (lanes 1–5) and *Bst*E II (lanes 7–11). Distinct gel banding patterns are seen for human (lanes 1, 2, 7 and 8) and bovine isolates (lanes 3–5 and 9–11). Nine other species of *Cryptosporidium* have been

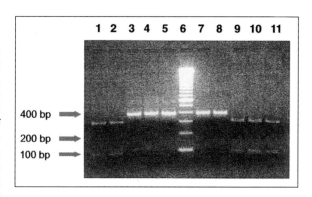

described, including parasites of other mammals, marsupials, birds, reptiles and fish.

Toxoplasmosis

645 Life cycle of *Toxoplasma gondii*

T. gondii has a very wide range of mammalian hosts, but the most important definitive host from the human point of view is the domestic cat (1). Within epithelial cells of the small intestine the organisms undergo a cycle of sexual reproduction that terminates in the production of oocysts (2), which are passed in the faeces and are remarkably resis-tant to environmental damage. Oocysts that enter the gut of wild rodents (3) form sporozoites that develop into cystic forms that eventually produce cysts (4) in the brain and other organs containing bradyzoites. When an infected rodent is consumed by a feline, the bradyzoites initiate a further cycle of sexual reproduction in that host. Humans and other mammals (including the cat) can become infected by direct intake of oocysts. Within the new host, a similar cycle of development occurs as in the rodent. Bradyzoites enter mononuclear cells (7) in which they rapidly undergo asexual schizogony to form pseudocysts containing tachy-zoites (8). These, in turn, further reproduce to form cysts (4), which contain numerous 'resting' stages—the brady-zoites. The cysts occur in all tissues, but are commonest in muscle and neural tissue, including the brain and eye. The commonest route of human infection is the consumption of bradyzoites from raw or undercooked, contaminated meat of domestic animals (5) or milk. Primary infection in humans (6), which may be associated with a mild, self-limiting, influenza-like fever, is extremely common, and positive serol-ogy may reach over 80% in many communities. The major

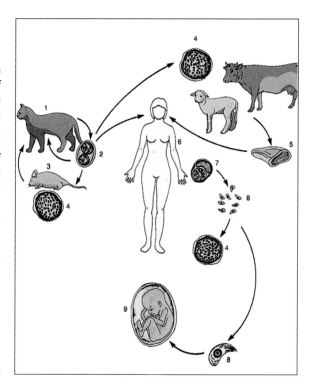

danger is infection acquired during early pregnancy, when tachyzoites (8) passing through the placental barrier to the foetus (9) may lead to heavy infection, giving rise to prema-ture abortion or severe congenital abnormalities.

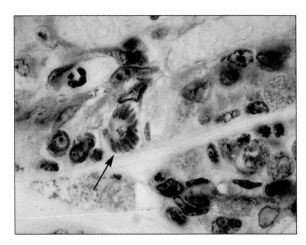

646 *Toxoplasma gondii* **schizont in epithelial gut cell of a cat**

Within 3–10 days of the consumption of cysts containing bradyzoites, an initial stage of schizogony (arrow) takes place in the epithelial cells of the small intestine, following which gametocytes are produced. These form oocysts, which are released into the lumen of the gut and passed with the faeces. (*Giemsa* × 900.)

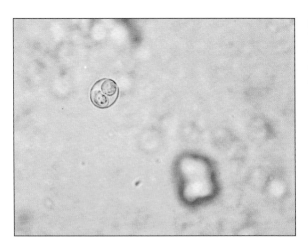

647 Sporulated oocysts of *Toxoplasma gondii*

The tiny oocysts (10 μm in diameter) are passed unsporulated. On maturation in the intestine of the normal intermediate host, the mouse, they produce two sporocysts, in each of which develop four sporozoites. (*Phase contrast* × 590.)

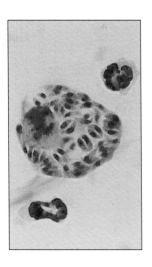

648 Tachyzoites of *Toxoplasma gondii* in a leucocyte

Asexual and sexual reproduction occur in the epithelium of the cat's intestine. In non-feline hosts, including humans, acute infection may result from ingestion of any stage, with the formation of tachyzoites which enter extraintestinal tissues such as lymph nodes. (*Giemsa* × 900.)

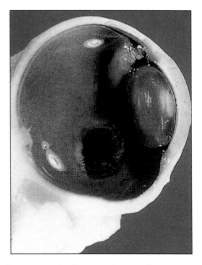

649 Eye in congenital toxoplasmosis

Acute toxoplasmosis in pregnancy seriously endangers the foetus. Transplacental infection, especially in the fourth month of pregnancy, produces congenital toxoplasmosis, which may result in abortion of a dead foetus or serious foetal lesions. The eye is a common target organ. This figure shows severe degeneration of the eye of a one-year-old child who died from congenital toxoplasmosis.

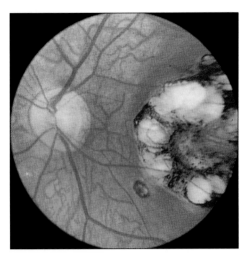

650 Fundal changes in congenital toxoplasmosis
Congenital toxoplasmosis may also produce choroidoretinitis in later years. A necrotising macular lesion with ectopic choroidal pigmentation is seen here. Defective vision and squint may result, or even blindness.

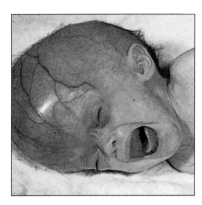

652 Hydrocephalus in congenital toxoplasmosis
Severe hydrocephalus, such as that seen in this infant, may result from congenital toxoplasmosis. The infection typically produces calcification of the subependymal tissues and sometimes dilation of the ventricles due to rapid proliferation of the parasites. There is usually serious cerebral damage in such cases.

651 Histology of lymph glands
Acute infection of older individuals may be cryptic or it may produce a prolonged low fever with lymphadenopathy. Lymph node biopsy shows follicular hyperplasia, with active germinal centres containing large, pale histiocytes. These contain ingested plasma cells, not parasites, but

Toxoplasma gondii may be isolated from such biopsy specimens by inoculation into mice. (*H&E × 20.*)

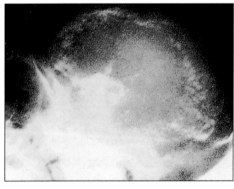

653 Brain radiograph in toxoplasmosis
Calcification is seen in the ventricles and subependymal tissues in this radiograph.

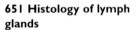

654 Appearance of brain at post mortem examination
Irregular areas of calcification in the lateral ventricles are seen in this brain of a seven-week-old child with toxoplasmosis. Mental disorders and blindness are common in children who survive. (*See also* **649** *and* **650**.)

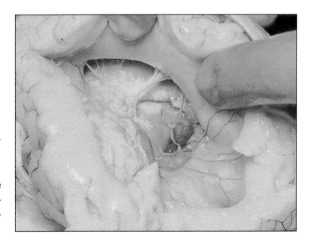

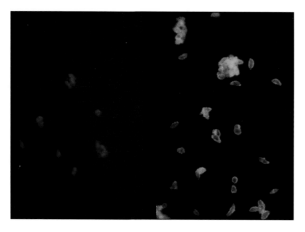

655 Serological tests for toxoplasmosis
(Negative control—left; positive—right). The Sabin Feldman dye test was formerly widely employed. Methylene blue stains *Toxoplasma gondii* tachyzoites obtained from mouse peritoneal exudate but, in the presence of antibody-containing serum, the uptake of dye is inhibited by 50% or more. High titres occur in acute infections, but a low positive titre remains indefinitely (*see comment in* **645**). Other useful serological tests are the complement-fixation test, direct agglutination test and toxoplasmin skin test. The most direct test is the indirect fluorescent antibody test shown here, in which antigen consists of cultured tachyzoites.

MICROSPORIDIOSIS

The medical importance of microsporidial infections in humans has only recently been highlighted by the frequent recognition of these parasites in material from patients with HIV infection and AIDS (see **Table 19**).

Table 19 Microsporidiosis in humans[1]

Genus and species	Sites	Geographical distribution	Notes
Pleistophora spp.	striated muscle	USA	two cases, immunocompromised ♂ ♂, one HIV+, one HIV–
Encephalitozoon cuniculi	brain, kidney, liver,	? global	very rare, four cases HIV– or HIV+
Encephalitozoon hellem	systemic spread to nose, eye, lung, kidney, etc.	? global	may be transmitted via sputum, urine, nasal aerosol; known only from HIV+ patients
Enterocytozoon bieneusi	small and large intestine, gall bladder, bile duct, lung, nasal epithelium	global	found in 6–30% of all AIDS patients with chronic diarrhoea; one case HIV–
Nosema corneum	eye		single case, HIV–
Nosema ocularum	eye		single case, HIV–
Nosema connori	striated and smooth muscle, generalised	USA	single, immunodeficient (athymic) infant
Septata intestinalis	small and large intestine, kidney, liver, gall bladder, bronchial epithelium, systemic spread	global	found in about 2% of all AIDS patients with chronic diarrhoea
'*Microsporidium africanum*'	eye	Botswana	single case, adult ♀
'*Microsporidium ceylonensis*'	eye	Sri Lanka	single case, 11-year-old ♂

[1]The classification of some species is still disputed.

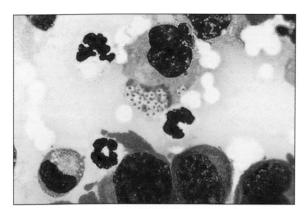

656 Microsporidia in a plasmacytoma cell
A clump of spores, probably of a species of *Encephalitozoon*, is seen in the cytoplasm of a macrophage in this bone marrow smear from a patient with a plasmacytoma. This is a rare case of microsporidiosis being detected in an immuno-compromised, but HIV-negative patient. (*Giemsa* × 1800.)

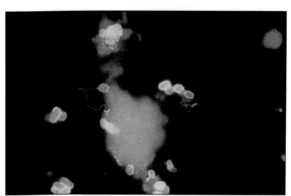

657 *Encephalitozoon hellem* **in cell culture**
This parasite produces a disseminated infection in immuno-compromised patients. *E. hellem* causes severe keratocon-junctivitis and has also been found in the urine in patients with signs of urinary tract disease. Spores have been identi-fied, moreover, in sputum, nasal swabs and faeces. Some of the spores seen here in tissue culture and stained with a specific antibody have extruded their polar filaments (*IFAT* × 2000). (*See also* **799**.)

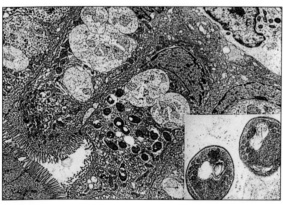

658 Mature spores of *Enterocytozoon bieneusi* **in human jejunal enterocyte**
Previously considered to be non-pathogenic in humans, infections are now being detected (particularly by biopsy) in individuals with chronic enteritis, cholangitis and cholecysti-tis who are immunocompromised, especially by AIDS (*see also* **800**). Their possible pathogenic role has, however, not yet been determined. Microsporidia are also suspected as a cause of ill-defined neurological manifestations. Note that the coils of the spiral filament of the spores seen in this biopsy lie in two rows in cross section. The parasite devel-ops in direct contact with the cytoplasm of the host's cell. (*Main section* × 2800; *inset* × 14 000.)

659 Mature spores of *Septata intestinalis*
This microsporidian is associated with nephritis and can also produce a similar clinical picture to that seen with *E. bieneusi*. Like that parasite, *S. intestinalis* develops in small intestinal enterocytes, but within a type of parasitophorous vacuole. The cross section of a spore shows the coils of spiral filament lying in a single row. (*Main section* × 2800; *inset* × 14 000.)

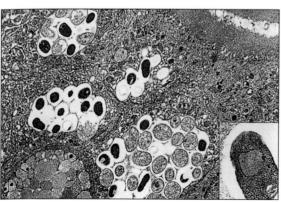

BALANTIDIASIS

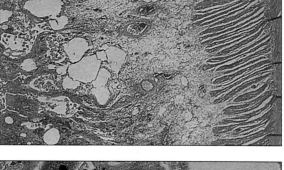

660 Balantidial ileitis

Balantidium coli is a common commensal of the large intestine of wild and domestic pigs but is pathogenic to humans and other primates, in which it causes severe diarrhoea. Active flagellated trophozoites and cysts are readily found in fresh faecal specimens. Numerous trophozoites are seen invading the submucosa in this section of human ileum. (*H&E × 10.*)

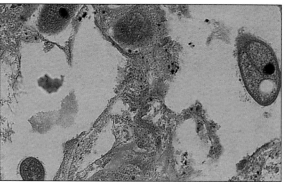

661 Trophozoites of *Balantidium coli*

Extensive ulceration of the ileum, colon and rectum may occur in severe cases. The characteristic morphology of *B. coli* trophozoites with their macronuclei and micronuclei is seen in this section. (*H&E × 160.*)

HELMINTHIASES—NEMATODES

(See **Table 11** for classification and **369–383** for eggs.)

TRICHINOSIS

662 Life cycle of *Trichinella spiralis*

This nematode is a zoonotic infection that circulates between rats (1) and various carnivores. Trichinosis in humans commonly results from eating raw or inadequately cooked pork or pork products such as sausages. Domestic pigs (2) and wild boar usually acquire the infection by eating infected rats (1). Cycles of infection also exist in wild Canidae and other carnivores that eat rodents. Infection is acquired by eating muscle (3) containing the encysted larvae (4). These excyst in the small intestine and develop into minute adults (5) in the mucosa. About five days after infection, the females, now mature, deposit larvae, which migrate through the tissues to reach skeletal muscles in which they again encyst. Larviposition may continue for a week or more. Finally the larvae become calcified. Three other species (or subspecies) that can infect humans have been described in this genus: *T. nelsoni* in parts of Africa and southern Europe, *T. nativa* in the Arctic region and *T. pseudospiralis*, which is now known to be widely distributed. In 1999

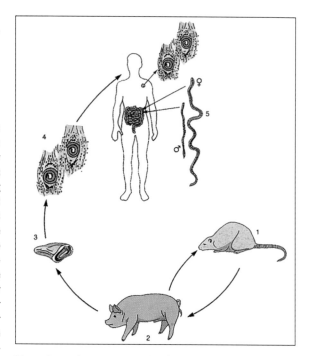

T. pseudospiralis was responsible for several human infections acquired from wild boar in the south of France.

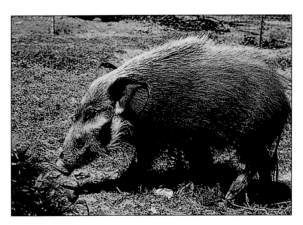

663 Wild reservoir of trichinosis

A common reservoir of infection is the wild pig, such as the African bush pig seen here. The flesh of other carnivores, such as the bear, has also served to initiate isolated outbreaks of human infection—after hunting parties, for example. Recent epidemiological surveys have shown that human trichinosis is increasing in all continents. In Chile, for example, calcified *Trichinella spiralis* larvae were found in 2% of all post mortem examinations in 1992.

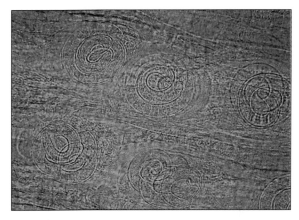

664 *Trichinella spiralis* larvae in crush preparation

The larvae are easily seen in pieces of muscle by crushing the tissue between two glass plates and inspecting it through a 'trichinoscope' (a simple magnifying system). (× 175.)

667 Patient with acute trichinosis

The four cardinal features of the disease are fever, orbital oedema, myalgia and eosinophilia.

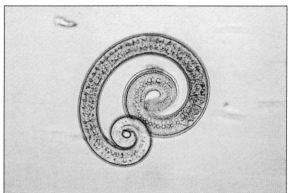

665 Larva free in gastric juice

The larvae can be freed for detailed examination by digesting a piece of contaminated muscle in artificial gastric juice. (× 175.)

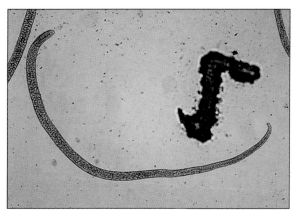

666 Parasitic female *Trichinella spiralis*

The adult female worm is about 2–3 mm long and 90 μm in diameter; the male 1.2 mm by 60 μm. (× 45.)

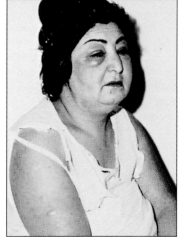

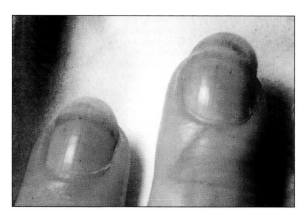

668 Splinter haemorrhages in trichinosis
Nail-bed haemorrhages are a common sign in acute trichinosis.

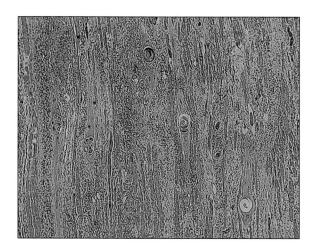

669 Larvae in muscle from a fatal human case
Many infections remain asymptomatic, but heavy infections may lead to fatal myocarditis or encephalitis. Encysted larvae are found in the muscles at biopsy (or post mortem examination). Calcification of the encysted larvae occurs after about 18 months in less severe infections and may be detected on radiography, but the encysted larvae remain alive for years. (*H&E* × *16*.)

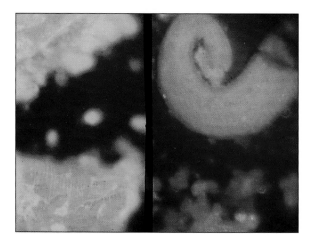

670 Fluorescent antibody test
Although immunity is largely cell mediated, circulating antibodies to *Trichinella spiralis* appear from 2–4 weeks after infection. Refined diagnostic antigens for their detection are currently being developed. For the present, a simple indirect fluorescent antibody test employing fragments of larvae as antigen is a useful diagnostic tool. Bentonite and latex tests with extracted larval antigens have also proved valuable in the acute stage, during which high antibody titres develop. An enzyme-linked immunosorbent assay is also available. (*Right*—negative control.)

CAPILLARIASIS

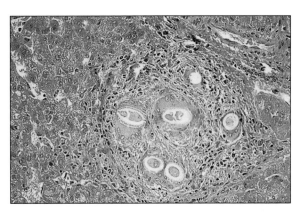

671 *Capillaria hepatica* in liver section
Human infection with this rodent nematode is very rare. In the rat, the worms have a direct life cycle resembling that of *Trichuris*. The adults live in the portal tracts. Eggs, also resembling those of *Trichuris* (see **378**), are infective only after undergoing maturation in the soil. Adult worms in the liver cause hepatic enlargement and severe parenchymal damage. Note the giant-cell reaction around the eggs. (*H&E* × *150*.)

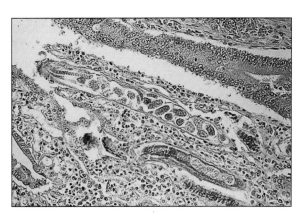

672 *Capillaria philippensis* invading small intestine
This species, the adults of which live in the upper small intestine, has occurred in epidemic form. A chronic malabsorption syndrome, which is sometimes fatal, develops in heavy infections. The parasites are acquired by eating raw, infected fish, which are the intermediate hosts. Monkeys seem to be the normal definitive host. Individual cases have been reported from a wide geographical area: from the Philippines, to as far westwards as Iran, the United Arab Emirates and Egypt. (*H&E* × *150*.)

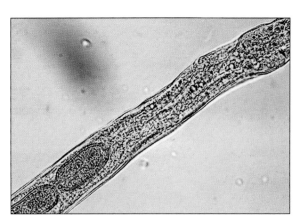

673 Female *Capillaria philippensis* from human faeces
The figure shows the vulval region of the female in which two typical eggs can be seen. (× *300*.)

OESOPHAGOSTOMIASIS

674 *Oesophagostomum bifurcum* in the human colon
Numerous human infections with this nematode occur in localised areas of West and East Africa. A recent survey in northern Togo and Ghana identified the larvae of *O. bifurcum* in the faeces of up to 30% of the inhabitants of 65 villages. The eggs, resembling those of hookworms, mature in the soil and produce infective third stage larvae that are morphologically distinct in stool culture from those of the common hookworms, which often co-exist. When swallowed, the larvae develop into adults in the mucosa and submucosa of the large intestine where they produce small abscesses. After maturation, the adults leave the abscesses to attach to the colonic mucosa. The figure, which shows part of the wall of the colon resected from a patient in Northern Ghana, is characteristic of the multinodular form of the infection,

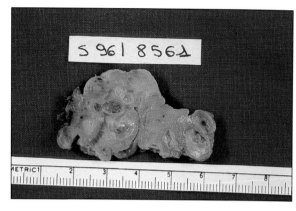

which can give rise to intestinal obstruction necessitating surgery. The numerous pea-sized nodules each contain a juvenile worm.

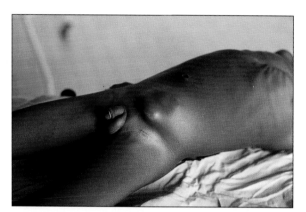

675 'Dapaong tumour' in a Togolese boy
At least 250 000 people are estimated to be infected with *Oesophagostomum bifurcum* in the north of Togo and Ghana, with a prevalence rate as high as 50% in some villages. In some individuals the worms cause large abdominal masses in the epigastric or periumbilical region, a condition known locally as 'Dapaong tumour.' These abdominal masses may be large, inflamed and painful as in the child seen here but are often smaller and less prominent. They characteristically contain a single juvenile worm about 10–12 mm long.

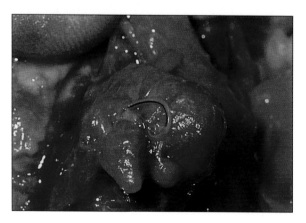

676 *Oesophagostomum* in a human appendix
The specimen seen here was found at operation for appendicitis in a Ugandan patient. The species was probably related to *O. stephanostomum*, which is a parasite of gorillas.

PARASTRONGYLIASIS AND EOSINOPHILIC MENINGITIS*

(*The species *Angiostrongylus cantonensis* and *A. costaricensis* have been reclassified in the genus *Parastrongylus*—see **Table 11**. The term 'Angiostrongyliasis' should, therefore, now be replaced by 'Parastrongyliasis.')

The main cause of eosinophilic meningitis is infection with larvae of the rat nematode, *Parastrongylus cantonensis*. This parasite has spread geographically in recent years with the dissemination of one of its best intermediate hosts, the giant African land snail (*Achatina fulica*), which is a popular item of food in some countries. Rats or humans are infected by eating infected molluscs or food contaminated by the snails' bodies.

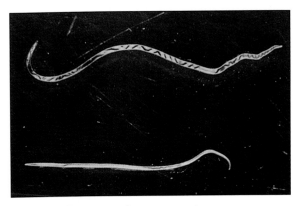

677 Adult *Parastrongylus cantonensis*
The adult worm, about 1–2 cm long, is a common parasite of rodents in the Far East and Pacific. It lives in the pulmonary arteries and arterioles. (Top, ♀, bottom ♂, × 3.5.)

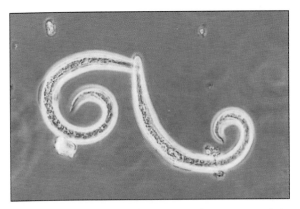

678 First stage larvae of *Parastrongylus cantonensis* in rat faeces
The eggs, passed in the blood stream, break through the pulmonary tract, are swallowed by the rodent and are passed in the faeces in which they may hatch to first stage larvae. (× 160.)

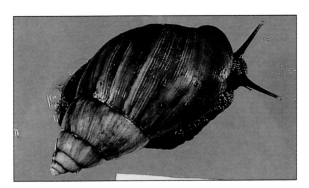

679 *Achatina fulica*, an intermediate host of *Parastrongylus cantonensis*
The first stage larvae in rat faeces are eaten by snails of various genera (including *Achatina*, *Cipangopaludina* and *Bradybaena*), as well as by some slugs and land planarians in which the larvae develop to the third stage. *A. fulica* is sometimes kept in vivaria as a 'pet,' or for educational purposes in schools. It is important to ensure that such molluscs are locally bred and not imported from countries where *P. cantonensis* is enzootic.

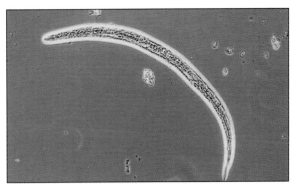

680 Third stage larvae in *Achatina fulica*
New rats become infested when they eat snails containing third stage larvae. (× 100.)

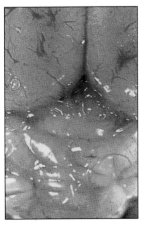

681 Larvae of *Parastrongylus cantonensis* in rat brain
The thread-like larvae can be seen in the subarachnoid space covering the base of this rat brain. Here, they mature to young adults, which migrate to the pulmonary arteries via the cerebral veins.

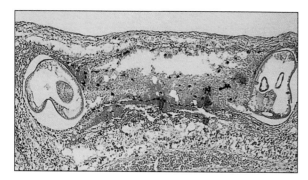

682 Section of *Parastrongylus cantonensis* larvae in meninges of human brain

Humans may be infested by eating freshwater prawns, but how these come to contain larvae is uncertain. Infection may also be acquired by eating molluscs that contain larvae or food contaminated with crushed molluscs. The larvae migrate to the brain where they cause eosinophilic meningitis or meningoencephalitis. The diagnosis is aided by the serological examination of paired specimens, using a specific antigen from adult worms. (× 60.)

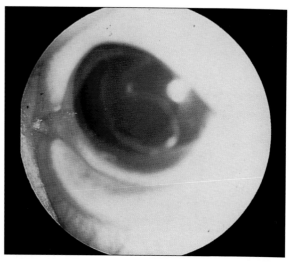

683 *Parastrongylus cantonensis* in the human eye

The adult nematode is seen floating in the anterior chamber of the eye of a 15-month-old Taiwanese child with eosinophilic meningoencephalitis.

684 *Parastrongylus costaricensis* in a mesenteric vessel

This enzootic nematode of cotton rats, black rats and other species of rodents as well as, on occasion, larger animals, is widely distributed in the New World and has also been found in Africa. Slugs are the intermediate hosts. Humans are occasionally infected by eating fruit or vegetables contaminated by infective larvae that have been shed by slugs with their mucus. In parts of Central America up to 85% of the slug *Vaginulus plebeius* have been found infected. In Costa Rica the prevalence of human infection has been estimated as 18 cases per 100 000 inhabitants. The larvae develop into adults in the mesenteric blood vessels (in contrast to *P. cantonensis*) and give rise to eosinophilic granuloma masses, a condition also known as 'Morera's disease'. The symptoms, which include abdominal pain, vomiting, diarrhoea and anorexia, are often mistaken for those of appendicitis whereas abdominal masses may arouse suspicion of a malignancy. The presence of a high eosinophil count is a guide to

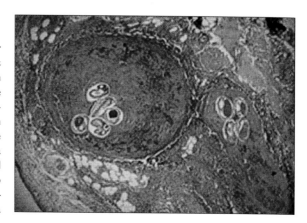

the diagnosis. This figure shows cross sections of adult worms in a mesenteric vessel occluded by a thrombus and surrounded by inflammatory exudate and eosinophils. (*H&E* × 25.)

ENTEROBIASIS

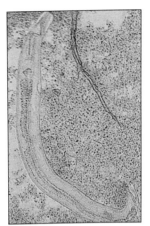 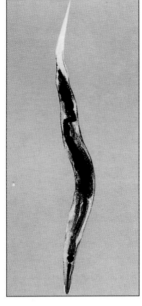

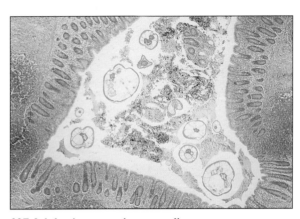

687 Adult pinworms in appendix

The worms are occasionally found in the appendix, but their role as a cause of acute appendicitis is uncertain. Sections of several adult worms are seen here. (*H&E* × *13.*)

685 & 686 Adult *Enterobius vermicularis*

These 'pinworms' are small, white and thread-like. The males (**685**, left) have coiled tails and measure 2.5 mm in length. The females (**686**, right), which are about 10 mm long, emerge to the perianal region, where they lay some 10 000–15 000 eggs and then die. In the process, they cause severe pruritus. The embryonated eggs, which are directly infectious on ingestion, hatch in the duodenum; the larvae pass to the caecum where they mature. (♂ × 20; ♀ × 8.)

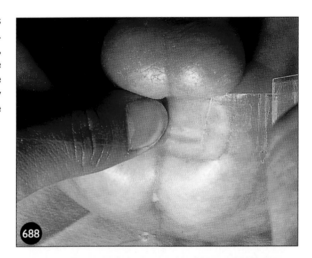

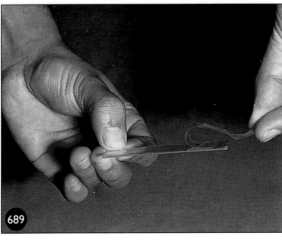

688 & 689 Scotch-tape swab to demonstrate perianal eggs

The eggs (see **379**) are found on the perianal skin. They adhere to the Scotch tape, which can then be placed on a slide and examined directly under a microscope. Because of severe pruritis ani, children often reinfect themselves from eggs under their fingernails. Bedding is also a source of infection, which tends to persist in households and institutions such as orphanages.

ANISAKIASIS

Anisakiasis is the term used for human infection with the larvae of *Anisakis simplex* or *Pseudoterranova decipiens*. These are common nematode parasites, the adults of which live in the stomach of marine mammals. There the worms produce eggs that are discharged with the faeces. The first stage larvae progress to the second stage in the egg, and these larvae hatch when the eggs are eaten by krill. In these invertebrates they mature to the third stage larvae, which encyst in the viscera or muscles of sea fish or squid that eat the krill. *A. simplex* infects numerous species of fish such as salmon, pollock, herring (hence the term 'herring worm' in Holland) and mackerel. *P. decipiens* mainly parasitises cod and halibut. Infection is acquired by consuming uncooked and even pickled fish—a custom that is very popular in countries such as Japan but that is no longer prevalent in Europe. In humans the larvae may moult to the fourth stage, but they do not mature into adults.

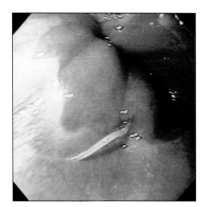

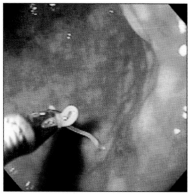

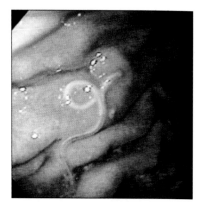

690 Third stage larva of *Anisakis simplex*

This figure shows the larva as visualised through an endoscope in the stomach of a 39-year-old Japanese woman. The consumption of raw fish is very popular in some countries of the Far East, especially Japan. Various symptoms may develop after infection with *Anisakis*, depending on the location of the larvae as they move further down the intestine. The most common site to be invaded is the gastric mucosa. This causes severe gastric pain within about six hours after the larvae are ingested. If the condition is diagnosed early, surgical removal is called for. The consumption of pickled herring in Holland used to be associated with anisakiasis ('green herring disease') but the compulsory freezing of all herring prior to consumption has now all but eliminated the condition there.

691 Removal of fourth stage larva of *Anisakis simplex*

The third stage larvae may moult to the fourth stage in the human host. The figure shows the removal with biopsy forceps through an endoscope of a fourth stage larva from the gastric mucosa of an 80-year-old Japanese woman.

692 Larval *Pseudoterranova decipiens*

The whitish coloured third stage larvae, about 2 cm long, are less invasive than those of *Anisakis simplex* but may invade the gastric mucosa, causing acute epigastric pain within a few hours of their being ingested. Typically they are vomited before invasion occurs. This third stage larva in the stomach of a 59-year-old Japanese woman has burrowed into the mucosa.

GNATHOSTOMIASIS

693 Life cycle of *Gnathostoma spinigerum*

Several species of the spirurid genus *Gnathostoma* are responsible for zoonotic infections in humans. The larvae of *G. spinigerum* are acquired mainly from various freshwater fish, especially in Thailand and Japan. Those of *G. hispidum* are acquired from inadequately cooked pork. In the definitive hosts, which are usually carnivores such as cats (1), tigers, leopards and dogs, the adult nematodes live in nodules in the stomach wall. Eggs (2) passed in the faeces develop, and sheathed first stage larvae hatch when they reach water; when these larvae (3) are ingested by species of *Cyclops* (4), they moult to produce second stage larvae in these first intermediate hosts. When the *Cyclops* are swallowed by fish (5) or frogs (6), the larvae pierce their gastric wall and develop into the third stage larvae, which become encysted. If eaten by the definitive hosts, the third stage larvae penetrate into their stomach walls and there mature to adults. If infected fish or frogs are eaten by other vertebrates that act as paratenic hosts (see **545**), such as herons (7), pigs (8) or

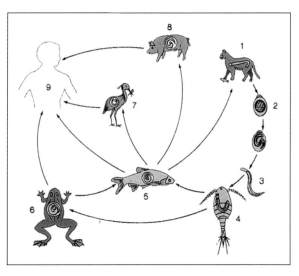

humans (9), they do not mature but migrate through the subcutaneous tissues where they are manifested as 'larva migrans.'

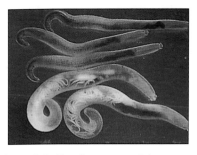

694 Living adult *Gnathostoma spinigerum*
The male worms have a red tail and the larger females a more curled one. (× *1.3*.)

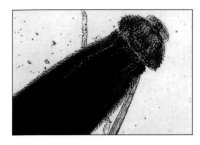

695 Head of adult *Gnathostoma spinigerum*
The adult usually lives in the stomach of dogs, cats and wild felines. It is found throughout Southeast Asia. There are two intermediate hosts. Humans acquires infection by eating fermented fish (a delicacy in Thailand) or any other form of raw fish. The parasite cannot mature in humans but migrates, causing cutaneous and visceral larva migrans. (× *30*.)

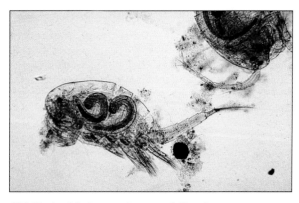

696 Early third stage larvae of *Gnathostoma nipponicum* in *Eucyclops serrulatus*
Several species of *Gnathostoma* have been incriminated in human infection in different continents. They include *G. nipponicum* for which a definitive host is the Japanese weasel. Larvae hatching from eggs that are passed with faeces into fresh water infect *Cyclops* water fleas and, later, fish that eat the *Cyclops*. The early third stage larvae develop in the body cavity of the copepod within seven to 10 days. They remain in this stage until the crustacean is ingested by a vertebrate host such as a freshwater fish, frog or possibly a small rodent. The larvae then penetrate from the intestine to take up a position in the new (second intermediate) host's muscles, where the late third stage larvae form cysts about 1 mm in diameter. (× *75*.)

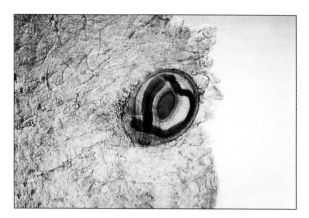

697 Third stage larva of *Gnathostoma spinigerum* encysted in fish muscle

Spiced raw fish known as 'somfak' or fermented fish, such as that sold in Thai markets, are a potential source of several helminths, including *G. spinigerum*. Infection may also be acquired from paratenic hosts that devour small fish that harbour the third stage larvae—for example, crabs, larger fish, amphibia, reptiles, rodents or chickens. Successive passages to paratenic hosts may occur including, of course, to humans who also serve (with rare exceptions when the adult stage develops in the stomach) as paratenic hosts if they consume, uncooked, any other animal harbouring third stage larvae. (× 20.)

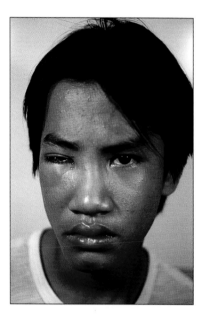

698 Periorbital larva migrans

One of the characteristic clinical features is a migrating, subcutaneous swelling associated with boring pain and eosinophilia. Third stage *Gnathostoma* larvae may be recovered surgically from swellings in suitable locations. Cerebral lesions with focal signs are not uncommon in Thailand.

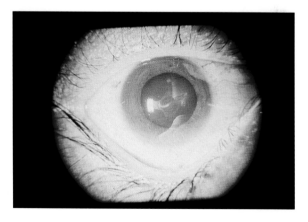

699 Late third stage larva of *Gnathostoma spinigerum* in the eye

The figure shows a migrating third stage larva of *G. spinigerum* in the anterior chamber of the eye of a Thai patient.

DRACUNCULIASIS (DRACONTIASIS, GUINEA WORM INFECTION)

The 'Medina worm,' so called because of its former frequency in that Arabian city, used to be widely distributed across Africa, the Middle East and South Asia. Small zoonotic foci also existed in parts of South America; in North America it is enzootic in various carnivores. Since the introduction of improved water supplies and the start of the recent global eradication campaign, its distribution and the numbers of cases in formerly afflicted regions have decreased rapidly. A major impact on transmission was made when a simple water filter was introduced to sieve out copepods from contaminated water (see **704**). In the 1980s, the annual global incidence fell from about 10 to two million, and it is now eradicated from Pakistan, India, Yemen, Senegal, Cameroon, Chad and Kenya. The numbers have decreased spectacularly also in some of the previously most highly infected parts of Africa where, in July 2000, only 855 cases were reported in the remaining 15 endemic countries.

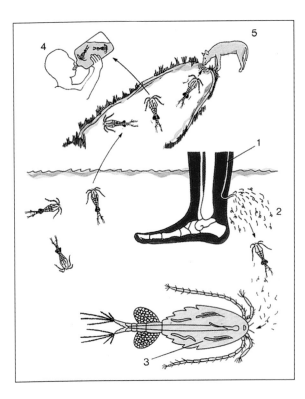

700 Life cycle of *Dracunculus medinensis*
(1) The mature female worm in the subcutaneous tissues of the human host causes the formation of a blister, which bursts when the skin is immersed in fresh water and from which the female's uterus releases large numbers of active, rhabditiform larvae (2). Larvae that are swallowed by copepods in the water penetrate the gut wall and enter the new host's body cavity, where they grow and undergo two moults (3). When infected water fleas are swallowed by humans in untreated drinking water (4), the larvae are released to penetrate the wall of the duodenum. They migrate through the body and, after undergoing two further moults, males and females mate in the subcutaneous tissues, with the males dying subsequently. Fertilised females migrate along the muscle planes and finally reach the subcutaneous tissues, commonly those of the lower limbs but sometimes the upper limbs or other parts of the body. They are ready to oviposit about one year after reaching the human host. Other animals that can be infected include dogs (5), horses, cows and some species of monkeys.

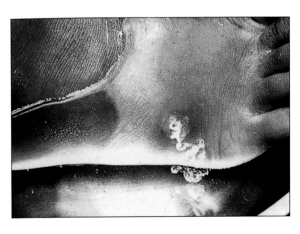

701 Contamination of surface water
A papule forms where the adult female worm reaches the skin surface; it ulcerates when the skin is immersed in water. A loop of the worm's uterus prolapses and ruptures, releasing large numbers of rhabditiform larvae into the water.

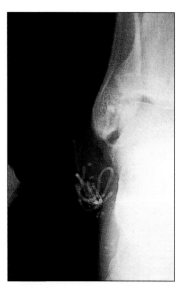

702 Radiography of calcified worms
The size of an adult female *Dracunculus medinensis* can be judged from this radiograph of a calcified worm in the ankle. Females attain a length of up to 100 cm, males only 10–40 cm.

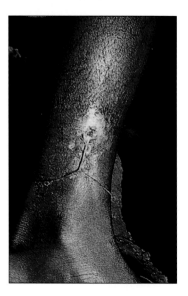

703 Extraction of female worm
Adult females are commonly extracted by progressively winding them round a matchstick as they emerge from the subcutaneous tissues. Chemotherapy has made the process easier and less hazardous.

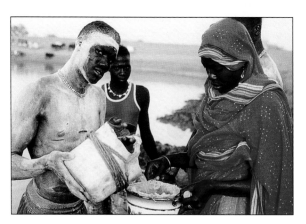

704 Filtering water for drinking through a nylon gauze sieve
The global campaign currently in operation is based on the provision of clean water supplies and the elimination of water fleas from drinking water. The latter is being achieved by a combination of simple filtration through a plastic mesh filter and the treatment of the water supply, where appropriate, with the organophosphate, Abate, which is non-toxic to humans in the very low concentrations required. Copepods that escape simple filtration, together with bacterial pathogens, will be killed by boiling.

HELMINTHIASES—CESTODES

(See **Table 20**.)

DIPHYLLOBOTHRIASIS (FISH TAPEWORM)

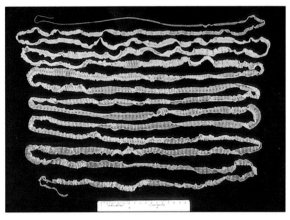

705 Intact adult *Diphyllobothrium latum*
A mature adult may reach 10 m in length. The head and mature proglottids are readily distinguished from those of *Taenia* in humans (see **731** and **732**). Mature worms may produce one million eggs daily (see **376**).

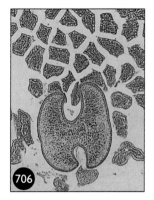 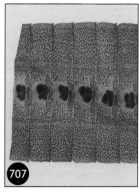

706 & 707 Cross section of head, and segments of adult *Diphyllobothrium latum*
This fish tapeworm is common around large lakes in Europe, North America and elsewhere. In Japan and countries of South America bordering the Pacific, zoonotic infection of humans occasionally occurs with *D. pacificum*, of which the adult is normally parasitic in seals. The plerocercoids (see **709**) live in marine fish. The classic clinical feature of the infection is the development of vitamin B12 deficiency, with a resultant macrocytic anaemia. (*Head × 16; segments × 6*.)

Table 20 Cestodes of medical importance and their prevalence[1]

Order	Family	Genus and species	Estimated Cases
PSEUDOPHYLLIDAE	Diphyllobothriidae	*Diphyllobothrium latum*	16 million
		D. pacificum	? hundreds
		Spirometra spp.	rare
		'Sparganum' spp.	rare
CYCLOPHYLLIDAE	Anoplocephalidae	*Bertiella* spp.	rare
	Davaineidae	*Raillietina* spp.	rare
	Linstowiidae	*Inermicapsifer* spp.	rare
	Mesocestoididae	*Mesocestoides* spp.	rare
	Dilepididae	*Dipylidium caninum*	rare
	Hymenolepididae	*Vampirolepis nana*[2]	36 million
		Hymenolepis diminuta	rare
	Taeniidae	*Taenia solium*	5 million
		T. saginata	76 million
		T. saginata asiatica	rare
		Multiceps multiceps	rare
		Echinococcus granulosus	thousands
		E. mulitilocularis	rare
		E. vogeli	rare
		E. oligarthrus	rare

[1] See footnote to **Table 11**.
[2] The species *Vampirolepis nana* was formerly known as *Hymenolepis nana*.

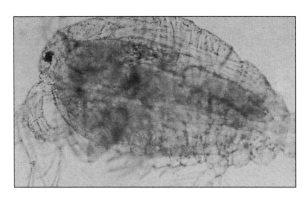

708 Copepod containing procercoids of *Diphyllobothrium latum*

From the operculated eggs, actively swimming, round, hexa-canth coracidia emerge. After ingestion by various species of water fleas, they form procercoid larvae in the haemocoel of the copepods. Among the species in which the larvae can develop are *Cyclops strenuus*, *C. brevispinosus*, *C. prasenus*, *Diaptomus gracilis* and *D. graciloides*. (× 185.)

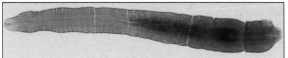

709 Plerocercoid in fish

When the copepod is ingested by a fish, the larva emerges to form a migrating plerocercoid (Sparganum), which comes to lie in the muscle. This develops into an adult in the gut of humans if the fish is consumed when incompletely cooked. (× 6.)

SPARGANOSIS

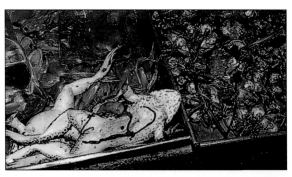

710 Edible frog and sea food on a Thai market stall

Sparganum occurs in a variety of amphibious animals (including frogs), and these also may be infective to humans if ingested. They are the larvae of tapeworms of the genus *Spirometra* that are common in various canines and felines. The first stage larvae are formed as procercoids in *Cyclops*. Ingestion of these larvae produces sparganosis in humans, since the larvae cannot mature in this abnormal host.

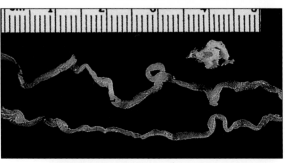

711 'Sparganum mansoni'

The Sparganum larvae proliferate, often in the subcutaneous tissues, where they become encysted in large nodules from which they can be removed surgically. The specimen shown here, for example, was found when a 'hernia' was opened in the groin of a Ugandan woman. When localised in the peri-orbital tissues or under the conjunctiva, severe oedema may result. In Vietnam and Thailand, this infection may follow the application of frogs as a poultice for inflamed eyes!

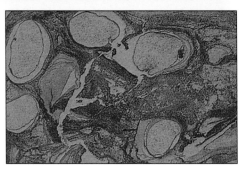

712 Section of Sparganum in a nodule

The larval cestode is walled off by an intense cellular and fibrotic reaction. (*H&E* × 7.)

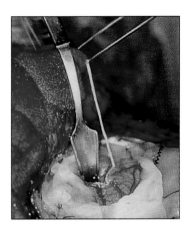

713 Sparganosis of the brain
A 10 cm long larva being removed from the subcortical area of the brain of a Japanese patient.

DIPYLIDIUM CANINUM (DOG TAPEWORM)

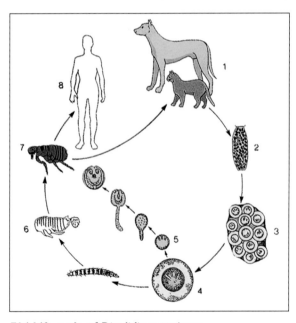

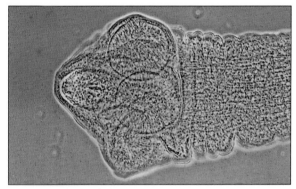

715 Scolex of *Dipylidium caninum*
This cestode, the adult of which reaches a length of 10–70 cm, is the common tapeworm of domestic and wild canines and felines. (× 15.)

714 Life cycle of *Dipylidium caninum*
(1) The adult cestode (10–70 cm long) in the small intestine of dogs, cats or wild canids, produces proglottids, which may be passed in the faeces intact (2) or may degenerate, releasing clusters of encapsulated eggs (3). Oncospheres (4) hatching from eggs ingested by flea larvae remain undeveloped until the larvae pupate, whereupon they develop into cysticercoids (5). The cysticercoids undergo a complicated metamorphosis in the body cavities of the pupal (6) and adult fleas (7) and (8, 1) pass into the small intestine of the definitive host when it accidentally ingests the fleas, there everting the hooked rostellum to attach to the gut wall where it will mature into an adult.

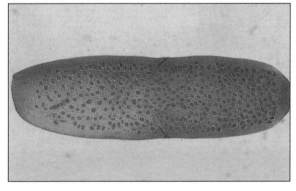

716 Mature segment of *Dipylidium caninum*
The cestode sheds whitish, mature segments, which are passed in the faeces or escape from the anus. The segments are visibly but slowly motile. (× 9.)

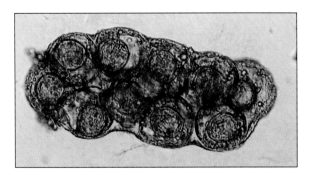

717 Egg capsule of *Dipylidium caninum*
In addition to mature segments, encapsulated clusters of eggs in which larval hooks may be seen are passed as the mature segments disintegrate. (× *240*.)

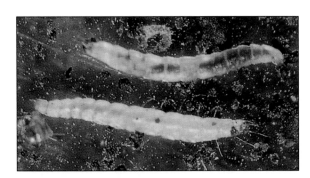

718 First instar larvae of *Ctenocephalides felis*
The eggs are ingested by larval cat, dog or human fleas. They develop first procercoid then cysticercoid larvae in the haemocoel of the insects, in which they remain when the fleas grow to the adult stage. These are cat flea larvae. (× *12*.)

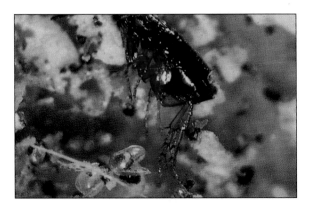

719 Male cat flea, *Ctenocephalides felis*
Humans become infected by inadvertently swallowing infected fleas from dogs or cats. (× *14*.)

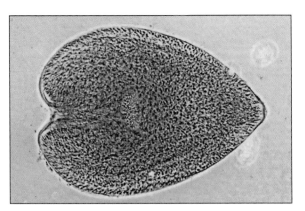

720 Immature cysticercoid from dog flea
(× *100*.)

VAMPIROLEPIS NANA (DWARF TAPEWORM)

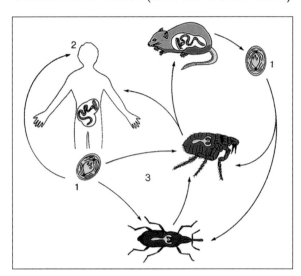

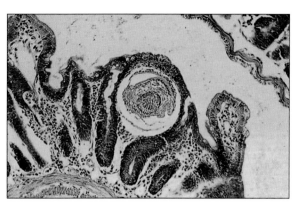

721 Life cycle of *Vampirolepis nana*
(1) Eggs released from mature proglottids in the upper ileum are passed in the faeces. (2) If ingested by another person, they hatch to yield hexacanth oncospheres, which burrow into the villi of the small intestine. There they mature into tailless cysticercoids (cercocysts), which migrate towards the ileum where the scolices become attached to commence the formation of proglottids. (3) Eggs that are ingested by such insects as fleas, beetles or cockroaches hatch to form tailed cysticercoids, which remain unmodified as long as they are within the insect's body cavity. If infected insects are accidentally ingested, the cysticercoids pass down the intestine to establish themselves in the ileum of the new vertebrate host. In this way rodents, as well as humans, may be infected, although the more common parasite of rodents is *V. nana* var *fraterna*.

723 Cercocyst in intestinal villi
In mammals the oncospheres penetrate into the villi of the small intestine. There they mature into tailless cysticercoids (cercocysts), which leave the villi, move further down the gut and become attached to other villi where they mature to adult tapeworms. (× 140.)

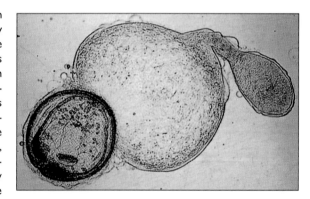

724 Cysticercoid in insect
If the egg is eaten by an insect, the oncosphere metamorphoses to form a tailed cysticeroid in the insect's body cavity. Further development takes place if the insect is ingested by a human. (× 90.)

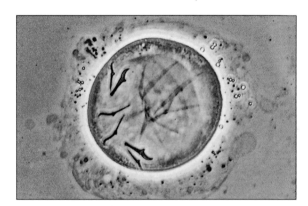

722 Hexacanth oncosphere
This cosmopolitan tapeworm reaches only 2.5–4 cm in length. Human infection is usually acquired directly by ingesting eggs. After ingestion by a mammal or by certain insects, the eggs (see **380**) hatch into the hexacanth oncospheres. (*Phase contrast* × 1150.)

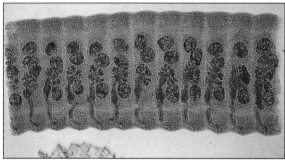

725 Mature proglottids
Humans are the only important source of human infection because rodents are parasitised normally by a strain that does not develop in humans. (× 25.)

HYMENOLEPIS DIMINUTA (RAT TAPEWORM)

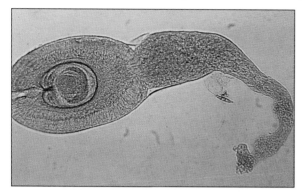

726 Cysticercoid of *Hymenolepis diminuta* in an arthropod

The adults of this, the common cestode of rodents, are 20–60 cm long. Their eggs (*see* **381**) resemble those of *Vampirolepis nana* but lack the polar filaments. An intermediate insect host is essential in this life cycle, and a wide variety of coprophagic arthropods serve as intermediate hosts. Occasionally humans are infected by accidentally swallowing infected arthropods (e.g. rat fleas, or larvae of grain moths and beetles). (× 90.)

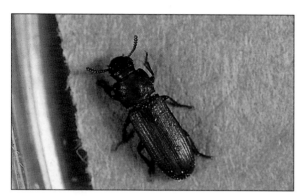

727 *Tribolium confusum*

These grain pests are typical intermediate hosts of *Hymenolepis diminuta*. (× 6.5.)

TAENIA SOLIUM (PORK TAPEWORM)

728 Life cycle of *Taenia solium* and *T. saginata*

The adults (1) of both species live in the small intestine of humans, the definitive hosts. The gravid segments (2) are very active and escape through the anus, releasing large numbers of eggs (3) in the perianal region or on the ground, where they can survive for long periods. Faecal egg loads are, therefore, relatively light. When ingested by pigs (4) (*T. solium*) or cattle (5) (*T. saginata*), the eggs hatch, each releasing an oncosphere that migrates through the intestinal wall and blood vessels to reach striated muscle within which it encysts, forming cysticerci (6). When inadequately cooked meat containing the cysts is eaten by humans, the oncospheres excyst (7), settle in the small intestine and develop there into adult cestodes (1) over the next three months or so. The segments of *T. solium* are somewhat less active than those of the beef tapeworm, but its eggs, if released in the upper intestine, can invade the host (autoinfection) (8), setting up the potentially dangerous larval infection known as cysticercosis in muscle, brain or any other site.

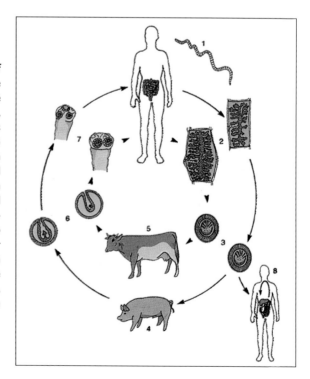

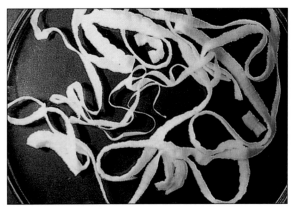

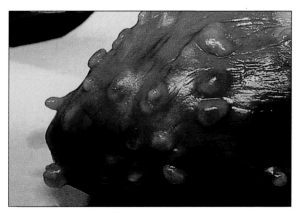

729 Head and part of segments of adult tapeworm
Taenia solium may reach 2–8 m in length, and multiple infections can occur.

730 Cysticercus in pork
The larval cysticercoid stage occurs in the pig, giving rise to 'measly pork.' Humans are infected by ingesting the meat when it is inadequately cooked. (× 2.0.)

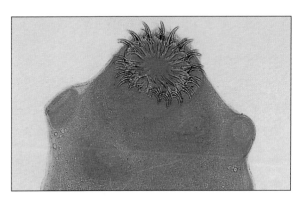

731 & 732 Scolices of *Taenia solium* and *T. saginata*
The head of *T. solium* (**731**, left) is armoured with hooks in addition to four suckers. *T. saginata* (**732**, right) has no hooks. (× 40.)

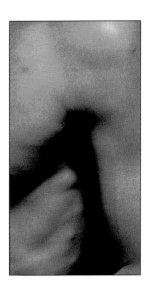

733 *Taenia solium* cysticerci in chest wall
Autoinfection can occur due to the release of eggs after the incorrect use of taeniacidal drugs. If regurgitation of gut contents carries mature segments with eggs into the stomach, the eggs can invade the human tissues just as those of the pig. The cysts (cysticerci cellulosae) may be formed in any tissue. This agricultural student was infected in Thailand.

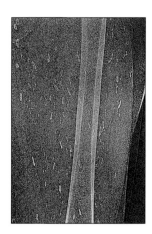

734 Radiograph of cysticercosis of soft tissues
When calcification occurs, the cysticerci are readily seen on a radiograph of the soft tissues.

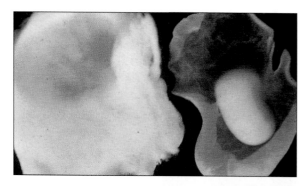

735 Cysticercus removed from subcutaneous tissues
This fibrous nodule containing a cyst is from the patient shown in **733**. (× 10.)

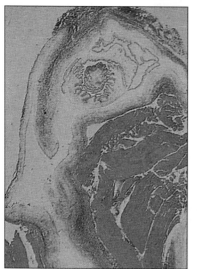

736 Section of cyst in human muscle
The figure shows a section of a typical cysticercus cellulosa removed from a chest wall. (× 6.)

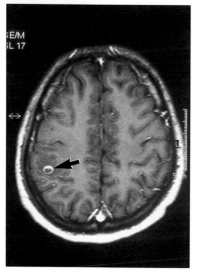

737 Computed tomography in cerebral cysticercosis
When cysticerci lodge in the brain calcification can occur, but usually much later than in tissues such as muscle and often after epilepsy has manifested itself. An early cysticercal lesion with surrounding oedema (arrow) is seen here in the right parietal region of a 22-year-old man who presented with focal convulsions of his left arm.

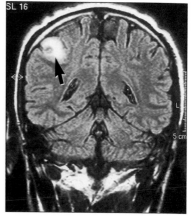

738 Coronal section of brain in cerebral cysticercosis
This is the same lesion as seen in **737**. In this magnetic resonance image the small cyst is seen clearly with its surrounding white area of oedema (arrow).

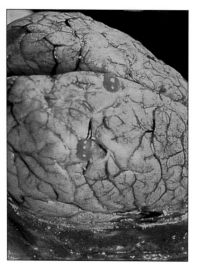

739 Fatal cerebral cysticercosis
At post mortem examination of such a case, the cysts are readily seen in various parts of the brain and brain stem.

TAENIA SAGINATA (BEEF TAPEWORM)

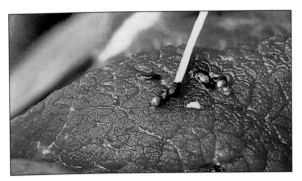

740 Cysticercus in beef
The cysticercal stage occurs only in cattle, humans becoming infected when they eat raw or partially cooked beef.

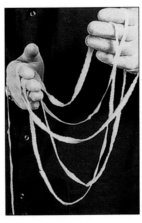

741 Adult *Taenia saginata*
The figure gives an impression of the size of this cestode, which can attain 10 m in length. This was only part of a worm passed after treatment with a taeniacide.

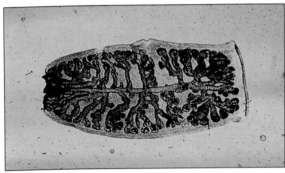

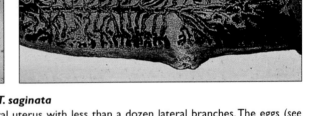

742 & 743 Mature proglottids of *Taenia solium* and *T. saginata*
The gravid segments of *T. solium* (**742**, left) contain a central uterus with less than a dozen lateral branches. The eggs (see **382**) are similar to those of other *Taenia* species. The gravid segments of *T. saginata* (**743**, right) contain a central uterus with 15–20 lateral branches. (× 6.)

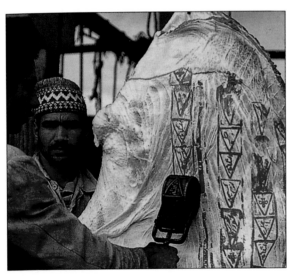

744 Meat inspection: certificate of health
Taeniasis is prevented by strict abattoir supervision, including adequate inspection of carcasses and condemnation of 'measly' meat.

HYDATIDOSIS

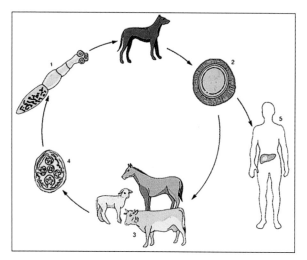

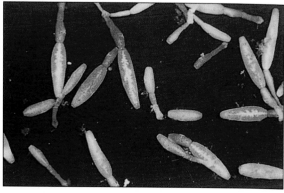

747 Adult *Echinococcus granulosus*
These tapeworms are about 5 mm long. Large numbers may be found in the small intestine of dogs, which are infected by eating offal of sheep, cattle or other animals containing hydatid cysts. The scolices in the cysts evaginate in the animal's intestine and mature into the adult worms. (× 7.)

745 Life cycle of *Echinococcus granulosus*
The adult tapeworm (1) inhabits the small intestine of dogs in the faeces of which typical taeniid eggs (2) (see **382**) are passed. Eggs ingested by herbivores (3) hatch in the duodenum, the hooked embryos entering the circulation where they are carried to various sites to develop into cysts (4). Dogs become infected when they eat the cysts contained in contaminated offal. Humans (5) are infected if they accidentally ingest eggs from infected dogs. The liver is the commonest site for the cysts. Nine distinct genotypes within the *E. granulosus* complex have been identified by molecular-based procedures and two in *E. multilocularis*, as well as two other species within this genus. Their full epidemiological importance has not yet been defined.

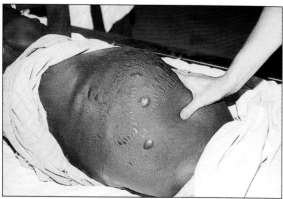

748 Massive hydatid cyst in a Kenyan boy
If humans accidentally ingest eggs, they become the host of the larval (hydatid cyst) stage, with the liver being most commonly affected. Hydatidosis is very common in the Turkana region of northern Kenya where there is a close association between dogs and humans. A local custom was to use 'nurse dogs' to guard the household where they were often encouraged to lick small infants clean, so encouraging infection with *E. granulosus* eggs. This young boy's abdomen bears the scars of local treatment aimed at alleviating pain over the grossly enlarged liver.

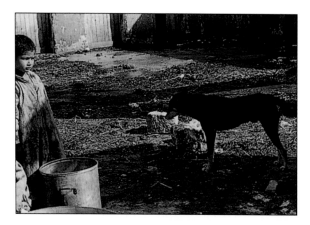

746 Dog in an insanitary abattoir
Hydatidosis can be largely prevented by strict control of abattoirs and disposal of infected offal. In some primitive rural communities that slaughter animals for food in an entirely uncontrolled and *ad hoc* fashion, hydatid disease is very common.

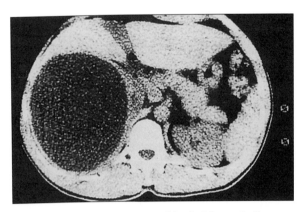

749 Computed tomogram of hydatid cyst in liver
The hydatid cyst is usually unilocular, with a double wall comprised of an outer laminated layer and an inner nucleated germinal layer. The figure shows a massive cyst in the right lobe of the liver of a 14-year-old Kuwaiti boy.

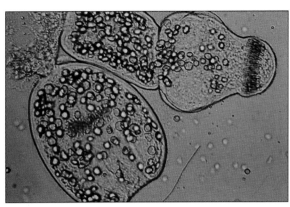

752 'Hydatid sand'
The daughter cysts are attached to the cyst wall of the parent or may float free in its milky fluid contents as so-called 'hydatid sand.' Rupture of a cyst into the tissues results in dissemination and further growth of the scolices. (× 250.)

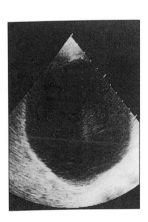

750 Ultrasound image of hydatid cyst
(Same case as **749**.) Diagnostically invaluable images can be produced in any of the many hospitals equipped with ultrasound imaging technology.

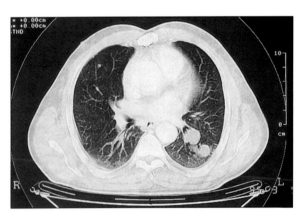

753 Computed tomogram of hydatid cysts of lungs
Hydatid cysts may occur in 20 to 30% of infections. This tomogram demonstrates the fluid content of several pulmonary cysts.

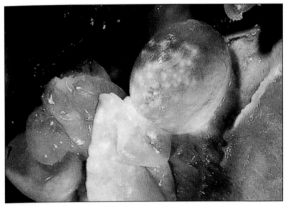

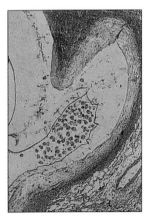

754 Hydatid cyst of lung
Section of cyst removed from a lung, showing the multilayered cyst wall and numerous daughter cysts produced by the germinal layer. (*H&E* × 30.)

751 Daughter cysts
The germinal layer produces brood capsules inside of which scolices grow.

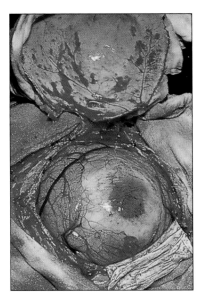

755 Hydatid cyst in brain
This cyst was found in the brain of a four-year-old girl.

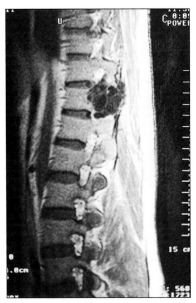

756 Medullary hydatidosis
In this magnetic resonance image of the spine taken in the longitudinal axis, the relation between the medulla and a hydatid cyst that caused hemiplegia is clearly seen. Serology in such cases often gives negative results.

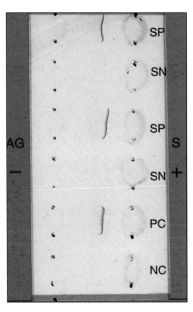

757 Immunodiagnosis of hydatidosis
The Casoni skin test employed formerly used crude hydatid fluid as antigen. This has been largely replaced by purified antigens such as 'arc 5,' which is employed in counter immunoelectrophoresis. [SP—positive sera; SN—negative sera; PC—positive controls; NC—negative controls; AG—antigen at cathodic ends; S—serum at anodic ends.]

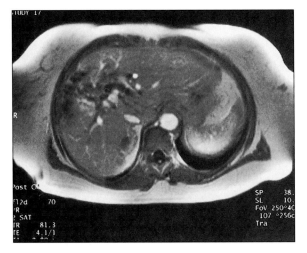

758 Magnetic resonance image of multilocular (alveolar) echinococcosis
Multilocular or alveolar cysts are caused by infection with *Echinococcus multilocularis*. The adult of this species is found in wild canines, especially foxes, and the usual larval hosts are rodents. The parasite is widely distributed in the Palaearctic region, and human infection is especially common in areas where domestic dogs also consume rodents. Between 2 to 5% of certain communities in China have been found infected, whereas the disease is reported to be hyperendemic in a number of Eskimo villages in North America. Treatment of this life-threatening condition is very difficult, although prolonged therapy with anthelminthic drugs is usually of benefit.

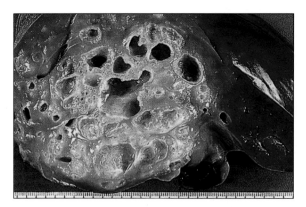

759 Multilocular hydatidosis in human liver
Prior to the use of modern imaging techniques, alveolar cysts in the human liver, which may mimic hepatic carcinoma, were usually discovered only at post mortem examination, as in this case.

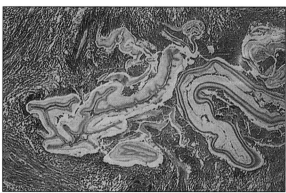

760 Section of alveolar hydatid cyst
Unlike *Echinococcus granulosus*, cysts of *E. multilocularis* in humans do not contain daughter cysts with scolices (× *40.*) (*c.f.* **754**.)

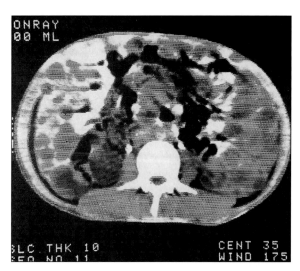

761 *Echinococcus vogeli*
This intestinal cestode of the bush dog (*Speothos venaticus*), and possibly domestic dogs in humid, tropical forest areas of South America, normally produces polycystic hydatidosis in pacas, agoutis and spiny rats, but zoonotic infection occasionally occurs in humans. The cysts are found most commonly in the abdominal or thoracic organs. This computed tomogram of a 20-year-old rubber tapper from Acre State, Brazil, shows large numbers of cystic masses in the abdominal cavity. The infection was probably acquired from his dogs, which were fed on the meat of infected pacas (*Cuniculus paca*). He was cured eventually with a combination of chemotherapy and surgery.

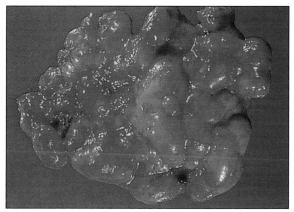

762 Polycystic mass of *Echinococcus vogeli*
This mass was removed surgically from a 22-year-old black Colombian complaining of repeated episodes of fever and purulent cough. At first he was suspected from a computed tomogram of having a neoplasm but was found at laparotomy to have polycystic masses on the surface of the liver. Subsequently, at thoracotomy, groups of cysts were removed from various sites, including the one shown here, which was in the pericardium.

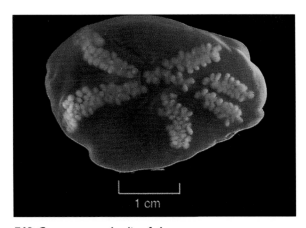

763 *Coenurus cerebralis* of sheep
This is the larval stage of *Multiceps multiceps*. The adult lives in the intestine of the dog and the 'bladder worm' larva is usually found in the brain of sheep. Fortunately, infection of humans is rare.

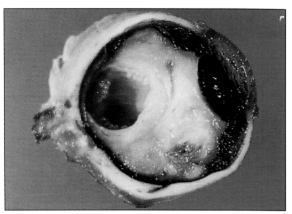

764 *Coenurus cerebralis* in human eye
This infection necessitated enucleation of the eye.

PENTASTOMIASIS

LINGUATULA SERRATA (TONGUE WORM)

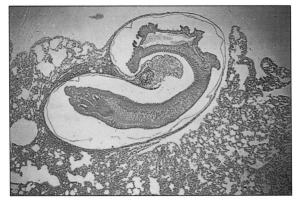

765 Third stage larva of *Linguatula serrata* in rabbit lung
These endoparasitic and highly specialised parasites have embryonic and ultrastructural affinities to the Arthropoda. Humans may be infected by eating inadequately cooked food containing third stage larvae. Other carnivores are also infected. (× 20.)

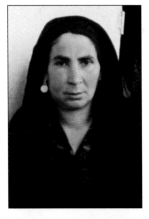

766 Halzoun syndrome
The parasites migrate to the nasopharynx where they produce large adults that block the airways and also cause deafness. Eggs are passed in the nasal secretions. Facial oedema is a common sign.

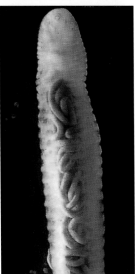

767 Adult *Linguatula serrata*
Cephalic third of a typical adult tongue worm. Note the oral opening and four hooks. (× 3.)

OTHER PENTASTOMIDS

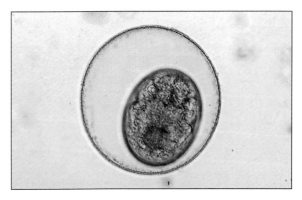

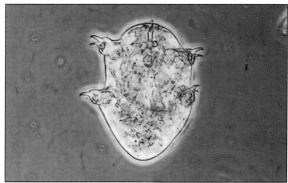

768 & 769 Egg and first stage larva of *Porocephalus*
The eggs and primary larvae with their four bifurcate legs point to the arthropod origin of this parasite of North American snakes (*Porocephalus crotali*). (**768**, left × *130*; **769**, right × *160*.)

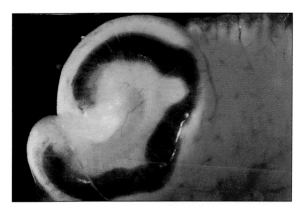

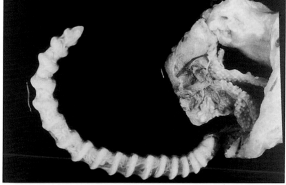

770 *Porocephalus crotali* third stage larva
After ingestion of eggs in food or water by a secondary host (usually a rodent), primary larvae emerge in the gut. They penetrate the gut wall and encyst in various tissues. This infective third stage larva lies subperitoneally in a rodent, the normal intermediate host. (× *4.5.*)

772 Adult males and a female *Armillifer armillatus*
This lungworm is a common parasite of several species of African snakes. The usual intermediate hosts are rodents, but humans are quite commonly infected with the larvae (× *0.7*). (AFIP No. 72–881.)

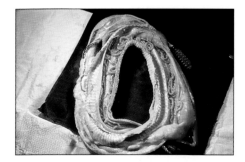

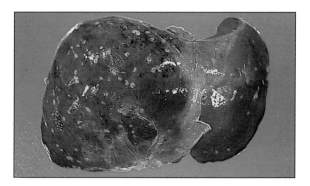

771 Adult *Porocephalus crotali* in rattlesnake lung
Eggs of this 'lungworm' are passed in saliva or faeces. The parasite is common in snakes, which acquire infection by eating rodents containing third stage larvae. (× *1/8.*)

773 Larvae of *Armillifer armillatus*
Third stage larvae are seen under the capsule of the liver of a Nigerian at post mortem examination.

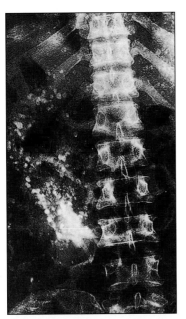

774 Radiograph of calcified nymphal cysts of *Armillifer annulatus* in a human

The C-shaped, encysted nymphs of pentastomids are often detected in diagnostic radiographs taken for unrelated symptoms. The heaviness of this widely disseminated infection is remarkable.

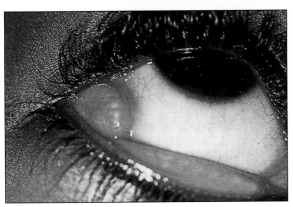

775 Pentastomid larva in eye

The eye is a rare site for pentastomid larvae, the abdomen being mainly affected in humans.

CHAPTER 5

Sexually Transmitted Diseases, including HIV/AIDS

Sexual promiscuity and unprotected sexual intercourse are the major factors in spreading a number of infectious diseases, including those caused by viruses, bacteria and protozoa. Although the problem is a global one, the burden of sexually transmitted diseases falls most heavily on many of the populations of the developing countries, except those among whom cultural and social factors tend to limit promiscuity or where safe sexual practices are advocated. Within a short period of two decades the world has witnessed the arrival of a pandemic of a previously unrecognised, mainly sexually transmitted, viral infection, caused by the human immunodeficiency viruses, HIV1 and HIV2. These retroviruses, first identified in 1983 and 1985, respectively, destroy the CD4$^+$ T-helper lymphocytes that form an essential compo-nent of the body's cell-mediated immune defence system against a wide spectrum of pathogens. Their destruction leaves an individual open to the growth of organisms that, normally absent or simply commensal, have proved to be opportunistic pathogens. The end result is AIDS. In 1990 WHO experts estimated that, by the year 2000, about 18.3 million people would be infected worldwide. In fact, by the end of 1999, 34.3 million people were estimated to have HIV/AIDS (*see* **776**), of whom 24.5 million were in Sub-Saharan Africa. Deaths from HIV/AIDS from 1980 to the end of 1999 were estimated at 18.8 million, of which 14.8 million were in people living in this region. Some 13.2 million orphans have been created. Southeast Asia and the Far East are now in the line of fire.

VIRAL INFECTIONS

ACQUIRED IMMUNODEFICIENCY SYNDROME (HIV, AIDS)

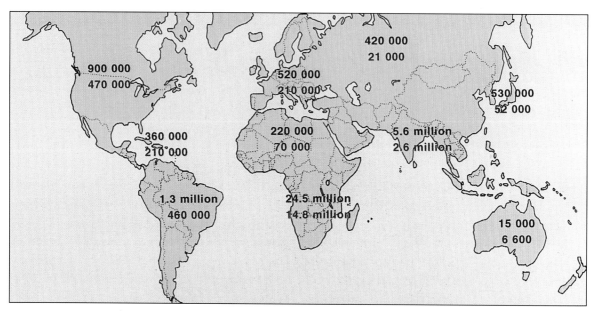

776 Prevalence of HIV/AIDS and mortality in adults and children

The human immunodeficiency viruses, HIV1 and HIV2, have assumed pandemic proportions since their first recognition in the 1980s. Although HIV1 was first identified as the cause of AIDS in homosexual males in Haiti, the USA and Europe, the virus is thought to have originated in Central Africa, where transmission is essentially heterosexual. Infection spread (possibly with migrant workers) to Haiti, from where it passed to the USA and direct to Europe. From Haiti, HIV1 is believed to have been carried mainly by male homosexuals to Europe and Australasia. Its routes of spread to Latin America were probably from the Caribbean and North America, and to Asia from Europe. Heterosexual transmission is now increasing in most countries. The virus is spreading rapidly through Thailand, India and parts of China. Some of the highest prevalence rates now occur in the countries of southern Africa where, for example, in Botswana in 1998, between 39 and 50% of all women attending antenatal care clinics were HIV positive. In parts of Central and East Africa especially, the AIDS epidemic caused mainly by HIV1 has already led to a devastating loss of life among adults, both old and young, whereas transmission from infected mothers to their infants is producing a rapidly escalating mortality among the youngest age groups. HIV2 has remained essentially an infection of West Africa. The map shows estimates made of the prevalence of HIV/AIDS at the end of 1999 (*blue*) and of the cumulative numbers of deaths (*red*) from the beginning of the pandemic in 1980 to that date. The most dramatic increase has been in Sub-Saharan Africa in some parts of which up to 36% of adults are infected with HIV. (Based on data from UNAIDS, 2000.)

Table 21 Common opportunistic infections and neoplasms associated with HIV/AIDS

Pathogen or neoplasm	Main syndromes	Relative frequency	
		HIV + patients in Africa	Others
VIRUSES			
Herpes simplex viruses	mucocutaneous lesions	+	+++
Cytomegalovirus	chorioretinitis, pneumonia, hepatitis, colitis, adrenalitis, disseminated infection	+	+++
Varicella zoster	primary varicella, local or disseminated herpes zoster	+++	++
Papovavirus (JC virus)	progressive multifocal leucoencephalopathy (PML)	+	+
? viral origin	hairy leucoplakia	++	++
BACTERIA			
Mycobacterium tuberculosis	pneumonia, disseminated tuberculosis	+++	++
M. avium-intracellulare	enteritis, disseminated infection	+	+++
Pneumococcus	pneumonia	+++	+++
Non-typhoid *Salmonella*	bacteraemia	+++	+
FUNGI			
Candida albicans	oropharyngitis, oesophagitis	+++	+++
Cryptococcus neoformans	meningitis, pneumonia, disseminated infection	++	++
Histoplasma capsulatum	disseminated histoplasmosis	++	+
Pneumocystis carinii	pneumonia	+	+++
PROTOZOA			
Toxoplasma gondii	encephalitis, brain abscess	+++	+++
Cryptosporidium parvum	enteritis, cholangitis	+++	+++
Isospora belli	enteritis	++	+
Trypanosoma cruzi	meningoencephalitis, myocarditis	–	+
Leishmania infantum	kala-azar	–	+
Encephalitozoon hellem	systemic spread in eye, nose, kidney etc.	?	+
Enterocytozoon bieneusi	enteritis	+	+
Septata intestinalis	systemic organ spread, enteritis	?	+
NEOPLASMS			
Kaposi's sarcoma[1]	mucocutaneous lesions, disseminated lesions in lung, gastrointestinal tract, lymph nodes, eye	++	++
Non-Hodgkin's lymphoma[2]	visceral and cerebral lymphoma	+	++
Squamous cell carcinoma of conjunctiva		+	–

[1] Associated with herpesvirus 8.
[2] Epstein–Barr virus is strongly associated with non-Hodgkin's lymphoma.
+, ++ and +++ indicate the relative, but not actual, frequencies of these conditions.

777 Human immunodeficiency virus

HIV1 is the major aetiological agent of AIDS. This type C retrovirus, formerly known as HTLV-III (human T-lymphotropic virus type III) or LAV (lymphadenopathy-associated virus), is one of several in the genus *Lentivirus* that grow in mammalian T cells. HIV1 is related to HIV2 (formerly known as HTLV-IV or LAV-2), which is found in humans in West Africa, as well as to SIV (the STLV-III group) of African Green monkeys (see 1018) and mangabeys. HIV1 and HIV2 are spread both by sexual contact and by the injection of virus in blood or blood products. The effect of the virus is to destroy the host's CD4+ helper T cells progressively. The fully developed 'acquired immune deficiency syndrome' (AIDS) produces death from a multiplicity of opportunistic infections (whether viral, bacterial, fungal or parasitic) or neoplasms. In southwest Europe, for example, between 1990 and 1998, 1440 cases of *Leishmania*/HIV co-infection (94% of them visceral) were reported to the WHO, 835 of them from Spain. Specific antiviral chemotherapy has made major advances but is still incapable of eradicating infection. Where used, specific antiviral

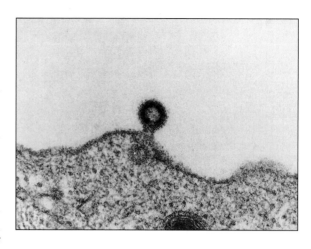

chemotherapy has dramatically reduced some of the secondary opportunistic infections that occur (see **Table 21**). The budding HIV1 particle seen here is growing in a lymphocyte cell line. (× *130 000*.)

778 Mature HIV particle in a cellular vacuole
(× *200 000*.)

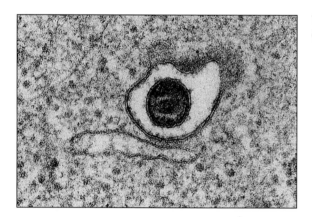

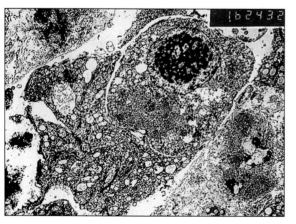

779 Cytomegalovirus in a human hepatocyte

This virus is the cause of death in up to 30% of patients with AIDS in the USA but, in contrast to Caucasians, is relatively uncommon as a cause of serious pathological changes in Africans. One of the herpesvirus group, it is present in the tissues of most normal adults, becoming pathogenic only in immunocompromised subjects in whom it can cause chorioretinitis, viral pneumonia, hepatitis or colitis among other conditions. (× *1500*.)

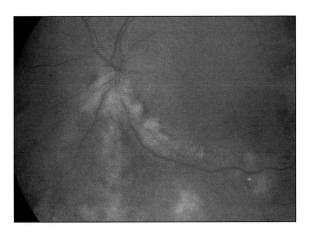

780 Cytomegalovirus chorioretinitis in AIDS

Extensive pathological changes caused by cytomegalovirus, such as those seen here, are relatively common in Caucasians. The retinal swelling, haemorrhages and necrosis that follow viral-induced retinal vasculitis are typical of this condition.

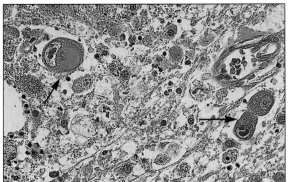

781 Cytalomegalovirus encephalitis

Large numbers of viral particles accumulating in the nuclei of enlarged infected cells, give rise to these dense, usually single, 'owl's eye' inclusions (arrows). (*H&E × 200*.)

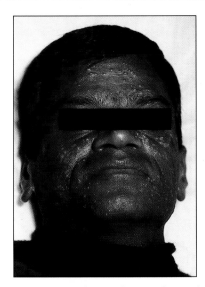

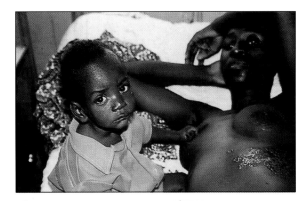

782 Molluscum contagiosum in a patient with AIDS

The numerous lesions with the classic umbilicated appearance seen here bear a superficial resemblance to those caused by smallpox. The condition is caused by infection with a DNA pox virus, which is spread by direct person-to-person contact and by fomites. Molluscum contagiosum can be extensive, as shown in this patient who is immuno-suppressed with HIV infection.

783 Perinatal transmission of AIDS

The virus in African communities, unlike the usual situation in other areas, is transmitted mainly by heterosexual contact, perinatally from infected mothers and by parenteral infection from contaminated blood in transfusions or dirty syringes. This woman with advanced AIDS had severe herpes zoster lesions. Her infant was also HIV positive.

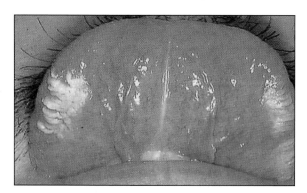

784 Hairy leucoplakia

This condition, which is possibly due to Epstein–Barr infection, consists of hairy projections of keratinised squamous epithelium along the sides of the tongue. It is commonly seen in AIDS.

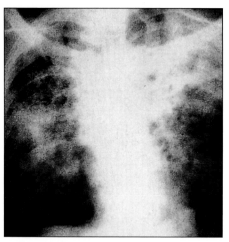

785 Advanced tuberculosis in AIDS

The HIV pandemic is responsible for a serious resurgence of tuberculosis in the Western World, as well as in the tropics and subtropics. Severe post primary pulmonary tuberculosis, such as that seen here, is common in AIDS patients, particularly in Africa.

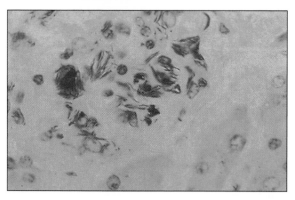

786 Hepatic infection with *Mycobacterium avium-intracellulare*

Foamy histiocytes filled with acid-fast bacilli are seen in a hepatic granuloma. Chronic inflammatory infection with this 'atypical' *Mycobacterium* and infection of various organs (e.g. the gastrointestinal tract) with other organisms in this group, is particularly common in the terminal phase of the AIDS illness. Paradoxically, no clear interaction has been detected so far between *M. leprae* and HIV infection. (*Kinyoun* × 1800.)

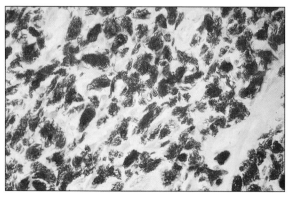

787 Atypical mycobacterial infection of the small bowel of a patient with HIV

The auramine stain shows masses of acid-fast bacilli which, on culture, were shown to be of the *Mycobacterium avium* complex, in this case *M. intracellulare*. (× 750.)

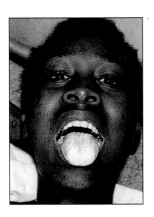

788 Oral candidiasis in an African man with AIDS
This patient with 'slim disease' (see **802**) had a very heavy *Candida albicans* infection of his buccal cavity.

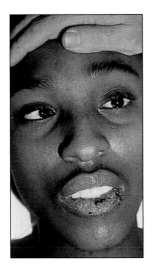

789 Cryptococcal meningitis in AIDS
Cryptococcus neoformans is an increasingly important concomitant pathogen in patients with AIDS in tropical areas. This HIV positive Zimbabwean man with cryptococcal meningitis has a left-sided abducent nerve paralysis. (© D.A. Warrell.)

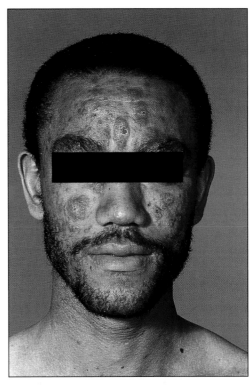

790 Cutaneous histoplasmosis
The typical lesions of cutaneous histoplasmosis are shown in this individual with HIV infection who came from the Carribean. *Histoplasma capsulatum* is a dimorphic fungus existing as a mould in organic matter and as a yeast in tissue. Disseminated infection occurs especially in the immunosuppressed

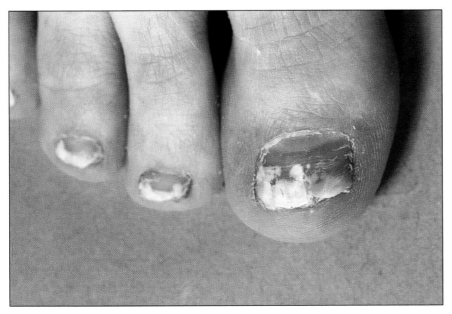

791 Onychomycosis (Tinea unguium) in an HIV positive patient
Fungal infection of the toe nails is most commonly caused by *Trichophyton rubrum*. In this individual who had been treated with zidovudine but no antifungal for four weeks, some clearing of the infection in the proximal toe nail, with residual distal infection, may be seen.

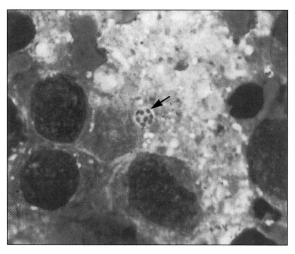

792 *Pneumocystis carinii* in lung smear
This organism, which is present as a commensal in many animals, is an opportunistic parasite in humans. It produces eight-nucleated cysts, which can be seen in smears of pulmonary aspirates (*Giemsa* × 2500). (*See also* **917**.)

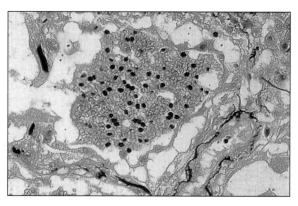

794 Silver stain of section of lung biopsy sample
The encysted *Pneumocystis carinii* is seen as black objects in the foamy exudate that fills the alveoli. (*Grocott stain* × 200.)

795 Magnetic resonance image in advanced cerebral toxoplasmosis
Encephalitis and brain abscess are common in AIDS. Typical changes with central necrotic areas surrounded by swollen, oedematous brain tissue are clearly visible here. Magnetic resonance imaging is even more sensitive than computed tomography for the detection of very early lesions.

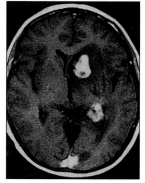

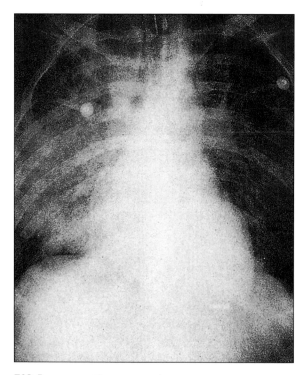

793 *Pneumocystis* pneumonia
Prior to the use of pneumocystis prophylaxis and highly active, antiretroviral treatment (HAART) in the Western World, but less so in Africa, massive pulmonary infection with pneumocystis was the commonest presenting opportunistic infection in patients with AIDS.

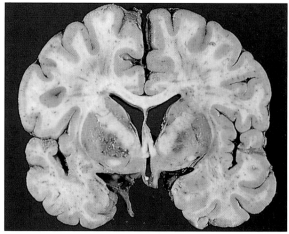

796 Gross appearance of cerebral toxoplasmosis at post mortem examination
Brain from a 33-year-old male with *Pneumocystis* pneumonia who died two months after manifesting neurological symptoms. This coronal section shows haemorrhagic foci in the white matter of the frontal gyrus, nucleus caudatum and putamen.

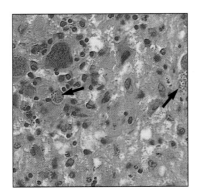

797 Toxoplasmal encephalitis

Several cysts (arrows) are seen in this section of brain from a patient with AIDS who died with acute encephalitis due to toxoplasmosis. This coccidian infection contributes to death in 15% or more of HIV-infected individuals worldwide. (*H&E × 250.*)

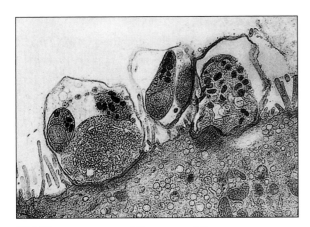

798 Ultrastructure of *Cryptosporidium*

In individuals with HIV infection, the existence of large numbers of *Cryptosporidium* on the surface of the intestinal mucosa can cause intractable, profuse, watery diarrhoea and weight loss. This coccidial infection is a major contributor to death in about 7% of people with AIDS in Western countries. The organisms in different stages of schizogony are seen surrounded by a membrane of host-cell origin in this electron micrograph, giving the parasites the false appearance of being extracellular. The section is from a biopsy of rectal mucosa from one of the earliest known patients with AIDS, who had lived in Zaïre. The parasites can colonise any part of the intestine from the pharynx to the rectum. The source of infection and the species of *Cryptosporidium* responsible for human infection are still unknown. (× 7500.)

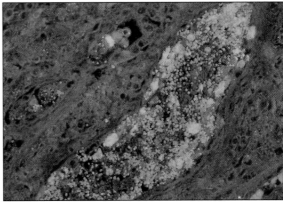

799 *Enterocytozoon hellem* in a kidney

Disseminated infection with this microsporidian in patients with AIDS can involve organs such as the kidneys, eyes or lungs. This section of kidney shows heavy infestation with *E. hellem* in a patient whose urine also contained numerous spores. (*IFA × 400.*)

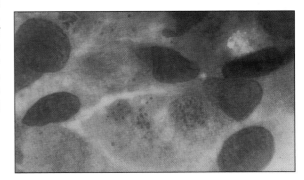

800 *Enterocytozoon bieneusi* in enterocytes

Three groups of encapsulated spores are present in this smear from a duodenal biopsy from a 35-year-old male AIDS patient with chronic diarrhoea. He subsequently developed generalised Kaposi's sarcoma from which he died. (*Giemsa × 300.*)

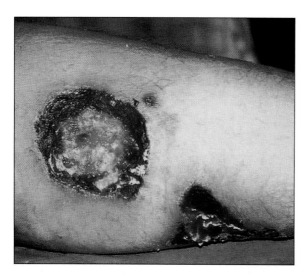

801 *Acanthamoeba castellanii* infection of the skin
Chronic ulceration with species of these facultatively pathogenic amoebae is seen in some patients with severe immunodeficiency such as that associated with AIDS. This 35-year-old man who presented with wasting and fever due to *Escherichia coli* septicaemia had a previous history of episodes of *Pneumocystis carinii* pneumonia and toxoplasmal encephalitis. During hospitalisation, two skin lesions appeared on the right arm and the left leg. Four months later, when the patient died of primary brain lymphoma, cutaneous lesions were present on all parts of his body. (*See also* **889**.)

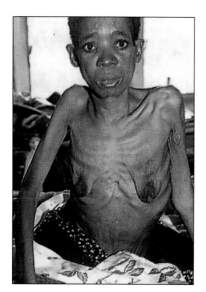

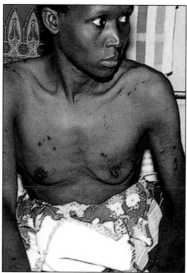

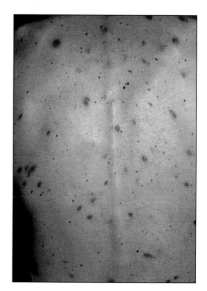

802 'Slim disease' in a 25-year-old African woman
This condition, which is the result of chronic diarrhoea that may be caused by *Cryptosporidium parvum* or other opportunistic intestinal parasites, is now recognised to be associated also with fulminating tuberculosis. Gross weight loss and a severe, itchy skin rash are characteristic of the condition, which is usually preterminal.

803 Kaposi's sarcoma in an African woman
Many patients with AIDS develop disseminated Kaposi's sarcoma thought to be due to human herpesvirus 8. In most patients with AIDS, the terminal stages are accompanied by a plethora of different infections. (*See also* **1034**.)

804 Generalised cutaneous Kaposi's sarcoma
This condition is common in patients of all racial origins. Unlike classic Kaposi's sarcoma previously seen in Africa, it is not restricted to the lower limb and may involve the internal organs, especially the gastrointestinal tract and lungs. It is often accompanied by lesions of the mucous membranes.

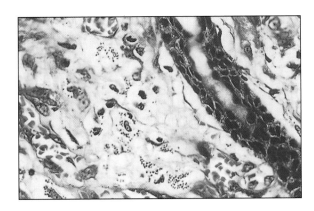

805 Biopsy of Kaposi's sarcoma in association with *Leishmania*
Large numbers of amastigotes were found in this section of a Kaposi's sarcoma lesion removed from the leg of a 35-year-old HIV positive male. The leishmanial infection, which was probably acquired in Greece, was identified as *L. infantum*. The man, who was afebrile, had an enlarged liver and spleen. Cryptic infection with this protozoan parasite often becomes activated in immunodeficient individuals. (*Giemsa–colophonium* × *350.*)

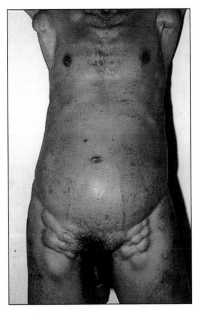

806 Non-Hodgkin's lymphoma
Visceral and cerebral lymphomas of this type are a fairly common feature in AIDS. This man had massive axillary and inguinal lymphadenopathy with gross hepatosplenomegaly and ascites.

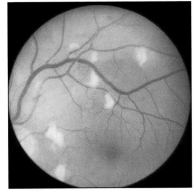

807 HIV-induced retinopathy
Any organism such as cytomegalovirus, *Toxoplasma gondii*, *Herpes simplex* virus and *Varicella zoster* virus can affect the eyes of HIV-infected individuals. This particular view shows the retinopathy caused by the HIV virus itself.

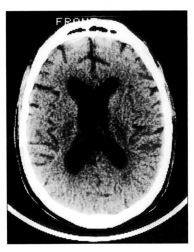

808 Cerebral atrophy in HIV infection
Numerous infections of the central nervous system can occur in HIV such as toxoplasmosis, cryptococcosis and progressive multifocal leucencephalopathy. This computed tomogram shows cerebral atrophy in a patient who presented with dementia, which was shown at post mortem examination to be due to the HIV virus itself. (*See* **Table 21**.)

BACTERIAL INFECTIONS

LYMPHOGRANULOMA VENEREUM (LYPHOGRANULOMA INGUINALE, CLIMACTIC BUBO, ESTHIOMÈNE)

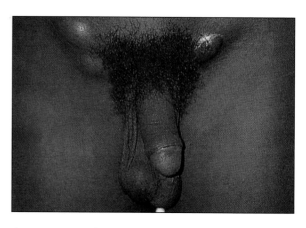

809 Inguinal adenitis

Lymphogranuloma venereum is a venereally transmitted infection due to L1, L2 and L3 serovars of *Chlamydia trachomatis*. It is particularly common in tropical countries but rare elsewhere. Inguinal lymphadenitis is a common feature, resulting in a large, sausage-shaped mass, over which the skin is shiny and purplish in colour. The intracytoplasmic elementary bodies can be identified in cultures made from the lesions (if necessary by aspiration of the bubos) and stained by Giemsa or monoclonal antibodies (see **839**). Serious genitoanorectal lesions can result from this infection. Formerly, the Frei test (a delayed hypersensitivity skin reaction) was of value in the diagnosis. Unfortunately it is used rarely now, as the antigen is no longer marketed; this renders an accurate diagnosis difficult other than on clinical grounds since an enzyme-linked immunosorbent assay based on the use of a specific monoclonal antibody is not yet available, and other laboratory diagnostic techniques are expensive.

CHANCROID (SOFT CHANCRE, ULCUS MOLLE)

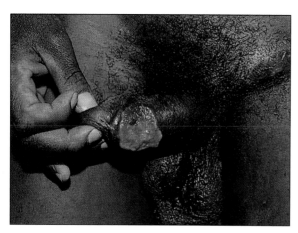

810 Chancroid ulcer of penis with inguinal lymphadenopathy

Chancroid (soft chancre, 'ulcus molle') is a venereal condition caused by *Haemophilus ducreyi*. It occurs most commonly among the poorer populations of developing countries among whom it is the commonest cause of genital ulcers. Although it occurs in both sexes it is most commonly observed in males. Papule formation commences after a short incubation period (often from 4–10 days) after exposure, the papule developing into a deep, very painful ulcer associated with inguinal lymphadenopathy. This is also painful and may be bilateral. The buboes may suppurate as seen here. In the female, the lesions, usually on the vulva or cervix, are often asymptomatic. The severe pain helps to differentiate chancroid from lymphogranuloma venereum, granuloma inguinale and syphilis.

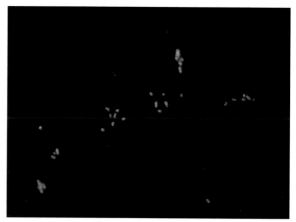

811 Indirect fluorescent antibody test of *Haemophilus ducreyi*

The small, Gram-negative bacteria may be seen on a smear or after cultivation on specialised media. They may also be identified by staining smears with a fluorescein-labelled, specific monoclonal antibody, as seen here. (*IFAT × 300.*)

DONOVANOSIS (GRANULOMA INGUINALE, GRANULOMA VENEREUM)

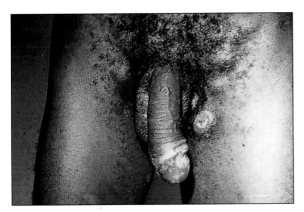

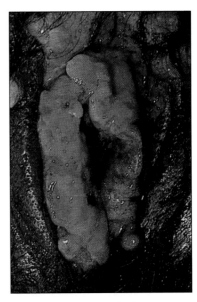

812 Donovanosis of penis and adjacent skin of leg
This venereal infection, which occurs mainly in the tropics and subtropics, is caused by a Gram-negative coccobacillus, *Calymmatobacterium granulomatis*. In the male it produces deep, punched-out ulcers of the penis. These are clean and painless initially but, with secondary bacterial infection, may become covered with a thick, offensive, purulent exudate and develop a marked granulomatous reaction; such lesions are painful. As seen here, secondary ulceration may appear on adjacent skin.

813 Donovanosis of female genitalia
The disease runs a very chronic course. As in lymphogranuloma venereum, mutilating ulceration of the genitalia may occur, and anorectal involvement is common. In comparison with lymphogranuloma venereum, the lymphatics are not primarily involved.

814 Donovan bodies in exudate
The encapsulated coccobacilli of *Calymmatobacterium granulomatosis* can be seen in Romanowsky-stained smears within the cytoplasm of macrophages. These are the so-called 'Donovan bodies' in which the bipolar staining gives the appearance of a closed safety pin. (*Wright–Giemsa* × 650.)

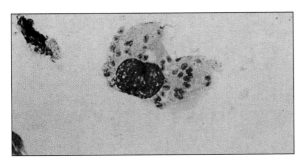

GONORRHOEA

815 Urethral discharge in gonorrhoea
Although gonorrhoea is prevalent worldwide, it is especially widespread in the tropics, where between 4 and 10% of the population may be infected. Chronic gonococcal salpingitis is a common cause of infertility in women. Gonorrheal urethral strictures are often seen in men.

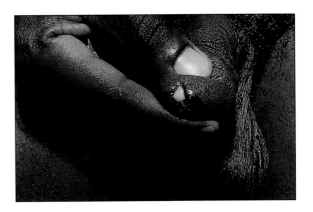

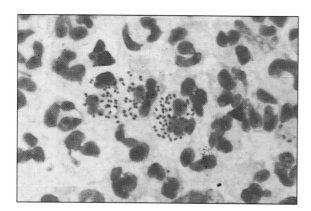

816 *Neisseria gonorrhoeae* in urethral exudate
The Gram-negative diplococci are readily seen in smears of the purulent exudate in the cytoplasm of polymorphs. (*Gram × 900.*)

SYPHILIS

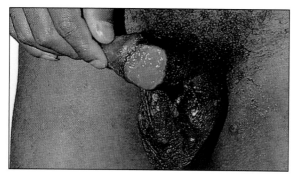

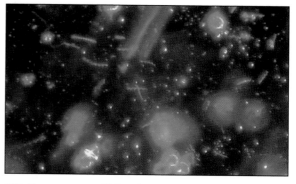

819 'Corona veneris' of secondary syphilis
Discoid lesions may develop on the face and head in secondary syphilis. The condition seen in this man is known as 'corona veneris.'

817 Primary syphilitic chancre and secondary rash
Syphilis, the venereally transmitted treponematosis caused by *Treponema pallidum*, is widespread in many parts of the tropics, but did not occur where yaws was endemic. The figure shows a typical primary chancre with associated secondary rash on the scrotal and abdominal skin. In contrast to chancroid, the primary chancre is painless and usually has a clean base and a rolled edge.

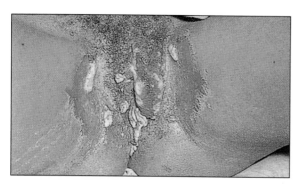

820 *Treponema pallidum* in dark-field microscopy
The spirochaetes can usually be seen in scrapings from serous fluid exuding from the chancre by simple dark-field examination. Their detection is facilitated by the use of a direct fluorescent antibody test for *T. pallidum*. The DFA-TP employs a fluorescein-labelled anti-*T. pallidum* globulin. (× *400.*)

818 Secondary syphilitic condylomata in the female
The condition is readily diagnosed by the demonstration of spirochaetes in a dark-field preparation. Late complications may be cardiovascular, gummatous or meningovascular.

PROTOZOAL INFECTIONS

(*See also* **Table 18**.)

TRICHOMONIASIS

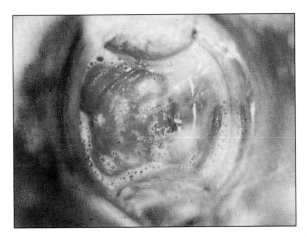

821 Vaginitis due to *Trichomonas vaginalis*

It has been estimated that the annual incidence of trichomoniasis in the female is approximately 180 million. Transmission is largely through sexual intercourse, but the infection in the male is often inapparent. The figure shows the typical appearance of vaginitis as seen through a vaginal speculum. Note the foamy, creamy discharge, which is often secondarily infected with *Candida albicans*. The motile, ellipsoid flagellates (*see* **632**) are found readily in the foamy vaginal discharge.

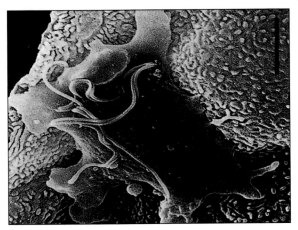

822 *Trichomonas vaginalis* on epithelial cells

When the flagellates make contact with vaginal epithelial cells they rapidly (within a few minutes) transform to a cytoadherent amoeboid form with thin lamellipodia that make multiple contact points with the cells. The axostyle disappears, but the flagella and undulating membrane remain on the free surface. The readiness with which this transformation occurs in different strains is apparently related to their virulence. (*SEM bar = 10 μm*.)

CHAPTER 6

Other Infections Acquired through the Skin and Mucous Membranes

The infective agents include viruses, bacteria, protozoa, helminths and arthropods. In one group, transmission of infection is by direct or indirect contact with contaminated people or objects. In the other group, infection may be acquired by exposure to infected soil (e.g. *Necator americanus*, *see* **Chapter 2**), water (e.g. schistosomiasis, *see* **Chapter 3**; leptospirosis, *see* **595–598**), by the bites of animals (rabies) or through wounds (tetanus).

In the first group are two diseases that are now mainly of historical interest: smallpox and yaws. The smallpox eradication campaign organised by the WHO resulted in the disappearance of the disease, with the last case being recorded in 1977. The virus itself, as far as is known, exists only in two, top security virology laboratories. However, other pox virus infections (e.g. monkeypox) are still present in some African foci. (Conditions associated with human immunodeficiency virus (HIV1) infection, which has attained pandemic proportions since its first identification in 1983, are described in **Chapter 5**.)

Following the mass treatment campaigns with penicillin in the 1950s, yaws is now almost a curiosity, although some cases still do occur (e.g. in the Solomon Islands). The chlamydial infection, trachoma, remains an important blinding disease, although considerable progress in its control has been made, especially in the Middle East. The venereal diseases (*see* **Chapter 5**) are more important in the tropics than has hitherto been appreciated, whereas the non-venereal treponematoses are widely distributed in the world.

The prevalence rate of leprosy in 32 endemic countries was 21.1 per 10 000 population in 1985. In 1991 a plan to eliminate leprosy by the year 2000 was set out by the WHO. A total of 3.1 million cases of leprosy were registered in 1992, a global prevalence of 5.7 per 10 000 people; this was already a distinct improvement over the 5.5 million registered during the previous year. By the start of 2000 the number of registered cases had fallen to 641 000, a global prevalence of only 1.25 per 10 000 people.

In 1989 the goal of eliminating neonatal tetanus by 1997 was established by the WHO, the two main weapons being the vaccination of pregnant women and the provision of clean services for the delivery of their babies. The target date was later postponed to 2000. Although the global numbers of reported cases fell from 510 000 in 1990 to 355 000 in 1997, that target date for the elimination of neonatal tetanus (i.e. less than one case per 1000 live births) could not be realised, and control efforts are now focussed on the countries at highest risk—notably in parts of Africa and Southeast Asia where, in 1997, there were still 95 000 and 86 000 deaths, respectively. Because *Clostridium tetani* is ubiquitous in the environment, the commitment to control neonatal tetanus will inevitably have to remain open ended.

A wide variety of fungi infect skin, hair and nails without deeper penetration of the host tissues.

Other fungi, however, particularly prevalent in the New World, cause deep mycoses that can result in some of the most disfiguring lesions seen in clinical medicine. *Pneumocystis carinii*, a common cause of death in individuals with AIDS, has now been classified among the fungi (*see also* **792–794, 917**).

Among the ectoparasitic arthropods, the cosmopolitan scabies mites, lice and bedbugs are particularly prevalent. Other cosmopolitan species of mites (*see* **Table 23**) that commonly cause local and/or systemic pathological changes are especially likely to be encountered in a tropical environment and are therefore considered here. Tungiasis is a major problem in many tropical areas. Although the myiases are rare and can be very serious or even lethal, the larvae of one species of fly are returning to favour as cleansers of contaminated wounds (*see* **949**).

VIRAL INFECTIONS

SMALLPOX

Twenty five years ago, smallpox was endemic in many tropical countries. The distribution of the rash, which was centrifugal and concentrated on the face, hands and feet, was accompanied by marked toxicity and left severe scarring ('pockmarks') in those who survived. Following a successful smallpox eradication campaign organised under the auspices of the WHO, this disease has now been eradicated, and vaccination is no longer carried out. As far as is known, the only *Variola major* virus surviving is in two top security virology research laboratories.

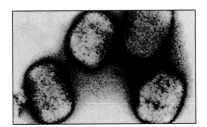

823 Ultrastructure of smallpox virus
One of the orthopox viruses, *Variola major* is a large, ovoid double-stranded DNA virus, which could readily be identified in fluid from the cutaneous lesions. (× 63 000.)

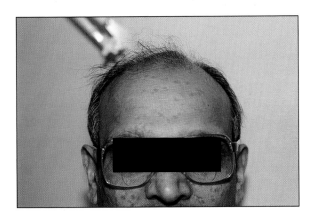

824 Residual scars ('pockmarks') of smallpox
Residual scarring is an unmistakable sign of past smallpox infection. The infection had a high mortality, and those who survived often had severe scars ('pockmarks'), as shown in this Indian man. The lesions, unlike those of chickenpox, were peripheral and appeared as a single crop.

ORF

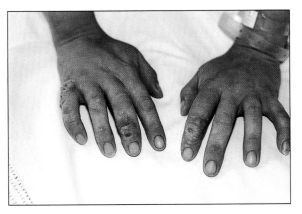

825 Bilateral digital lesions of orf ('contagious pustular dermatitis')
This infection of worldwide distribution is caused by a DNA parapox virus and is usually seen in people working in the meat industry. Two lesions are seen here on the fingers of an abbatoir worker who became infected from newly born lambs. Infection is acquired from the mouth and nose of sheep and goats. After an incubation period of three to four days, a macular rash develops, which turns papular or nodular and then passes through several stages until it slowly regresses. The entire process takes about 35 days. Treatment is symptomatic. A closely related poxvirus is responsible for the skin condition known as molluscum contagiosum (see **782**).

MONKEYPOX

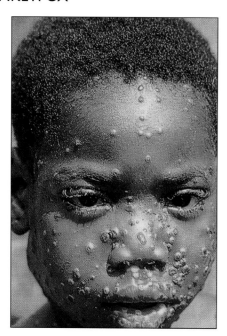

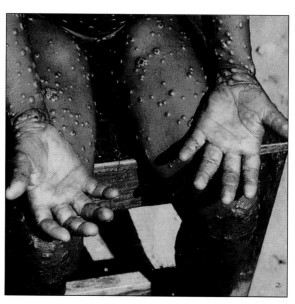

826 & 827 Rash of monkeypox

This zoonotic infection, caused by an orthopox virus morphologically indistinguishable from that of smallpox, produces a relatively benign infection in humans in parts of the tropical rain forest areas of West and Central Africa. The rash is very similar to that of smallpox. This seven-year-old girl from central Zaire showed large numbers of papules (some forming pustules) on the trunk, head (including eyelids and tongue) (**826**, left), extremities (including the palms and soles) and external genitalia. Marked cervical and inguinal lymphadenopathy (**827**, right), typical of monkeypox, can also be seen. Infection is acquired by handling or eating infected monkeys. The lesions in most patients heal within two weeks, leaving no complications. Secondary human to human transmission is unusual, and epidemics are not recorded. As smallpox vaccination gave cross protection against monkeypox but is no longer deployed, it is possible that cases of monkeypox will now increase.

VARICELLA

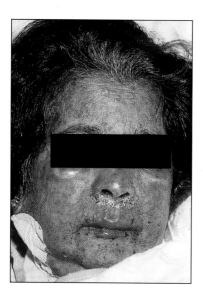

828 Fulminating varicella (chickenpox) with encephalopathy

Although the pock-like lesions of varicella bear some resemblance to those of smallpox and monkeypox, the varicella zoster virus belongs to the alpha subfamily of *Herpesviridae*. Severe infections, especially in adults such as the Sri Lankan patient seen here, may be complicated by encephalitis, pneumonitis and hepatitis. Herpes zoster (shingles) is usually seen in adults and may be especially severe in patients with HIV infection (see **783**).

RABIES

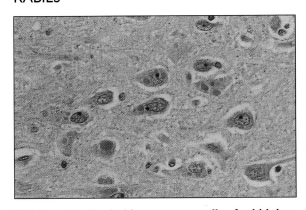

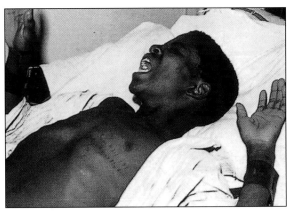

829 Negri bodies in hippocampus cells of rabid dog
Rabies is a zoonotic disease of the nervous system caused by infection with a bullet-shaped RNA rhabdovirus. Although the dog, and to a lesser extent the cat, is the main urban transmitter of infection, foxes and other feline species, as well as vampire bats, are natural hosts and may also transmit the disease to humans. Intracytoplasmic inclusion bodies ('Negri bodies') in brain cells are pathognomonic of rabies. Rabies can be prevented by pre-exposure or rapid post-exposure vaccination. However, the established clinical condition is invariably fatal. (*H&E × 200*.)

830 'Furious rabies'
A 14-year-old Nigerian boy with hydrophobia following dog bites on the wrist and knee. Inspiratory spasms occurred spontaneously or were induced by the sight of water. The condition developed despite his receiving a 14-day course of anti-rabies vaccine. (© D.A. Warrell.)

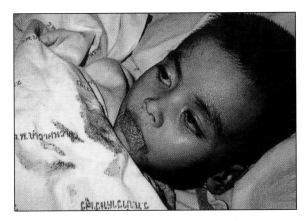

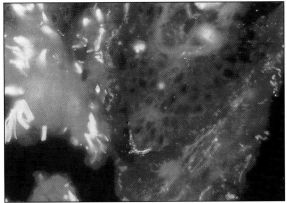

831 Autonomic nervous disorders in rabies
Hypersalivation, profuse sweating due to autonomic nervous system lesions and haematemesis characterised the infection in this Thai boy. (© D.A. Warrell.)

832 Fluorescent antibody staining of rabies virus
The presence of virus may sometimes be detected with the aid of a fluorescent antibody in a biopsy of the corneal epithelium during the incubation period. Here a nerve is seen fluorescing bright green in such a specimen. (× 440.)

HERPES SIMPLEX

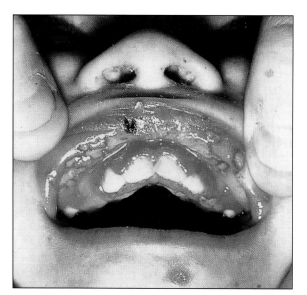

833 Acute herpetic ulcerative gingivostomatitis
This condition, due to herpes simplex virus in children with severe protein-calorie malnutrition, causes a serious illness seen only uncommonly in the developed world.

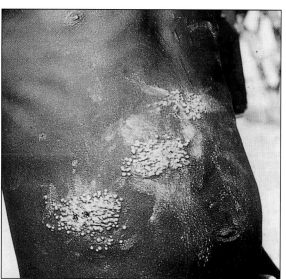

834 Herpes simplex of skin following meningitis
Any debilitating illness that causes a depression of immunity may be followed by an extensive herpetic rash, as in this boy who had recovered from meningococcal meningitis.

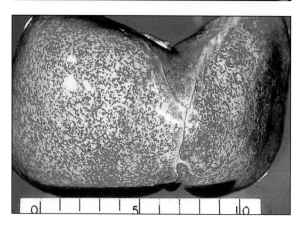

835 Liver in disseminated herpes simplex infection
Disseminated infection may affect the internal organs (e.g. liver, brain, heart, etc.). This complication, which is usually fatal, occurs in patients with AIDS.

BACTERIAL INFECTIONS

CHLAMYDIA TRACHOMATIS INFECTIONS

The genus *Chlamydia* contains three species, of which *C. trachomatis* includes several distinctive groups of serovars. Serovars A, B, Ba and C cause endemic trachoma, B and D–K cause genitourinary disease and L1, L2 and L3 cause lymphogranuloma venereum. *C. psittaci* is the agent of avian (and occasionally human) ornithosis, whereas *C. pneumoniae* is a respiratory pathogen. The pathogens invade host cells as infectious elementary bodies, which develop within phagosomes into reticulate bodies. These, in turn, replicate and then condense into the familiar elementary bodies, which eventually erupt to release a new generation of infective elementary bodies.

Trachoma

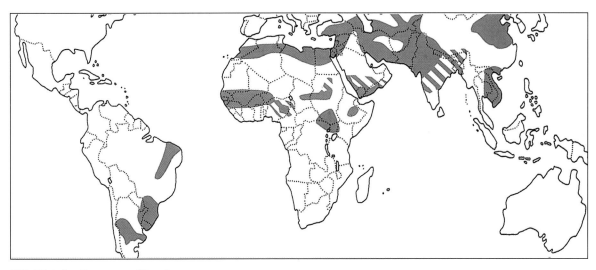

836 Distribution map of trachoma
Trachoma is particularly common in the Middle East and Africa, as well as in other parts of the tropics. The infection is spread both by contact with infective material via soiled hands, clothing, etc., and by flies that feed on lachrymal fluids. Prevention must include improved health education and the use of appropriate antibiotics. (Solid colour on the figure indicates high incidence, lines indicate lower incidence.)

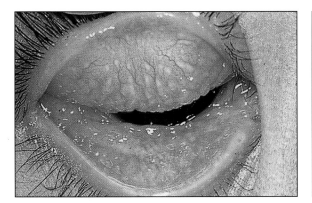

837 Early lesions of trachoma
Small, pinhead-sized, pale follicles beneath the epithelium over the tarsal plates, especially in the upper lid, are a characteristic feature of the disease. The infective agents may be identified in epithelial scrapings at this stage and up to the time scarring commences.

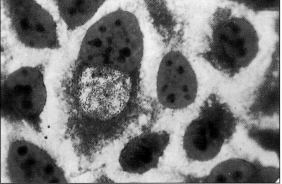

838 Granular inclusion bodies of *Chlamydia trachomatis*
Giemsa-staining demonstrates the typical granular appearance of groups of elementary bodies in this cell monolayer. (*Giemsa × 660.*)

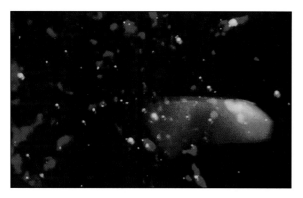

839 Direct immunofluorescence of *Chlamydia trachomatis*
The use of a specific monoclonal antibody facilitates the demonstration of the elementary bodies in tissue smears. (× 590.)

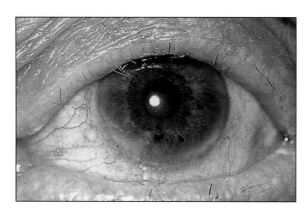

840 Entropion and trichiasis
Scarring of the tarsal plates may be extensive and result in entropion of the edge of the lid. The eyelashes point inwards and rub against the cornea (trichiasis), adding to the damage already done by the virus.

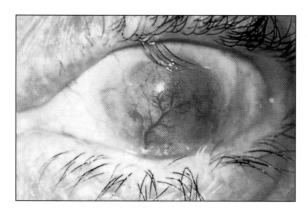

841 Late corneal scarring and trichiasis
The end point of trachoma is often blindness due to corneal scarring and other complications.

LEPROSY

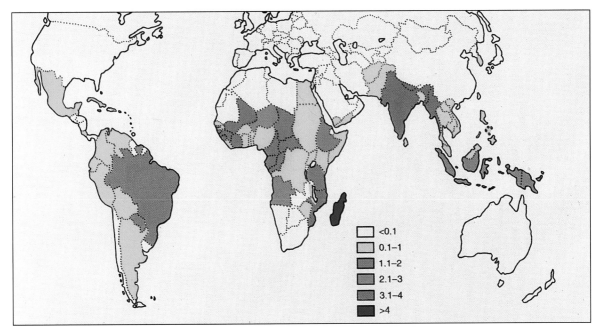

842 Distribution map and prevalence rates of leprosy
The numbers indicate prevalence rates per 10 000 population. The greatest concentration of people infected with leprosy by early 2000 was still in Southeast Asia, which had 77% of the world's cases and a prevalence rate of 4.3 per 10 000 people. The prevalence rates in Africa varied widely from less than two cases per 10 000 population in most of the continent to 4.7 in the worst affected country. Of the Latin American countries, the highest prevalence rate, 4.3 per 10 000 people, was reported from Brazil. Europe, the Eastern Mediterranean and Western Pacific represented only 2.8% of the world total of patients. Hopes are high for the eventual elimination of this disease with the aid of early detection, multiple drug treatment and the prevention of disabilities. Vaccination is still an elusive target. (Adapted from WHO *Map No. 97417* and *WHO Weekly Epidemiological Record* (2000) **75**, 226–231.)

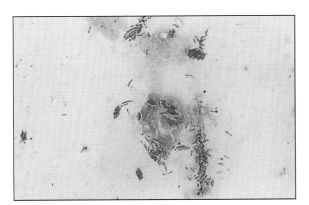

843 *Mycobacterium leprae*
The acid-fast and alcohol-fast bacterial agent of leprosy in a smear preparation. (*Ziehl–Neelsen* × 770.)

Tuberculoid leprosy

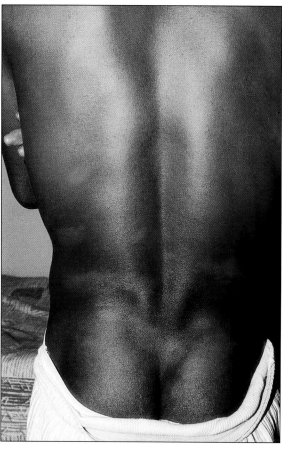

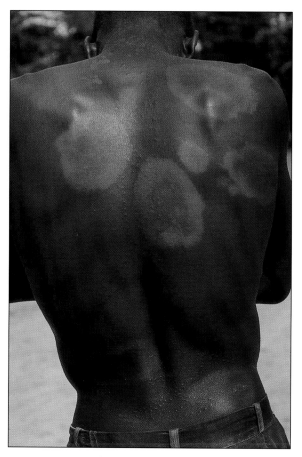

844 Early macules
The disease shows a broad spectrum depending on the patient's immune response, from healing tuberculoid at one pole to non-resolving lepromatous at the other. These responses are reflected in the histopathological picture (*see* **861–863**). An early sign of leprosy, the *indeterminate* macule, is slightly hypopigmented and ill defined. It retains tactile sensitivity, sweating function and hair growth.

845 Tuberculoid leprosy
The early tuberculoid lesion is characterised by macules showing loss of sensation and hypopigmentation.

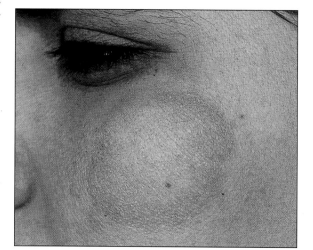

846 Tuberculoid lesion of face
The cooler, peripheral parts of the body are common sites for tuberculoid skin lesions. This patient's face had a large, dry, annular patch that was anaesthetic.

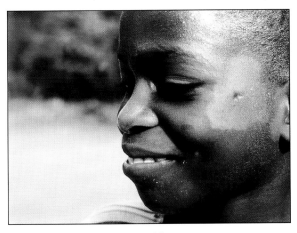

847 Tuberculoid macules of face
A large, depigmented macule with a small necrotic centre and a smaller, preauricular lesion are seen on this West African boy.

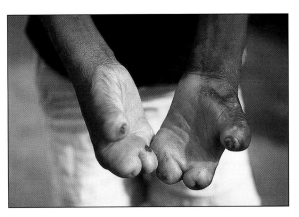

850 Loss of extremities in late tuberculoid leprosy
Neurotrophic atrophy eventually leads to the loss of phalanges, especially following trauma resulting from the anaesthesia. The hands, as seen in this Liberian man, or feet may be affected.

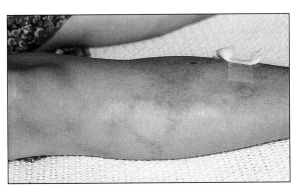

848 Borderline (dimorphous) leprosy
The skin lesions on the right shin of a patient who presented with a depigmented hypoanaesthetic patch with an erythematous periphery.

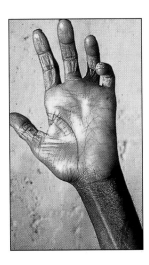

849 Bilateral ulnar nerve lesions
Damage to the ulnar nerve in tuberculoid leprosy leads to weakness and wasting, followed by complete paralysis and atrophy of the ulnar-innervated hand muscles, resulting in the characteristic picture of the 'main de prédicateur.'

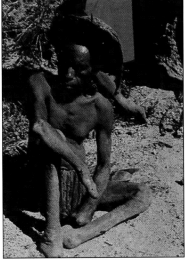

851 Total deformity in late tuberculoid leprosy
This New Guinea highlander had completely lost his hands and feet and was totally incapacitated.

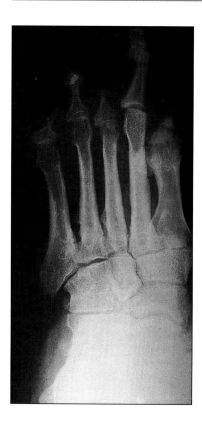

852 Atrophy of toes in tuberculoid leprosy
The partial loss of the bony structures of the toes can be seen in this radiograph of a patient with advanced tuberculoid lesions.

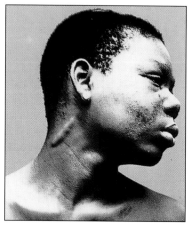

853 Nerve thickening
Thickening of the great auricular nerve is a common feature in tuberculoid leprosy.

Lepromatous leprosy

854 Early lepromatous leprosy
This adult female patient has numerous, small, lepromatous nodules on the face.

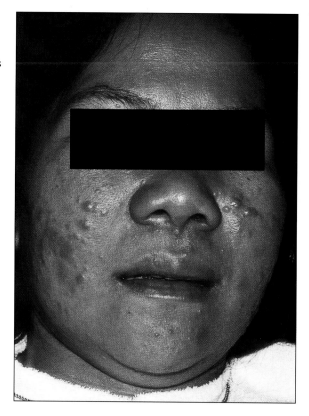

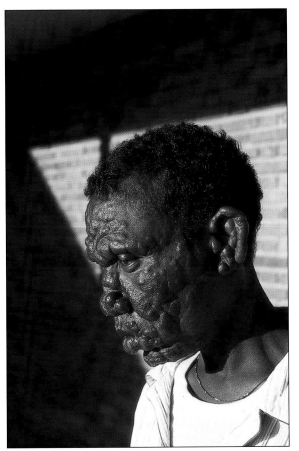

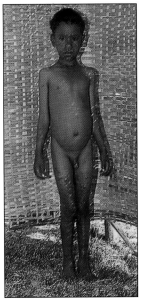

857 Young boy with lepromatous leprosy
This Ethiopian youngster had multiple nodules on the face and extremities, including the penis, but his trunk was clear.

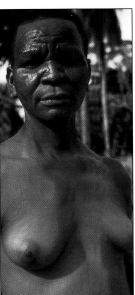

858 Gynaecomastia in leprosy
This condition, which is relatively common in adult males with long-standing lepromatous leprosy, follows testicular atrophy.

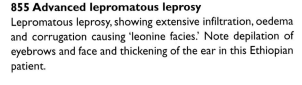

855 Advanced lepromatous leprosy
Lepromatous leprosy, showing extensive infiltration, oedema and corrugation causing 'leonine facies.' Note depilation of eyebrows and face and thickening of the ear in this Ethiopian patient.

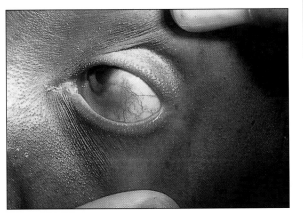

856 Lepromatous nodule in eye
Leprosy is a common cause of blindness in the tropics.

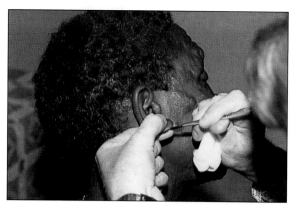

859 Preparation of skin smear
A biopsy is taken from a nodule and smeared for staining with Ziehl–Neelsen stain (*see* **843**).

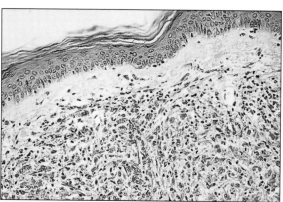

860 Organisms in skin biopsy stained by TRIFF method
Mycobacterium leprae is readily seen, staining deep red in skin sections stained by this method (*TRIFF* × *150*). In dubious cases, the application of polymerase chain reaction can be useful in confirming the presence of bacterial DNA.

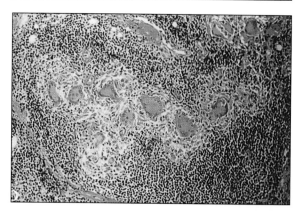

861 Histopathology of active tuberculoid leprosy
The presence in this biopsy of granulomata containing numerous epithelioid cells and Langhans' giant cells is characteristic of the healing response in cases of tuberculoid leprosy. No bacilli are visible. (*H&E* × *30.*)

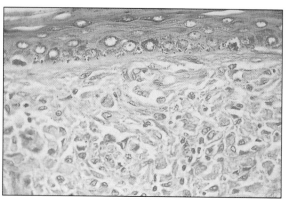

862 Histopathology of lepromatous leprosy
Very large numbers of acid-fast bacilli in vacuolated macrophages are present in this skin biopsy of a nodule from a patient with lepromatous leprosy. The infiltrate does not extend to the basal layer of the skin (*H&E* × *200*). (AFIP No. 74–2725.)

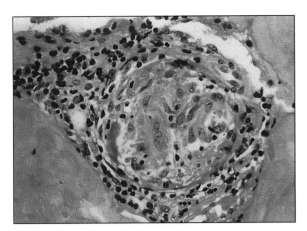

863 Biopsy of nerve in tuberculoid leprosy
Cellular infiltration of the neural sheath leads to destruction of the nerve fibres, resulting in sensory and motor loss in the areas affected. This slide shows an epithelioid granuloma of a nerve. (*H&E* × *200*.)

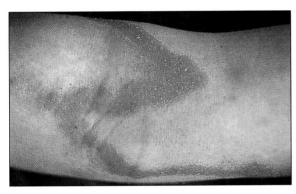

864 Lepromin test
The 'Mitsuda' reaction, which usually attains its maximum in 4–5 weeks, indicates the sensitivity of the patient to the mixture of antigens (prepared from leprosy bacilli) that have been injected. The reaction is expressed in millimetres, with or without ulceration, and is read on about the 21st day after injection. In patients with lepromatous leprosy, the reaction is completely negative. In patients with tuberculoid leprosy, it is variably positive.

MYCOBACTERIUM ULCERANS AND M. MARINUM

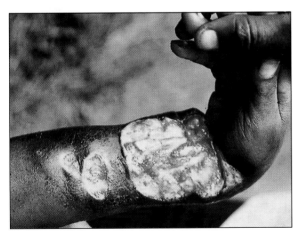

865 Typical 'Buruli' ulcer in a Nigerian child
The condition is characterised by gross, necrotising skin ulcers in which numerous acid-fast bacilli are present (*Mycobacterium ulcerans*). The disease occurs in localised tropical areas in all continents.

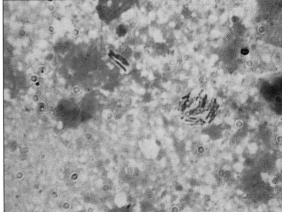

866 *Mycobacterium ulcerans* in section of ulcer
Acellular necrosis occurs involving the dermal layers and subcutaneous fat. Acid-fast bacilli are found in the necrotic material. (*Ziehl–Neelsen* × *1000*.)

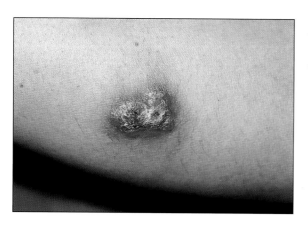

867 'Fishtank granuloma'
The purplish lesion of a patient who kept tropical fish as a hobby. *Mycobacterium marinum* was grown from a biopsy of the chronic, nodular lesion.

OTHER TROPICAL ULCERS

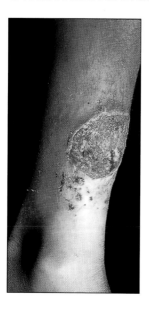

868 Tropical (phagedaenic) ulcer
Chronic necrotising ulcers involving the skin and subcutaneous tissues are common in country areas in the humid tropics. They contain a mixed bacterial flora including *Bacillus fusiformis* and *Treponema vincenti*.

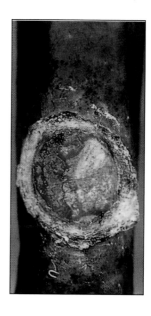

869 Bone involvement in tropical ulcer
Sequestra result when bone involvement occurs, as is seen here.

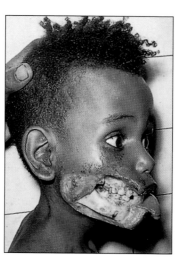

870 Cancrum oris ('Noma')
This gangrenous condition of the facial region associated with poor oral hygiene and the presence of *Treponema vincenti* plus Gram-negative organisms may follow any acute systemic disease (e.g. measles) in malnourished infants in the tropics. Gross disfigurement usually results. Half a million new cases are believed to occur every year.

ANTHRAX

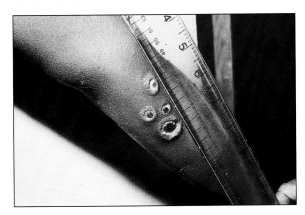

871 Cutaneous anthrax

Four discrete lesions on the arm of an African patient infected with *Bacillus anthracis*. The black eschars are associated with direct inoculation through a break in the skin after contact with infected animal material or from transmission by flies. The lesion is painless without pus but is often surrounded by an arc of oedema and ultimately heals, leaving a scar.

TROPICAL PYOMYOSITIS

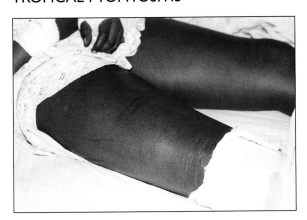

872 Tropical pyomyositis

The right thigh is swollen with infection by *Staphylococcus aureus*. Such infections are common in tropical Africa but uncommon in temperate climates. It is not understood why the organism selects muscle rather than any other tissue in which to multiply. This suppurative muscle infection may occur in as many as 1 per 1000 people in tropical countries.

TETANUS

873 Estimated incidence of neonatal tetanus

Neonatal tetanus remains an especially important infection in several tropical countries where the basic health service infrastructure is still unable to implement the simple measures (vaccination of pregnant women and clean delivery services) on an adequate scale. The figures shown represent the numbers of infant deaths per 1000 live births as estimated in 1992 (based on data from *WHO Weekly Epidemiological Record* 1993, **38**, 279). Reported deaths fell by 39% from 1990 to 248 000 in 1997, but the areas of highest incidence still remained much as shown in this figure by 2000. The greatest decreases have been in the New World where the disease has been eliminated from most countries, in Egypt, North Africa and the Middle East, Myanmar, Sri Lanka, Vietnam, China and Indonesia.

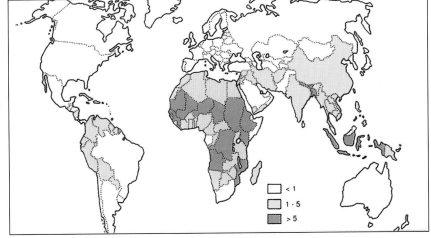

□ < 1
▨ 1 - 5
▥ > 5

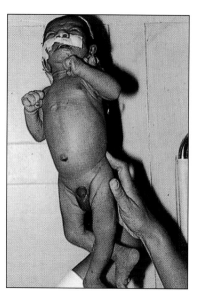

874 Tetanus neonatorum

Infection through the umbilical cord with *Clostridium tetani* is common where poor facilities for childbirth are available. One of the characteristic features is the 'risus sardonicus' resulting from spasms of the facial muscles.

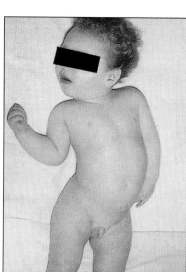

875 Opisthotonos in neonatal tetanus

The generalised muscle contraction leads to arching of the back and limb rigidity; in the conscious patient it is extremely painful and distressing. Urgent treatment with anti-tetanus immunoglobulin, appropriate muscle relaxing agents and, if indicated, positive pressure ventilation are essential. Protection by the immunisation of mothers and improved delivery services has greatly diminished the incidence of neonatal tetanus in developing countries. For example, the number of cases prevented in 1997 has been estimated to be in the order of 1.2 million.

NON-VENEREAL TREPONEMATOSES

(*See also* **Table 4**.)

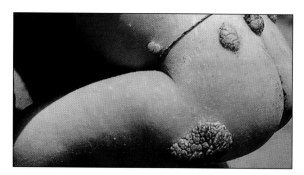

876 Secondary framboesiform yaws

Thanks to the mass, penicillin-based eradication campaign of the 1950s, yaws is now a relatively rare disease in the humid tropics, although a new outbreak was recently recorded in Ghana. This Papuan child shows classic framboesiform lesions, caused by *Treponema pertenue*. Secondary lesions are common also at mucocutaneous junctions.

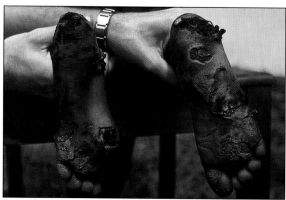

877 Plantar hyperkeratosis

Hyperkeratosis of feet and hands is a common secondary phenomenon in yaws. This man's feet were seriously eroded.

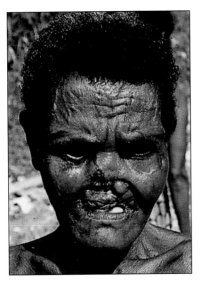

878 Gangosa
The most advanced and destructive lesions affect the maxillary bones and hard palate, resulting in a condition known as 'gangosa.'

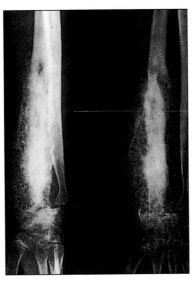

879 Radiograph of forearm with yaws osteitis
Focal cortical rarefaction and periosteal changes are seen, especially in the tibia ('sabre tibia') but also in other long bones.

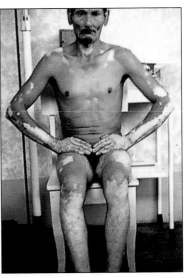

880 Depigmented lesions of Pinta
Pinta is endemic in the New World from Mexico to the Amazon. 'Pintids' start as small papules and develop into plaques with actively growing edges, which become confluent. In the late stages the 'pintids' become depigmented. The causative organism of pinta, *Treponema carateum*, is morphologically indistinguishable from that of syphilis and bejel.

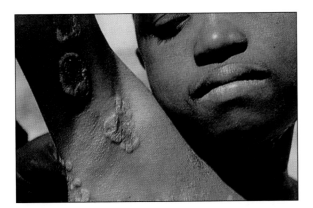

881 Secondary rash in endemic syphilis
These non-venereal spirochaetoses ('endemic syphilis') occur mainly in dry parts of Africa, the Balkans and Australia. A florid, secondary, maculopapular eruption and associated adenitis is usually the first sign. Tertiary complications including gangosa may develop. In the Middle East the condition is known as bejel. Other forms of non-venereal 'endemic syphilis' are njovera (Zimbabwe), skerlievo (Borneo), dichuchwa (Botswana) and siti (Gambia).

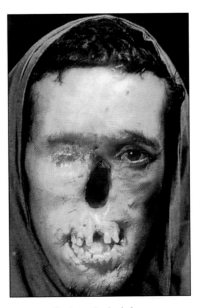

882 Gummatous lesions in bejel
If left untreated, bejel can produce severe, gummatous changes of the bone, cartilage and skin as seen in this unfortunate patient from the Middle East.

PROTOZOAL INFECTIONS

(*See also* **Table 17**.)

INFECTION WITH 'FREE-LIVING' AMOEBAE

(*See* **Table 17**.)

A number of free-living amoebae that are widely distributed in soil and water are also facultative parasites in humans. They are responsible for three disease syndromes: primary amoebic meningoencephalitis (PAM), granulomatous amoebic encephalitis (GAE) and chronic amoebic keratitis (CAK). GAE is seen in immunocompromised individuals.

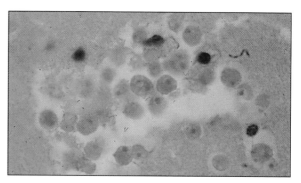

884 *Naegleria fowleri* in the brain of a patient with primary amoebic meningoencephalitis
Numerous trophozoites are seen in this brain section taken at post mortem examination from a patient who died of primary amoebic meningoencephalitis in Texas. (*H&E* × *100*.)

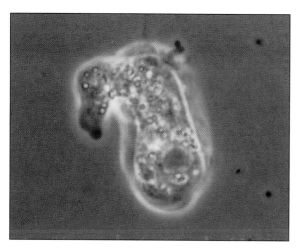

883 Living trophozoite of *Naegleria fowleri*
Several species of *Naegleria* (Vahlkampfiidae) have been incriminated as the causative pathogens of amoebic meningoencephalitis, a condition with a high fatality rate that is usually acquired from bathing in warm water. *N. fowleri* has been isolated from such water in various swimming places, including thermal baths. Infection seems to be acquired through the cribriform plate of the nasal cavity after immersion in contaminated water. As its cysts are susceptible to dessication, its dispersal may be more restricted than that of *Acanthamoeba* species. *N. fowleri* develops a biflagellate form in water. (*Phase contrast* × *1200*.)

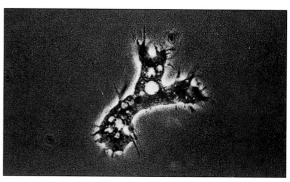

885 Living trophozoite of *Acanthamoeba castellanii*
The 'prickly' appearance of the surface membrane from which these organisms acquire their name is seen clearly; a large vacuole is also present. Various species have been incriminated as the causative agents of granulomatous amoebic encephalitis and infections of the eye (see **886**), with *A. culbertsoni* being the most notorious. The cysts, which are resistant to dessication, are probably airborne (see *also* **801**). (*Phase contrast* × *1000*.)

886 Corneal infection with *Acanthamoeba* species
This condition, previously rare, is increasing with the more frequent use of 'soft' contact lenses. A recent study of contact lens infections revealed *A. polyphaga* in 15 cases and one each of *A. hatchetti* and *A. castellanii* in the series. Over 200 such cases have been reported in the past two decades.

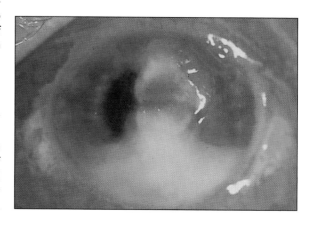

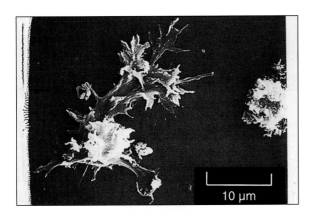

887 Trophozoite of *Balamuthia mandrillaris*

This leptomyxid amoeba was first isolated from a baboon and has since been found in several cases of granulomatous amoebic encephalitis in humans. The patients are always immunodeficient in some way (e.g. through extremes of age or with HIV infection). The living trophozoites in culture are extremely irregular in shape and readily distinguished from those of *Naegleria* or *Acanthamoeba*. (*SEM*)

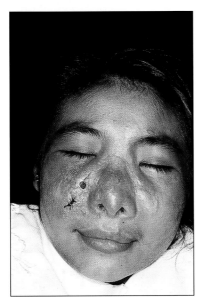

888 *Balamuthia mandrillaris* infection in a Peruvian girl

This girl was believed to have become infected from swimming in ponds in northern Peru. The organism causes a necrotising, granulomatous encephalitis in humans and animals in the New World, as well as in Europe, Australia and possibly Africa (see **889**). Parasites were recovered from the biopsy site seen on the right cheek. A bilateral, granulomatous lesion was present on the face and computed tomography revealed extensive, intracranial masses, which were presumed also to be caused by this pathogen. (© D.A. Warrell.)

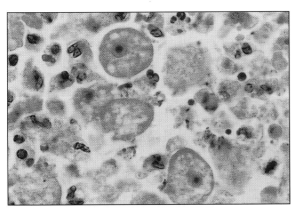

889 Section of brain with granulomatous amoebic encephalitis

This section is from a Zambian patient who died from AIDS. The parasites, which were first believed to be an *Acanthamoeba* species, failed to react with a specific antiserum and are probably attributable to a *B. mandrillaris*. In this section, the nuclear structure of the invasive trophozoites is clearly seen. The amoebae of both *B. mandrillaris* and *Acanthamoeba* species are also quite often found in skin abscesses in patients with AIDS (*H&E × 260*.) (*See also* **801**.)

SUPERFICIAL MYCOSES

(*See* **Table 22**.)

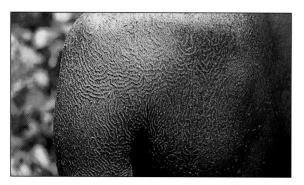

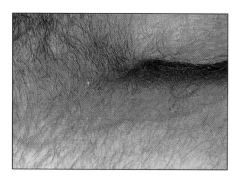

890 Tinea imbricata

Trichophyton concentricum produces characteristic, superficial, scaly lesions in parallel lines and concentric circles. Although it is common in the South Pacific and parts of the Far East, it is occasionally seen in other hot, humid areas.

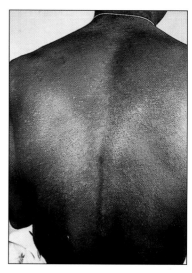

891 Tinea cruris

This infection, which is very common in young males in hot, humid areas, is usually caused by *Epidermophyton floccosum*, *Trichophyton rubrum* or *T. mentagrophytes* var *interdigitale*. The red, slightly raised margin of the lesion in this patient can be seen to be advancing down the inner thigh.

892 Pityriasis versicolor

Infection with *Malassezia furfur* is a common cause of hypopigmentation in dark-skinned young adults. Fluorescence of the patches in Wood's light helps to differentiate the condition from vitiligo and other depigmenting lesions.

SYSTEMIC MYCOSES

(*See* **Table 22**.)

893 Mycetoma ('Madura foot')

This chronic and disabling condition may be caused by a wide variety of organisms ranging from *Actinomycetes* to various *Fungi imperfecti*. This patient was seen in The Sudan where mycetoma is common.

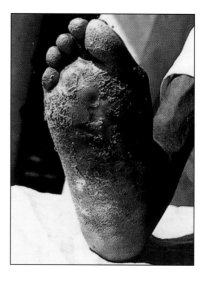

Table 22 Superficial and systemic mycoses

Group	Clinical syndrome	Causative agents
SUPERFICIAL (dermatomycoses)	Mainly hair affected	
	Black piedra	*Piedraia hortae*
	White piedra	*Trichosporon beigelii*
	Favus	*Trichophyton schoenleinii*
	Tinea barbae	*Trichophyton* spp.
	Tinea capitis	*Microsporon* spp.
	Hair not affected	
	Tinea cruris	*Epidermophyton* spp.
	Tinea pedis	*Trichophyton* spp.
	Tinea unguium	*Trichophyton* spp.
	Tinea corporis	*Microsporum* spp.
	Pityriasis versicolor	*Malassezia furfur*
	Tinea imbricata	*Trichophyton concentricum*
	Otomycosis	various genera
	Superficial candidiasis	*Candida albicans*[1]
SYSTEMIC	Actinomycosis	*Actinomyces israelii*
	Madura foot (Mycetoma)	wide variety of organisms including *Nocardia* spp. *Streptomyces* spp., *Pseudallescheria* spp. etc.
	Chromomycosis	*Phialophora* spp., *Cladosporium carrionii*
	Keloidal blastomycosis (Lôbo's disease)	*Lôboa lôboi*
	Blastomycosis	*Blastomyces dermatitidis*
	Paracoccidioidomycosis	*Paracoccidioides brasiliensis*
	Coccidioidomycosis	*Coccidioides immitis*
	Cryptococcosis (Torulosis)	*Cryptococcus neoformans*[1]
	Systemic candidiasis	*Candida* spp.[1]
	Sporotrichosis	*Sporothrix schenckii*
	Histoplasmosis	*Histoplasma capsulatum*[1]
	African histoplasmosis	*H. duboisii*
	Zygomycosis	various genera
	Rhinosporidiosis	*Rhinosporidium seeberi*
	Aspergillosis	*Aspergillus fumigatus*
	Pneumocystosis	*Pneumocystis carinii*[1]

[1] Mycotic infections can become fulminant in immunocompromised subjects. Those marked [1] are especially associated with AIDS.

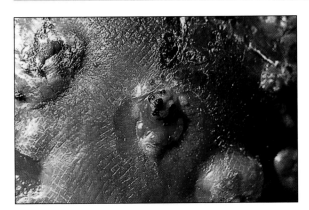

894 Fungal grains discharging
Close-up of **893** showing the coloured fungal grains being discharged from multiple sinuses.

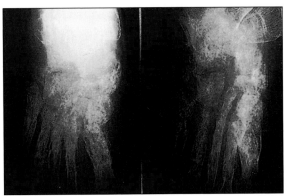

895 Radiographs of Madura foot
Infiltration of the tarsals and metatarsals occurs in late cases.

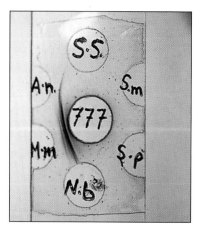

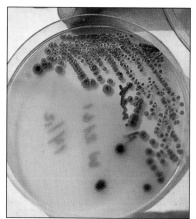

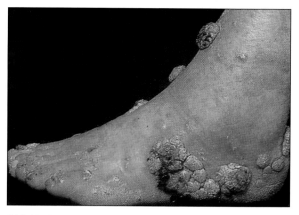

896 Serological diagnosis

Fungal species identification can be made serologically. This serum contains antibodies to *Madurella mycetomae*.

897 & 898 Culture diagnosis

Madurella mycetomae (**897**, left) and *Streptomyces pellietieri* (**898**, right) on Sabouraud medium show typically shaped and pigmented colonies.

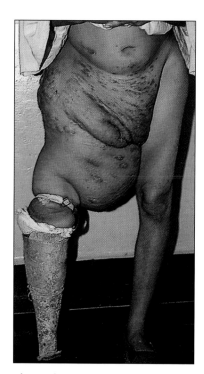

900 Early chromomycosis

The early lesions show a violet discolouration. The primary ulcer spreads slowly and is followed by verrucous lesions. This condition is seen in many tropical areas, including Queensland, where this man was infected.

899 Chronic maduromycosis due to *Streptomyces somaliensis* infection

Extensive sinus formation and osteitis have led to gross disfigurement in this Sudanese man.

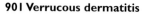

901 Verrucous dermatitis

This is the late stage of chromomycosis. The lesions are very chronic, and are usually painless but irritating. Lymphoedema follows lymphatic stasis.

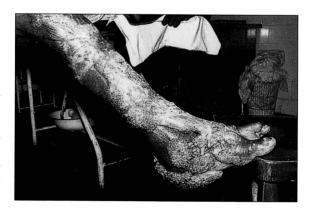

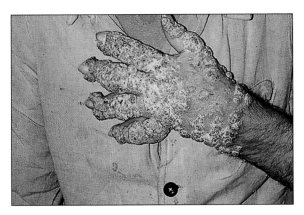

902 Chromomycosis of the hand
The infection can also cause severe but usually superficial lesions on the hands, as in this man from the northeast of Brazil.

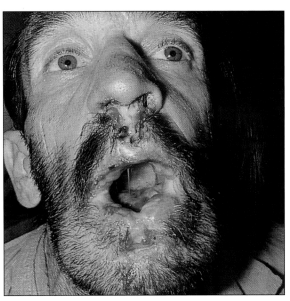

905 Mucocutaneous lesions in paracoccidioidomycosis
In adults, gross infiltration of mucocutaneous and mucous surfaces by *Paracoccidioides brasiliensis* may spread to the pharynx and larynx. The diagnosis is made by demonstrating the fungi in smear or biopsy preparations, or by serological testing.

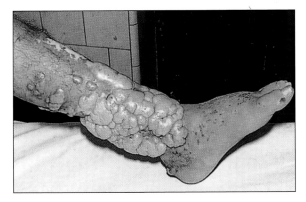

903 Lôbo's disease
This condition, usually presenting with shiny, keloid-like lesions, produces a general picture similar to late chromoblastomycosis and occurs in the northeast of Brazil. It is caused by *Lôboa lôboi*.

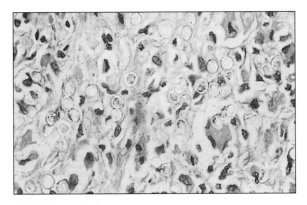

904 *Lôboa lôboi*
The typical spores of this fungus are seen in this biopsy specimen from the keloidal lesions. (*H&E* × *350.*)

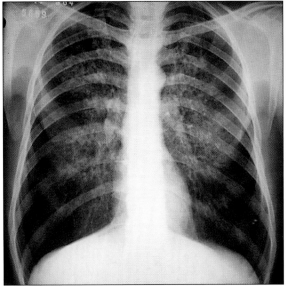

906 Radiograph of chest in paracoccidioidomycosis
Chronic pulmonary infiltration may result in fibrosis and eventual death from respiratory insufficiency in infections with *Paracoccidioides brasiliensis*.

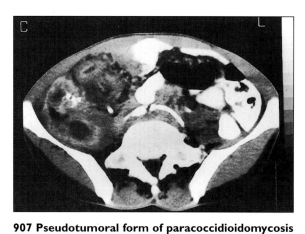

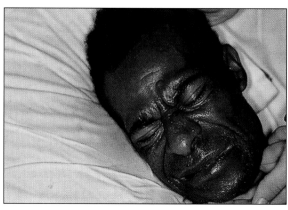

907 Pseudotumoral form of paracoccidioidomycosis
Computed tomogram of the abdomen of a 57-year-old Brazilian man who presented with right lumbar pain and massive weight loss 15 years after having oropharyngeal infection. Physical examination suggested the presence of a colonic carcinoma but radiography and computed tomography revealed the presence of abcesses involving the psoas muscle as well as calcification and thickening of the ileocaecal region of the intestine. Material removed during radical surgery confirmed that the lesions were caused by infection with *Paracoccidiodes brasiliensis*.

909 Chronic cryptococcal meningitis
Infection with *Cryptococcus neoformans* or its tropical subspecies, *C. neoformans gattii*, is most often manifested as a chronic meningitis, but may localise in the lungs or disseminate to other organs, especially in individuals who are immunocompromised; it is seen especially in HIV positive individuals in Africa. This Papuan man with chronic meningitis shows marked meningism. In disseminated disease, cutaneous and lytic bone lesions are common. (*See also* **789** *and* **Table 21**.) (© D.A. Warrell.)

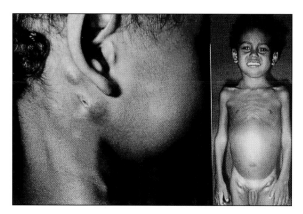

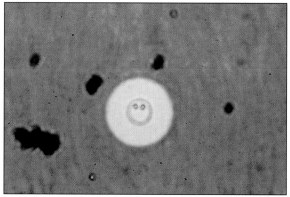

908 Paracoccidioidomycosis in a Brazilian child
In children, *Paracoccidiodes brasiliensis* infection is a widely disseminated disease affecting macrophages and causing generalised lymphadenopathy and hepatosplenomegaly. Although it is uncommon prior to adolescence, this boy was aged only four and a half years. Ultrasound may help to locate intra-abdominal lymphadenopathy, which was present in this case. Infection of the macrophages results in a state of immunodeficiency, which was reflected here by a negative skin test result. Note the general emaciation associated with an enlarged abdomen, generalised lymphadenopathy and ulcerating cervical lymph nodes. In this boy, a titre of 1/1280 against *P. brasiliensis* was recorded.

910 *Cryptococcus neoformans* in cerebrospinal fluid
The organisms are readily visualised in Indian-ink preparations of infected CSF from patients with meningitis infection. They may also be cultured from CSF, blood or urine in some cases. The prostate gland is believed to be an important reservoir for the organisms, which may lead to reactivation of the disease after therapy in some patients. (× 500.)

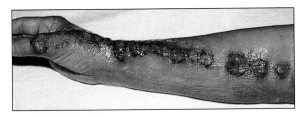

911 Lesions of sporotrichosis
The primary lesion on the thumb, and the lymphatic spread (with ulceration) of secondary nodules on the arm, seen here in a Brazilian woman in São Paulo, are characteristic of this mycotic infection.

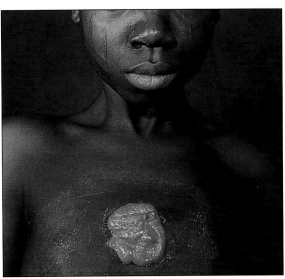

914 African histoplasmosis
Histoplasmosis caused by *Histoplasma duboisii* commonly produces large destructive lesions of the skin and subcutaneous tissues. Bones are often involved in the invasive process. Histoplasmosis has been reported as an opportunistic infection in patients with AIDS in the Caribbean.

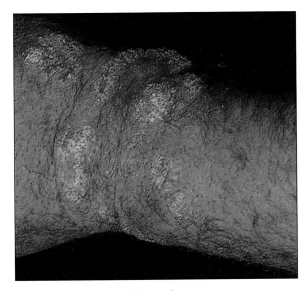

912 Sporotrichosis of the wrist
This patient was infected in Queensland. Like other deep mycoses, infection with *Sporothrix schenkii* occurs in a number of tropical regions.

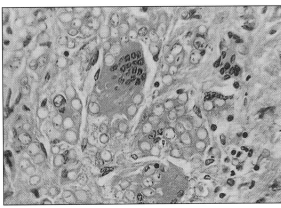

915 *Histoplasma duboisii* in biopsy
The typical giant-cell reaction to the presence of *H. duboisii* spores is seen in this figure. (*H&E × 350.*)

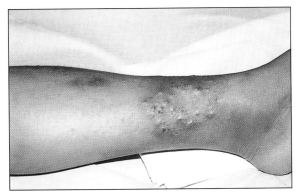

913 Early lesions of sporotrichosis
Characteristic nodular lesions caused by *Sporothrix schenkii* on the lower leg of a patient from Mauritius.

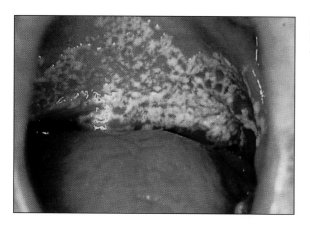

916 *Candida albicans* of the palate
Severe candidiasis of the mouth and gastrointestinal tract is commonly seen in AIDS patients.

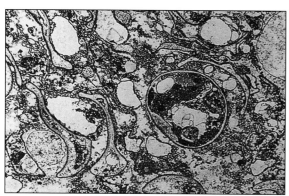

917 Ultrastructure of *Pneumocystis carinii*
Comparison of the DNA and ribosomal RNA of *P. carinii*, which is an opportunistic parasite commonly found in immunocompromised individuals (*see* **792–794**), with that of a wide range of protozoa and fungi, has confirmed that it is one of the group of ustomycetous red yeast fungi. The ultrastructure of the organisms is shown here. (× *26 500*.)

ECTOPARASITIC ARTHROPODS

PARASITIC MITES

(*See* **Table 23**.)

918 *Ornithonyssus bacoti*, the tropical rat mite
Gamasid mites of the family Dermanyssidae are ectoparasites of birds and small mammals. Humans are accidental hosts but several gamasid species transmit human pathogens (*see* **Tables 1, 23**), as well as causing severe cutaneous reactions. Despite its name, *O.bacoti* is a cosmopolitan species found commonly in sea ports. It often bites humans and produces large, irritating, papular lesions. Most species feed nocturnally, and all those that affect humans tend to produce a similar response consisting firstly of itching, the onset of which may be delayed by some hours, followed by a rash. This varies in character from simple macules, papules or wheals to a vari-celliform reaction. The history of exposure, which may be

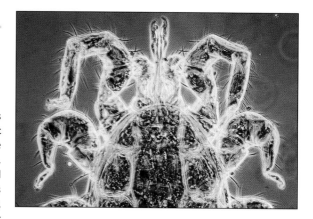

related to the individual's occupation, gives a clue to the diagnosis of the condition. The mites are relatively large (many about 1 mm long) compared with Astigmata (including sarcoptid and trombiculid mites) and Prostigmata.

Table 23 Acari (ticks and mites) of medical importance[1]

Order	Family	Genus and species	Notes
TETRASTIGMATA	(red mites)	*Holothyrus* spp.	may be toxic if ingested
METASTIGMATA	(ticks—see **Tables 1, 2, 3**)		
MESOSTIGMATA	(gamasid mites) Dermanyssidae	*Dermanyssus gallinae*	poultry red mite, infests humans
		Liponyssoides sanguineus	carries *Rickettsia akari*
		Ornithonyssus bacoti	tropical rat mite
		O. sylviarum	northern fowl mite
		O. bursa	tropical fowl mite
		Androlaelaps casalis	in nests of birds and small mammals, may carry Q fever
ASTIGMATA	Acaridae (*sensu lato*)	*Tyrophagus putrescentiae*	causes 'copra itch'
		Suidasia nesbitti	causes 'wheat-pollard itch'
		Acarus siro	causes 'baker's itch'
		Carpoglyphus lactis	causes dried-fruit dermatitis
		Glycyphagus domesticus	causes 'grocer's itch'
		G. destructor	common in hay, causes allergy
		Goheria fusca	in flour, causes allergy
	Pyroglyphidae	*Dermatophagoides* spp.	feed on skin detritus, birds, mammals, common in house dust
		D. pteronyssinus	main house dust allergen
		D. farinae	common house dust allergen
		Euroglyphus maynei	common house dust mite
	Sarcoptidae	*Sarcoptes scabiei*	scabies, Norwegian scabies
PROSTIGMATA	Pyemotidae	*Pyemotes ventricosus*	grain, straw mite, causes dermatitis
	Cheyletidae	*Cheyletiella parasitovorax*	in dog fur, causes dermatitis
		C. blakey	mainly in dog fur
		C. yasguri	in dog, cat, rabbit fur
		Cheyletus eruditus	predator of grain mites etc.
	Demodicidae	*Demodex folliculorum*	in human hair follicles
		D. brevis	in sebaceous glands
	Trombiculiidae	*Eutrombicula* spp.	causes 'scrub-itch'
		Schoengastia spp.	causes 'scrub-itch'
		Neotrombicula autumnalis	'harvest mite'
		Leptotrombidium akamushi	vector of *Orientia tsutsugamushi* (scrub typhus)
		L. deliense	vector of scrub typhus
	Anystidae	*Anystis* spp.	'whirligig mites'

[1] Adapted from Alexander (1984) and Lane and Crosskey (1993).

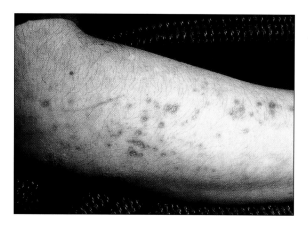

919 Varicelliform reaction to bites of *Dermanyssus gallinae*
Note the scratch marks due to the intense irritation on the skin of this man who was bitten by the red poultry mite, another of the gamasid mites, while plucking turkeys.

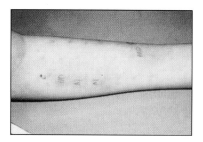

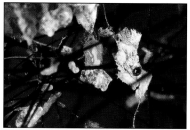

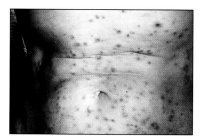

920 Skin test for hypersensitivity in a patient with urticaria and hay fever
The reaction can be seen to allergens derived from (HD) house dust, (M) house dust mites and (CP) pollen, compared with the control (C). *Dermatophagoides pteronyssinus* and *D.farinae* are commonly found in house dust and have been associated in recent years with the common 'stuffy nose' syndrome that afflicts many people at night. They feed mainly on dead epithelial scales and other organic matter in house dust. The presence of protein from dead mites, which is probably responsible for allergic reactions to these mites, can also precipitate paroxysms of asthma in sensitised individuals and may cause atopic skin eruptions including eczema in others. Over 100 mites/g of dust have been recovered from the house dust of some asthmatic individuals whose condition may improve if they can be moved to a mite-free environment.

921 *Cheyletiella parasitivorax*
The Cheyletidae are parasitic on small mammals, living in their fur and feeding mainly on dead epidermis, hair and other fur mites. Humans are affected by handling infested dogs or cats. This figure shows hair combings from a puppy. Three species in this genus are now recognised to cause lesions in humans. (× 25.)

922 Rash caused by *Cheyletiella parasitivorax*
The lesions developed in a woman who had recently acquired a puppy. The lesions consisted of small, erythematous papules with haemorrhagic, vesicular centres, which were intensely irritating. They may become pustular and may be excoriated by scratching. Management of cases should include the use of acaricides to rid pet animals and their bedding of the mites.

SCABIES

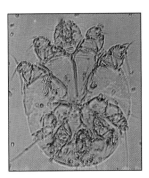 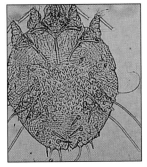

923 & 924 Male and female scabies mites
The gravid female *Sarcoptes scabiei* (**924**, right) burrows into the epidermis, lays its eggs and dies at the end of the tunnel. It is cosmopolitan in distribution (**923** left, *ventral view* ×115; **924** dorsal view × 85.)

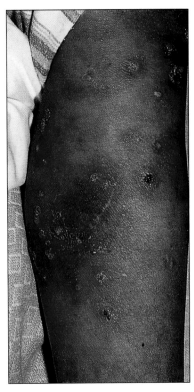

927 Secondary erythema in scabies
Secondary infection is common, and erythrema may be associated with bacterial invasion of the sarcoptic tracks.

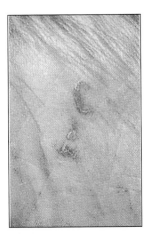

925 Scabies burrows
These are seen here on the instep of the foot of an infant. The foot is the second commonest site of early infection at this age, with the axillae and neck also being invaded in some cases. The darker colouring represents the inflammatory reaction to the mites and their detritus.

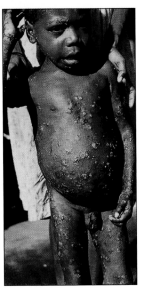

926 Infected scabies in a Papuan boy
Intense local pruritus and dermatitis appear within a few days of infection. The tortuous tunnels may extend for several centimetres.

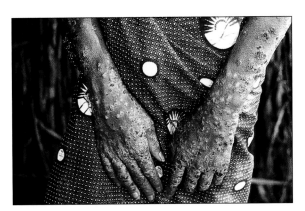

928 Chronic eczematous scabies in a Gambian woman
The backs of the hands and arms are heavily infested in this woman. Constant scratching owing to the intense itching may result in lichenification of the dry skin. The condition would need to be differentiated from onchocerciasis where both conditions are present.

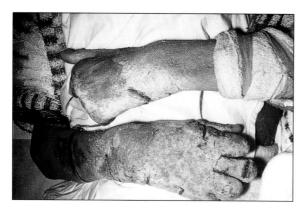

929 Hyperkeratotic ('Norwegian') scabies in a patient who had had a 70% burns injury
This condition is often associated with immunosuppression, which may result, among other causes, from severe burns, and includes HIV infection. The dorsum of the hands and fingers are most affected in this patient.

OTHER MITE INFESTATIONS

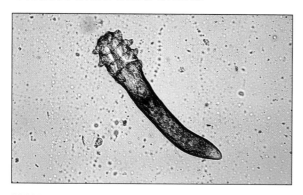

930 Ventral view of *Demodex folliculorum*
This species inhabits human hair follicles, especially on the head and ears. It is believed that the mites can be found if carefully looked for in most healthy adults in whom they cause no pathological changes. The follicles of the nose, nasolabial folds and malar prominences are most commonly infested, whereas the eyelashes often shelter numerous mites. Details of their life cycle are still obscure but they seem to undergo several moults in rather rapid succession. Infection is probably acquired during infancy from close physical contact with the infected mother. The mites are especially common in sebaceous glands and may cause a condition on the head of some individuals known as pityriasis folliculorum. The condition is confirmed by expressing the mites from individual nodulopapules or pustules. In recent years a second species has been identified in human sebaceous glands, *Demodex brevis*. (*Phase contrast* × 25.)

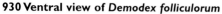

932 Bullous lesions following 'chigger' bites
The larvae do not ingest blood but feed through the 'stylostome' on host tissue that has been dissolved by salivary secretions. After feeding the larvae develop into free-living, predatory nymphs.

931 Larval *Trombicula autumnalis*
These 'harvest mites' are common in grassland in temperate climates. The larvae, which normally feed on small mammals and birds, also attack humans causing intense irritation (× 75). (*See also* **39**.)

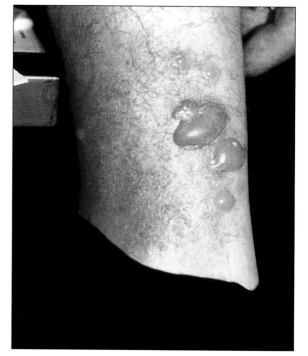

LOUSE INFESTATION

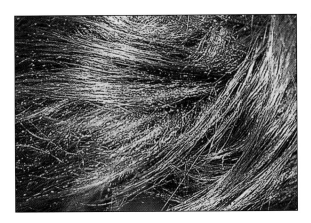

933 *Pediculus capitis*
The head louse, *P. capitis*, is very common, and heavy infestations such as that seen here in an Indian girl can cause severe irritation. The eggs ('nits') are attached to the hairs and appear as masses of white dots. Unlike *P. corporis*, *P. capitis* is not known to be a disease vector.

934 Severe pediculosis corporis
Heavy infestation is common where people live in un-hygienic conditions. Body lice spread rapidly wherever suitable ecological conditions prevail and are common in soldiers and refugees during wartime, in institutions for the mentally subnormal, prisons, etc. Formerly known also as 'vagabond's disease,' severe dermatitis due to the presence of heavy louse populations and the scratching that the bites stimulate, especially at night, is often accompanied by pigmentation of the affected areas, restlessness causing loss of sleep and, in chronic cases, lichenification and eczema. As in

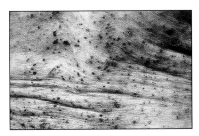

this patient, thousands of lice may be present on patients' bodies and in their clothes.

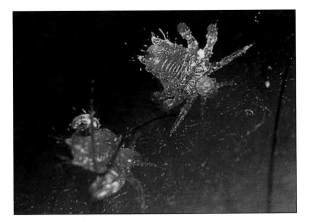

935 *Phthirus pubis*
The pubic or 'crab' louse is commonly spread during sexual intercourse. Sites infected other than the pubic area include the eyelashes. (× 7.)

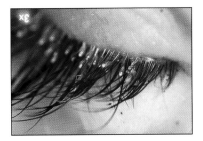

936 Eggs of *Phthirus pubis* attached to the bases of eyelashes
As seen here the infection load can be severe in this location.

BED BUGS

937 *Cimex lectularis*

This species and the tropical bed bug, *Cimex hemipterus*, frequent houses where they feed on the blood of the inhabitants at night. Multiple bites are very common and may be due to interrupted feeding by a single bug. Blood is actively sucked up by the pumping action of the hypopharynx once the stylets have pierced a small blood vessel, from 10 to 20 minutes being required for the bug to become fully engorged. The bite itself is not painful but erythema and itching develop later. Bedbugs are a considerable pest but probably of no major importance in disease transmission. It is believed that their numbers are increasing in some western countries due to their unobserved importation with the possessions of

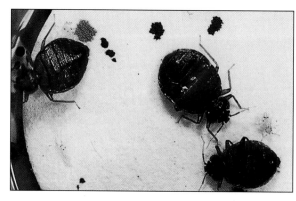

returning 'back packer' tourists who sleep in insanitary accommodation, especially in tropical areas. (× 3.)

FLEA INFESTATIONS

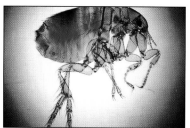

939 Extensive papular urticaria caused by massive flea infestation

The intense irritation in the lumbar region caused this man to scratch incessantly, producing marked excoriation of lesions that were accessible.

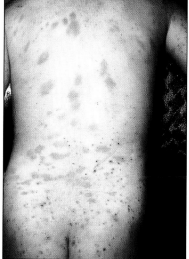

938 Female *Pulex irritans*

The 'human flea' is a cosmopolitan species that is becoming uncommon in houses in many temperate countries. Under especially favourable climatic and environmental conditions, fleas may appear in almost epidemic proportions. Humans are most commonly bitten by cat and dog fleas of the genus *Ctenocephalides*. (× 20.)

TUNGIASIS

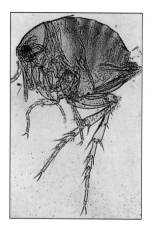

940 Male *Tunga penetrans*

The 'jigger' or 'chigger' flea occurs in tropical areas of South America and Africa. The male, which has a characteristically angular head, is free living. (× 28.)

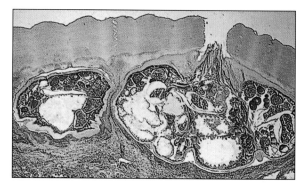

941 Section of female *Tunga penetrans* in the skin

The gravid female buries itself in the skin, often under the toenails, and swells up to the size of a small pea. Eggs are laid through the entry hole. (H&E × 75.)

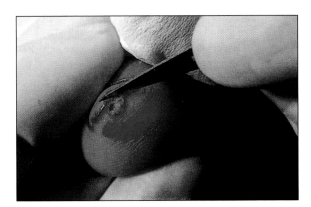

942 Jigger flea being removed from toe
Habitual carriers shell the gravid females out of the skin with a pin or sliver of bamboo, usually scattering eggs in the process. Tetanus is a common sequel to this type of self-treatment. The larvae mature to adulthood on the ground.

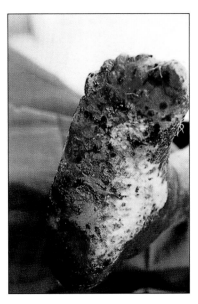

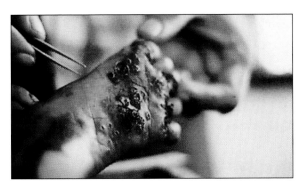

943 Tungiasis in the foot of a Yanumami Indian
Numerous females buried under the feet and toes of this Amerindian man causing considerable pain and difficulty in walking. Secondary infection commonly aggravates the condition.

944 Severe tungiasis in the foot of a man with leprosy
The feet and toes of this African patient, who had lost all sensation and had partial amputations of the toes due to tuberculoid leprosy, were riddled with *Tunga penetrans*.

MYIASIS

(*See* **Table 24.**)

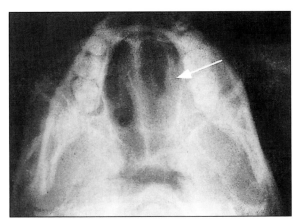

945 Radiograph of nasal sinuses invaded by larvae of *Chrysomya bezziana*
The patient was a 14-year-old girl from the eastern province of Saudi Arabia who complained of recurrent nose bleeding and pain of five days' duration. Radiography showed that the lateral wall of her left nasal cavity (*arrow*) had been destroyed. More than 80 larvae were removed surgically from the sinuses, and the patient recovered.

Table 24 Myiasis-producing diptera of medical importance[1]

Family/Subfamily	Genus and species	Other names	Notes
CALLIPHORIDAE Calliphorinae			
'metallic group'	Chrysomya bezziana	Old World screw worm	feed on living tissue in wounds
	Cochliomyia hominivorax	New World screw worm	
	Lucilia spp.	greenbottles,	feed on dead tissue in wounds
	Calliphora spp.	bluebottles, blow flies	
	Phormia regina	'black blow fly'	can cause dermal, enteric myiasis
	Cynomopsis cadaverina		invades wounds
'non-metallic group'	Auchmeromyia senegalensis[2]	Congo floor maggot	sucks blood from skin
	Cordylobia anthropophaga	Tumbu, mango fly	causes subcutaneous boils
Sarcophaginae			
	Wohlfahrtia spp.	flesh flies	invade wounds or normal tissue, especially on head
	W. magnifica		commonest species in humans
	Sarcophaga haemorrhoidalis		may occur in gut
CUTEREBRIDAE	Dermatobia hominis	human bot fly	causes subcutaneous boils
	Cuterebra spp.	North American bot flies	skin and eye lesions
GASTEROPHILIDAE	Gasterophilus spp.	stomach bot flies	invade skin and may migrate to eye
HYPODERMATIDAE	Hypoderma spp.	warble flies	cause dermal, eye or nasopharyngeal lesions
	H. lineatum	lesser cattle warble	
	H. tarandi	reindeer warble	ophthalmomyiasis
	Cephenemyia ulrichii	moose throat bot fly	
OESTRIDAE	Oestrus ovis	sheep nasal bot fly	invades nasopharynx and eye

[1] Modified from Zumpt (1965) and Lane and Crosskey (1993). This Table does not include facultative parasites such as larvae of the family Syrphidae, which may be found in the lower intestine or urogenital tract, faeces or urine. Species of Muscidae, genera *Fannia, Musca* and *Muscina* may also be found in faeces

[2] Formerly known as *Auchmeromyia luteola*.

946 Male *Cochliomyia hominivorax*

The family Calliphoridae contains six metallic-coloured flies in the subfamily Calliphorinae of which two species, the screw worms, have carnivorous larvae that are obligatory feeders on living flesh, and four that are essentially scavengers of decaying flesh. The New World screw worm is a notorious parasite of domestic livestock, and its depravations have caused huge economic losses in North, Central and South America amounting to over $100 million in the 1950s and 1960s. Humans are frequently infected. Fortunately the female only mates once and this has made possible a control campaign using mass reared, irradiation-sterilised males, which has pushed the frontier southwards from the USA towards Mexico. The fly was discovered for the first time in Africa in Libya in the 1980s (probably having been imported with cattle from South America), where it infected over 2000 cattle and 200 people before its presence was exposed. Since adult females can fly over 200 km, it was feared that the species could spread across North Africa and perhaps south across the Saharan trade routes. However, a

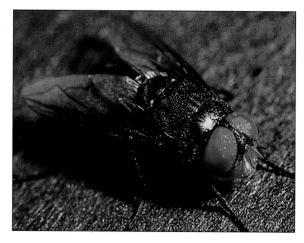

mass international campaign using sterilised males (reared and imported from the USA) was successful in eradicating it. The larvae also attack open wounds on humans, feeding on living as well as dead tissue. (× 8.2.)

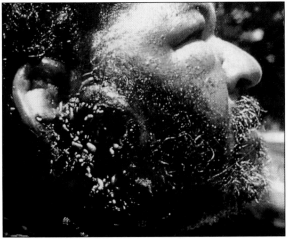

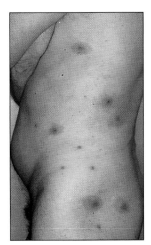

950 Tumbu fly lesions
Multiple infections with
larvae of *Cordylobia
anthropophaga* caused
painful boils on this man's
trunk.

947 Brazilian man infected with screw worm
A large number of larvae of *Cochliomyia hominivorax* can be
seen in a gaping wound beneath the ear of this man, an
escaped convict who had been attacked while hiding in the
jungle. A heavy infection can kill a large animal such as a cow
in 10 days.

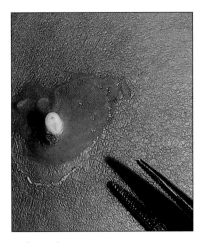

**948 Adult female *Lucilia
sericata***
'Greenbottles' the larvae
of which are opportunistic
feeders on carrion and
other dead organic matter,
sometimes invade wounds but
feed only on dead tissue.

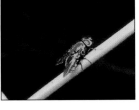

Another species that sometimes invades wounds is *L. cuprina.*
(× 3.2.)

951 Extracting a larva
The larva leaves the skin if it is covered in oil that blocks the
spiracles. It can then be removed easily with forceps.

**949 Third instar larvae
of *Lucilia sericata***
Note the fleshy posterior
appendages known as 'anal
lobes.' Because they do not
invade healthy tissue, the
larvae of this calliphorid fly
have been used to help in the
cleaning of infected wounds,
for example under occlusive

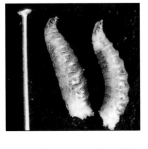

952 Larva of Tumbu fly
The figure shows the
powerful hooks with which
the larvae feed inside the
skin. (× 20.)

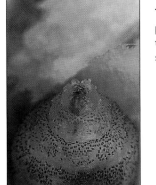

plaster of Paris splints in patients with osteomyelitis. This
practice is currently becoming more popular, especially in
the presence of antibiotic resistance. The larval stages,
however, last only about one week, after which the insects
pupate. The adults hatch in about a week to 10 days. (× 5.)

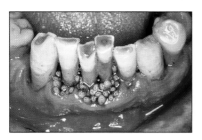

953 Mouth of an old man infested with larvae of an unidentified *Wohlfahrtia* species

The larvae of this genus of 'flesh flies' of the subfamily Sarcophaginae are essentially scavengers in decaying flesh, faeces, rotting food, etc. but occasionally are found in wounds and sores. The females are larvivorous, producing batches of 20 to 40 first instar larvae, which develop rapidly, the third instars burying in soil to pupate. This man was infected while asleep under a tree in a Middle East country. The spiracles of the numerous larvae are very obvious in this view. Normally they are not easily seen because they are situated within a larval pit.

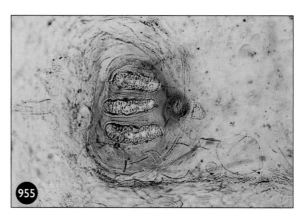

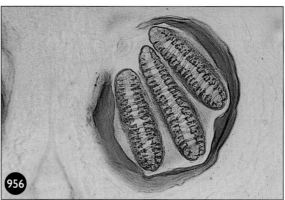

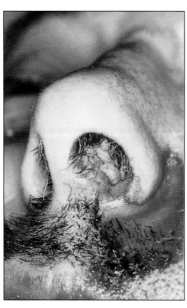

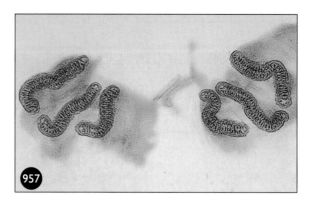

954 Larvae of *Sarcophaga* in the nose of a man with a nasal tumour

The spiracles, concealed in the spiracular pits, are not visible in this figure. Like *Wohlfahrtia*, the larvae of flies in this closely related genus are normally found in decaying organic matter but may be laid in malodorous wounds or tumours, as in this case. The species may be *S. carnaria*.

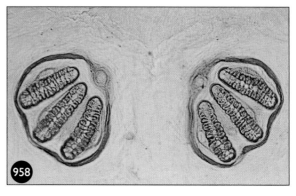

955–958 Larval spiracles of calliphorid flies
Auchmeromyia senegalensis (= *luteola*) (**955**), *Chrysomya* (**956**), *Cordylobia* (**957**), *Lucilia* or *Calliphora* (**958**). *A. senegalensis*, the 'Congo floor maggot,' feeds on humans by sucking blood nocturnally but does not remain attached. The adult is similar to that of the Tumbu fly. The larva is separated from that of other calliphorid flies by the distinctive posterior spiracles. With the increased use of beds, infection with this fly has greatly decreased. ($\times$ *approximately 100.*)

◀ ——————————————————

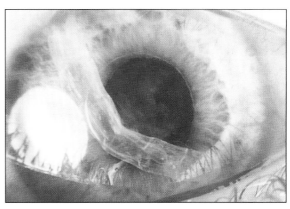

961 Ophthalmomyiasis due to larva of *Hypoderma bovis*
Migrating larvae in humans usually remain in the subdermal tissues but can make their way to various organs, including the eye. In this case the larva was in the anterior chamber of the eye (a condition known as opthalmomyiasis interna anterior); the larva was subsequently removed surgically.

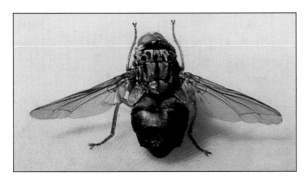

959 *Dermatobia hominis*
The larvae of this fly are a cause of serious cutaneous myiasis in Brazil and other tropical areas of the New World. ($\times$ *2.5.*)

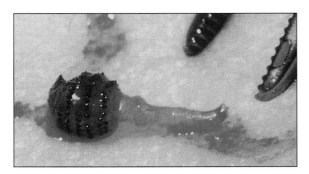

960 Second instar larva of *Dermatobia hominis*
The immature stages have characteristic rows of dark spines. This larva was extracted from the skin of an entomologist! ($\times$ *5.0.*)

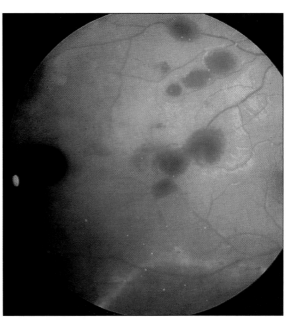

962 Ophthalmomyiasis caused by *Hypoderma tarandi*
Severe retinal haemorrhages in a 13-year-old Norwegian boy caused by a migrating first instar larva of *H. (Oedemagena) tarandi*. The female fly lays eggs on the fur of reindeer. Humans are probably infected by accidentally transferring first instar larvae to the conjunctival sac when handling infected animals. The larva was removed surgically from the eye in this patient.

963 Periorbital oedema and severe conjunctivitis in an Iranian patient with ophthalmomyiasis due to a first instar larva of *Oestrus ovis*

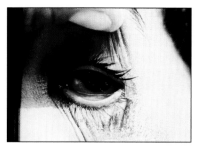

The sheep nasal bot fly, which is a parasite of the nasal cavities and sinuses, is now found wherever sheep are raised on a large scale. The females, which are viviparous, swarm round the heads of their victims and deposit first instar larvae in the nostrils or sometimes orbit of sheep. Ophthalmomyiasis externa is not uncommon among shepherds and others working closely with sheep. The larvae do not grow beyond the first instar but cause a painful inflammation within the conjunctival sac for several days. Occasionally the larvae are deposited in the ears, nose or mouth, and they can invade the nasal sinuses.

CHAPTER 7

Airborne Infections

Infections of the upper respiratory tract are acquired mainly by the inhalation of pathogenic organisms for most of which humans are reservoirs. Carriers play an important role and may represent the major part of the reservoir (e.g. in meningococcal meningitis). The three main media for the transmission of airborne infections are droplets, droplet nuclei and dust. Mass vaccination campaigns have reduced the incidence of some of these diseases that previously caused a very high toll in infant and child morbidity and mortality.

Measles tends to be a severe disease in malnourished children and, in some epidemics in the rural tropics, mortality has been as high as 50%. The infection not infrequently precipitates 'kwashiorkor.' Whooping cough is another important cause of infantile mortality in some areas of the tropics.

Massive pandemics of meningococcal meningitis due to *Neisseria meningitidis* continue to occur periodically in the so-called 'meningitis belt' of tropical Africa (*see* **969**). In this zone, the pandemics come in waves followed by periods of respite. Over 300 000 cases were reported between 1996 and 2000, and this figure was almost certainly an underestimate. Overall, at least 1.2 million cases of bacterial meningitis occur of which 0.5 million are due to *N. meningitidis*, with a mortality of about 10%.

Tuberculosis is increasing as a major health problem, not only in many tropical countries, where it is aggravated by poor sanitary conditions and dense overcrowding in urban slums, but also in the Western World, where the problem is aggravated by the development of multiple drug-resistant strains of *Mycobacterium tuberculosis*. The infection presents a wide variety of clinical forms, but pulmonary involvement is the commonest and most important epidemiologically, because it is the form mainly responsible for transmission of the infection. Whereas in the developed countries tuberculosis is seen with increasing frequency in HIV-positive individuals, in Africa it and pneumococcal pneumonia are among the commonest causes of death in people with AIDS (*see* **Table 21**). It is estimated that three million people die worldwide from tuberculosis each year.

MEASLES

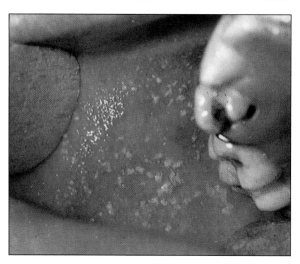

964 Koplik's spots
Koplik's spots are pathognomonic of measles. They are found on mucous membranes during the prodromal stage and are easily detected on the mucosa of the cheeks opposite the molar teeth, where they resemble course grains of salt on the surface of the inflamed membrane. Histologically, the spots consist of small necrotic patches in the basal layers of the mucosa, with exudation of serum and infiltration by mononuclear cells.

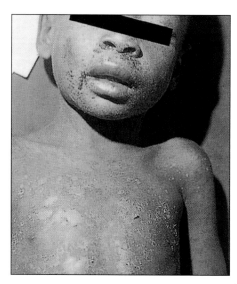

966 Measles in an African child
The desquamating skin rash of measles was accompanied by herpes simplex stomatitis and rhinitis in this child, who died from respiratory complications.

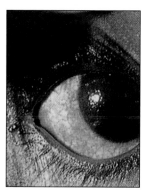

967 Keratoconjunctivitis and xerophthalmia in measles
In malnourished children, these complications are commonly seen.

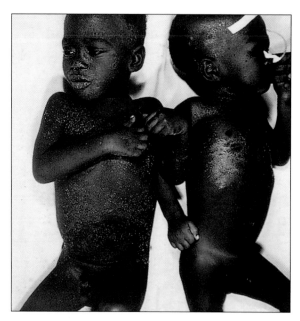

965 Measles in twins
Measles is one of the most important causes of childhood mortality in the tropics. The twin on the left shows typical post-measles desquamation, but is otherwise recovering. The other twin has post-measles encephalitis.

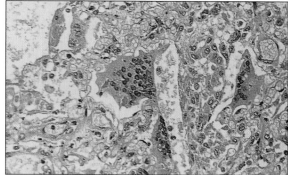

968 Lung in giant cell pneumonia
Mortality is commonly associated with giant cell pneumonia during the prodromal stage. This section was from a 10-year-old girl who contracted measles while receiving steroid therapy for treatment for nephrotic syndrome. (*H&E × 375.*)

MENINGOCOCCAL MENINGITIS

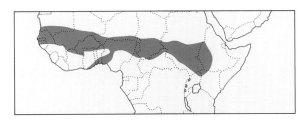

969 Distribution map of meningoccocal meningitis in Africa
Meningococcal meningitis occurs in epidemic or pandemic form in the 'meningitis belt' of tropical Africa, the zone lying approximately between 5° and 15° north of the Equator, which is characterised by an annual rainfall of between 300 and 1100 mm. In a pandemic of serogroup A *Neisseria meningitidis* infection in this zone, over 300 000 people were affected between 1996 and 2000. The disease, however, is not limited to Africa, and overcrowding enhances the risk of acquiring the infection; nearly 3000 people died from menin-gitis in two Brazilian cities in 1974. Other epidemics occurred in Nepal in 1983 and 1984 and in Pakistan and India in 1985. Effective vaccines against serogroups A and C are now available.

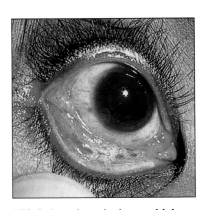

970 Rash of acute meningococcaemia
The rash consists typically of irregular, scattered, non-blanching petechiae, which tend to be peripherally distrib-uted. The lesions, which vary in size, may be macular, papular or clearly purpuric.

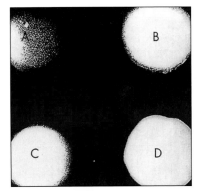

971 Meningococcal septicaemia
Non-blanching and necrotic lesions on the hand of an African patient with meningococcal septicaemia.

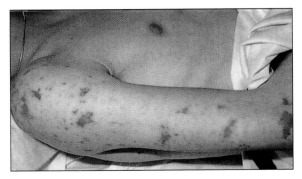

972 Subconjunctival petechial haemorrhages
This Nigerian boy with meningococcal meningitis had numerous subconjuncti-val petechiae. (© D.A. Warrell.)

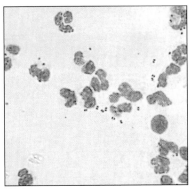

973 Smear of cerebrospinal fluid
Neisseria meningitidis is a Gram-negative, bean-shaped diplococcal organism. In the 'meningitis belt' of Africa, group A is the causative agent of epidemics. (*Gram stain* × 900.)

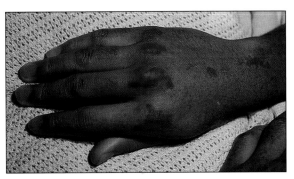

974 Latex agglutination test
This sensitive serological test is valu-able for the differentiation of meningo-coccal from pneumococcal and other types of meningitis. [A—meningo-coccus antigen; B—pneumococcus antigen; C—*Haemophilus influenzae* antigen; D—negative control.]

TUBERCULOSIS

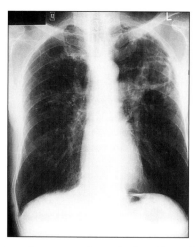

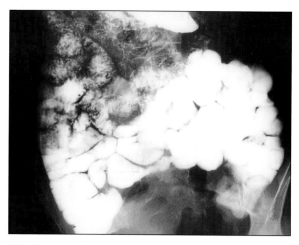

975 Acute pulmonary tuberculosis with cavitation
Tuberculosis remains one of the major health problems in the tropics. Tuberculosis can affect all organs in the body. The lungs are the most common, being the route of entry, and the most important as infection of the lung is responsible for transmission of the disease. As less than one in every 10 people infected develops disease, an infectious case needs to infect at least 20 people for transmission to continue. The characteristic pulmonary lesion is the cavity, as shown here in the left upper lobe. Patients with cavities on radiography are more likely to have positive sputum smear results and hence are infectious to others. The most important risk factor for tuberculosis is infection with HIV. The incidence of fulminating tuberculosis in Africa parallels that of AIDS, which is the underlying cause of the immunological breakdown in many individuals.

976 Ileocaecal tuberculosis
The barium follow-through shows a fixed stricture of the terminal ileum in a patient with ileocaecal tuberculosis. Diagnosis was unfortunately only confirmed at laparotomy after a period during which the patient had been treated as a case of Crohn's disease.

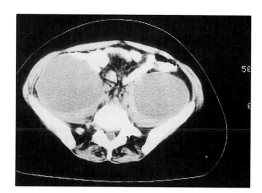

977 Bilateral psoas abscesses
The computed tomogram shows large hypodense areas in both psoas muscles in a patient who was found to have bilateral psoas abscesses due to *Mycobacterium tuberculosis*. There is also involvement of the lumbar vertebra.

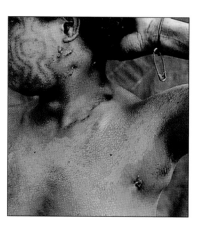

978 Tubercular glands
Glandular enlargement due to human tuberculosis is not uncommon in many tropical areas, as seen in this Fijian woman.

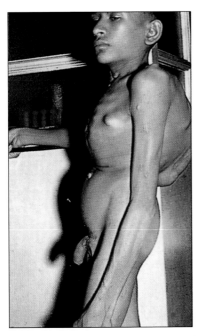

979 Tuberculosis of the spine (Potts disease)
Vertebral involvement, as seen in this young Indian, causes severe deformity.

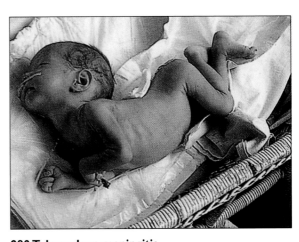

980 Tuberculous meningitis
In infants, miliary tuberculosis and meningitis have a high mortality. This three-month-old Nepalese infant with tuberculous meningitis and demonstrating pronounced head retraction, died despite intensive chemotherapy. Tuberculous meningitis in infants results in permanent neurological sequelae in at least 50% of cases.

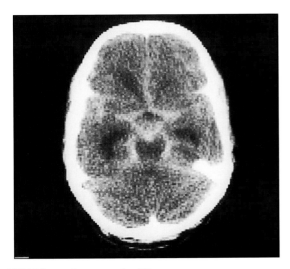

981 Tuberculous meningitis
A computed tomogram of the brain showing increased uptake of contrast around the vessels at the base of the brain in the circle of Willis in a patient with tuberculous meningitis.

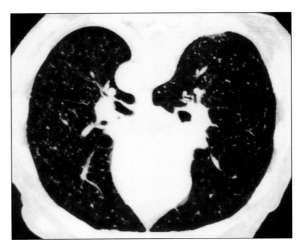

982 Computed tomogram of chest in miliary tuberculosis
A transverse section through the midzone of the lungs showing typical miliary seedlings in a patient with miliary tuberculosis. These can sometimes be missed on straight chest radiograph.

WHOOPING COUGH

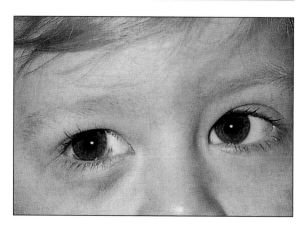

983 Child with whooping cough
Whooping cough is an important cause of infantile mortality in the tropics. Subconjunctival haemorrhages are a common accompaniment of the severe coughing spasms. The haemorrhages resolve rapidly once the child recovers.

PSITTACOSIS

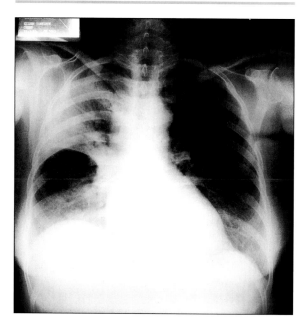

984 Radiograph of patient with psittacosis (ornithosis)
Infection with *Chlamydia psittaci* is usually acquired from pet birds, e.g. parrots, but also occurs widely throughout the animal kingdom. The organism is closely related to *Chlamydia pneumoniae*, which is responsible for a high proportion of respiratory infections, especially in children living in poor urban communities in tropical countries. This radiograph shows dense consolidation of the right upper lobe in a patient who presented with pneumonia due to *C. psittaci*. She was an avid collector of tropical birds and had recently acquired a new bird.

CHAPTER 8

Nutritional Disorders

Hunger, as manifest through famines or chronic undernutrition, has been recorded from prehistoric times. In large areas of the tropics, malnutrition, especially that affecting young children, is one of the principal causes of morbidity and mortality. The problem of feeding the populations of the world and therefore maintaining an adequate status of nutritional health, is a serious one, which has again come to prominence, especially in parts of Africa, in recent years. Its magnitude and severity have still not received adequate attention, and there is no completely reliable assessment of it in quantitative terms.

Human malnutrition is an ecological problem, and the following intimately related factors may be involved in its pathogenesis:

- Food production and distribution
- Food storage and processing, including contamination, e.g. with aflatoxins
- Demographic problems related to food—the rate of increase of the population in most developing countries is over 2%, and yet the rate of increase of food production in most areas has not kept up with the population increase
- Education and sociocultural factors
- Food preparation and consumption
- The role of infection.

The United Nations agencies have estimated that about one third of the world's population goes to bed hungry every day, mostly in the countries of Asia, Africa and Latin America. The most 'vulnerable' groups are infants, preschool children, and pregnant and nursing mothers. Protein-calorie malnutrition is the name for a disease syndrome which includes kwashiorkor (believed to be largely due to an interaction between protein deficiency and other factors) and nutritional marasmus (which is due to a general deficiency of all nutrients, especially calories). In tropical communities, cases range from one extreme to the other.

Among adults, acute periods of undernutrition may occur in large populations because of natural or man-made disasters. The failure of food crops because of drought, pestilence (locust plagues, for example, have been known since time immemorial and remain a serious threat) and catastrophes (such as those caused by floods and earthquakes) are unavoidable. Advance planning of relief operations by the more affluent nations and the deployment of that relief are still grossly inadequate. However, mass civil disruption by warfare as seen in all too many countries even today (with its consequent interruption of normal agricultural practices and food distribution) plays a major part both in the increase of undernutrition and in the spread of infectious diseases, especially, but not exclusively, in the tropics and subtropics. Further detrimental climatic changes associated with global warming imply that an increase in problems due to malnutrition in the inhabitants of many of the world's poorest countries is very likely in the coming years.

Overall, the background of ill health caused by nutritional deficiency is very diverse and can be seen to be more dependent on the socioeconomic level of an individual community than practically any disease resulting from specific pathogens. Protein-calorie malnutrition is the most important nutritional problem of the whole world, although deficiencies of vitamins A, B complex and D are also quite common. The nutritional deficiencies in many cases are complicated further by additional stress imposed by multiple parasitic infections, such as intestinal helminthiases and malaria.

Many tropical diets are based on some staple carbohydrate foodstuff to which other substances are added fortuitously. These diets consist mainly of yams, cassava, rice, plantains, breadfruit and maize. Maize is a poor staple food at any time, but when in addition the crop fails because of insect pests or drought, famine may result. Such diets are badly balanced at the best of times and lack total protein and other essential substances. They result in quantitative and/or qualitative deficiencies, which are prejudicial to health and to normal body growth. Stunting in the 24-month to 59-month age group was estimated in 1980–90 to be present in 65% in India, 39% in Sub-Saharan Africa and 26% in Latin America and the Caribbean, compared with 2% in Britain and the USA. Malnutrition also leads to anaemia, which was estimated to exist during the 1970s and 1980s in 88% of pregnant women in India, 41% in Sub-Saharan Africa and 35% in Latin America and the Caribbean, as compared with only 17–19% in Britain and the USA (data from World Bank, 1993).

KWASHIORKOR AND MARASMUS

985 Oedema and hypopigmentation

The presence of oedema may give a false impression that an infant with kwashiorkor is well nourished. General hypopigmentation, together with some haemorrhagic skin lesions, are seen in this infant who died shortly after the photograph was taken. The exact cause of kwashiorkor is still debated. Rather than being due to simple protein-energy malnutrition, it is suggested that it is related to a deficiency in the diet of the trace element selenium, which is essential to glutathione peroxidase-mediated oxidation-reduction processes in the

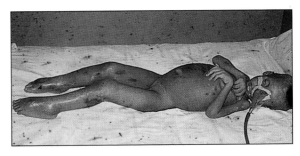

tissues. Aflatoxins and other, so far, unidentified factors may also play a part.

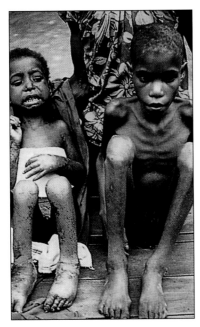

986 Kwashiorkor and marasmus in brothers

Compare the miserable expression, pale hair, generalised oedema and skin changes in the child on the left who has kwashiorkor with the marasmic wasting of his older brother. Kwashiorkor often follows acute infection and/or diarrhoea in a child during the weaning period.

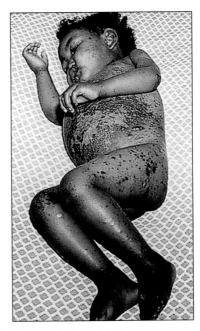

987 Skin changes in kwashiorkor

Serious skin changes including erythema, followed by hyperpigmentation, 'black enamel skin' and peeling, may terminate in serious ulceration and gangrene. Note the ulceration where desquamation has occurred in this child.

NUTRITIONAL MARASMUS

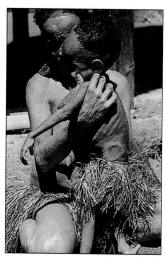

988 Papuan child with nutritional marasmus
Note the obvious wasting and dehydration in this marasmic infant, an all too common picture in times of famine when the total calorie intake is grossly insufficient. (The mother has tinea imbricata of the skin; see **890**.)

AVITAMINOSES

VITAMIN A

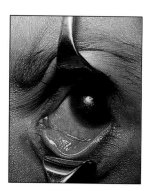

989 Xerophthalmia
Vitamin A deficiency is a common cause of blindness among preschool children in the tropics, especially in Asia. The dryness of the cornea and conjunctiva give the eye a dull, hazy appearance.

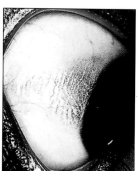

990 Bitot's spots
These are silver-grey, foamy spots, usually external to the cornea and often bilateral. They are thought to be due to avitaminosis A.

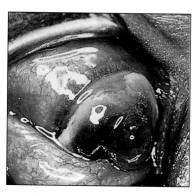

991 Keratomalacia
A softening or coagulative necrosis of the cornea occurs in chronic, severe vitamin A deficiency. As for kwashiorkor, vitamin A deficiency may be precipitated by acute infections in undernourished children.

VITAMIN D

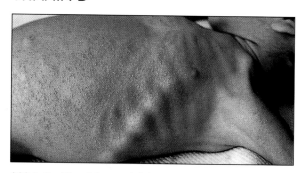

992 Infantile rickets—'rickety rosary'
This is a disease of infants and children due to insufficient vitamin D. Infants are sometimes over-protected from the sun by their mothers to avoid too-rapid pigmentation of the skin; rickets occurs in this situation when it could easily be avoided. Rounded swellings that appear over the costochondral junctions near the sternum give rise to the term 'rickety rosary.'

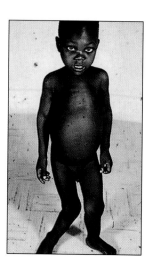

993 Infantile rickets
Note the gross deformity of the legs and pigeon chest of this boy.

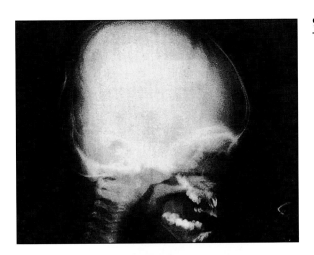

994 Skull of two-year-old infant with rickets
The anterior fontanelle remains open and its edges are soft.

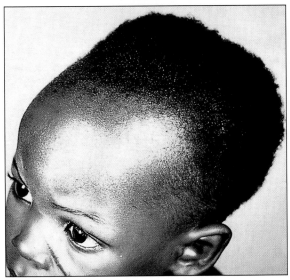

995 Bossing of the skull
Bossing of the frontal and parietal eminences occurs.

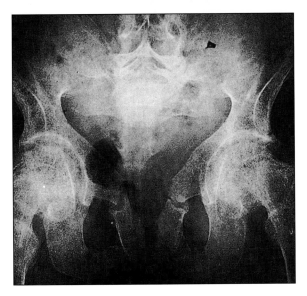

996 Osteomalacia
The increased demands of pregnancy may result in gross deformity of the pelvis. This occurs, for example, in mothers kept in purdah.

THE B VITAMINS

Thiamine (Vitamin B1)

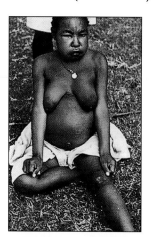

997 Beri beri oedema
'Wet' beri beri is a disease characterised by generalised oedema, peripheral neuropathy and sometimes heart failure, associated with thiamine deficiency.

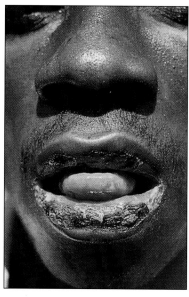

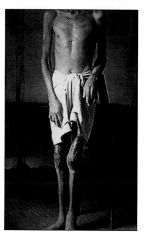

998 Peripheral neuropathy
Wrist drop and marked wasting of the lower extremities occur in some patients.

1000 Cheilosis
A sore, cracked condition of the lips occurs in association with riboflavin deficiency.

Riboflavin (Vitamin B2)

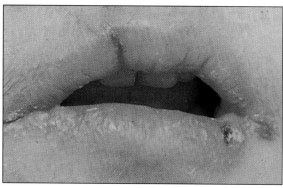

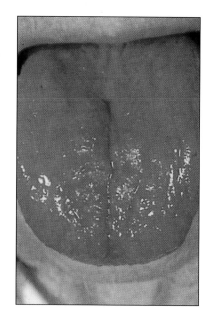

1001 Glossitis
The tongue is sore, smooth and an abnormally deep-red colour. This sign may also occur with other nutritional deficiencies.

999 Angular stomatitis
This consists of grey-white fissures at both angles of the mouth due to riboflavin deficiency. This patient also has sore, cracked lips (cheilosis).

Folic acid

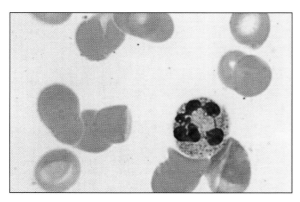

1002 Anaemia of folic acid deficiency
Folic acid deficiency results in a macrocytic megaloblastic anaemia. Shown here is a characteristic, hypersegmented neutrophil. (*Giemsa* × *1350.*)

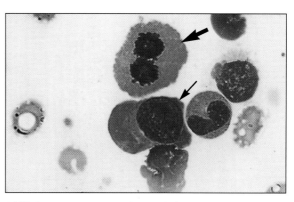

1003 Bone marrow in folic acid deficiency
The appearance in this marrow is characteristic of folic acid deficiency, with megaloblastosis of erythroid precursors (*large arrow*) and large leucocyte precursors (*small arrow*). (*Giemsa* × *900.*)

Nicotinic acid (PP)

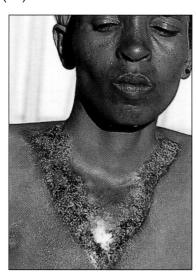

1004 Pellagra
The diagnostic triad of pellagra is dermatitis, diarrhoea and dementia. The rash of pellagra is a combination of symmetrical skin lesions with sharp demarcation and distribution in parts exposed to the sun. Shown here is the so-called 'Casal's necklace,' a ring of dermatitis around the neck. Pellagra is relatively common in people whose diet is composed predominantly of maize. It also commonly accompanies the emaciation of 'slim disease,' which is associated with AIDS in Africans.

Vitamin C

1005 Scurvy
Vitamin C deficiency is rare in the tropics. Severe gingivitis and loosening of the teeth occur in scurvy.

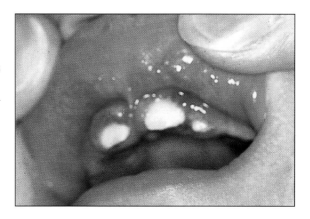

IODINE DEFICIENCY

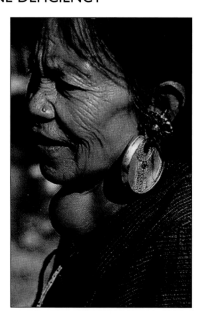

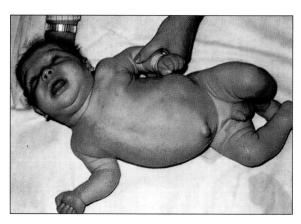

1007 Cretinism
Endemic cretinism is often seen in areas where endemic goitre occurs. These children have gross mental retardation, short stature, squint, gait disturbances and variable deaf mutism.

1006 Nepalese woman with goitre
Endemic goitre, which is common in many parts of the tropics, especially in mountainous areas, is probably due directly or indirectly to iodine deficiency.

CHAPTER 9

Miscellaneous Disorders

In this section are included some of the most prevalent and lethal diseases known to humans. The zoonotic viral haemorrhagic diseases (**Table 25**), fortunately uncommon, include a number, such as Lassa fever, Marburg fever and Ebola fever, that have only been recognised in recent years. On the contrary, acute viral hepatitis (which is parenterally acquired) is one of the most prevalent and dangerous cosmopolitan infections of the present day. Hepatitis B virus (HBV) is present in over 300 million active carriers, of whom over 40% will become chronic carriers as adults. Chronic infection with this potentially oncogenic virus can result in hepatic cirrhosis in up to 80% of those infected, and this, in turn, is associated with hepatocellular carcinoma. With an incidence of over 250 000 per year, 85% following chronic cirrhosis, this is one of the 10 commonest malignancies worldwide; Africa alone has more than 50 million chronic carriers. HBV infection, which kills more than one million infants and children each year, is now preventable by vaccination.

Numerically of less importance but probably of global distribution are infections caused by hantaviruses of the Bunyaviridae family (**Table 25**). They are responsible for three syndromes in humans: haemorrhagic fever with renal syndrome, nephropathia epidemica and hantavirus pulmonary syndrome. The viruses are enzootic in rodents from which humans probably acquire infection mainly via aerosol spread of rodent excreta.

Among the neoplasias that are prevalent in the tropics are Burkitt's tumour, nasopharyngeal carcinoma and hepatoma. The first two are related to the presence of Epstein–Barr virus in individuals who are immunocompromised by malaria or other diseases, and the latter, as stated above, to infection with HBV and, in some cases, to HCV.

A number of genetic blood dyscrasias are especially common in some tropical areas. Some, such as the sickle-cell trait, may have afforded a positive selective advantage in areas highly endemic for falciparum malaria. However, as they are well documented elsewhere, only passing reference is made to these conditions here.

Injuries from the bites or stings of venomous invertebrates and vertebrates are particularly hazardous in warmer climates. A number of examples from the main animal orders are presented in this chapter, which concludes with figures of a few conditions that are of uncertain aetiology.

Table 25 Classification and causes of haemorrhagic fevers and Hantavirus syndromes[1][2][3]

Virus (Family: genus)	Disease	Transmission	Vector(s)	Reservoir(s)
Flaviviridae *Flavivirus*	Dengue HF	mosquito bite	*Aedes aegypti* and other mosquitoes	mosquitoes[4]; ? monkeys
	Kyasanur Forest disease	tick bite	*Haemaphysalis* spp.	rodents; ? monkeys
	Omsk HF	tick bite	*Dermacentor* spp.	ticks[4]; muskrats
	Yellow fever (Africa)	mosquito bite	*Aedes* (*Stegomyia*) spp.	mosquitoes[4]; monkeys
	Yellow fever (S. America)	mosquito bite	*Haemagogus* spp.	mosquitoes[4]; forest rodents
Togaviridae *Alphavirus*	Chikungunya fever	mosquito bite	*Aedes* (*Stegomyia*) spp.	monkeys; ?rodents
Bunyaviridae *Phlebovirus*	Rift Valley fever	mosquito bite	various culicine spp.	domestic livestock; ? rodents
Nairovirus	Congo-Crimea HF	tick bite	*Hyalomma* spp.	ticks[4]; wild and domestic animals
Hantavirus	HFRS[5] (Korean HF)	rodent excreta aerosol ?; tick bite?		*Apodemus agrarius*; other rodent spp.
	Balkan HFRS (Porogia virus)	rodent excreta aerosol ?		*Apodemus flavicollis*
	Seoul HFRS	rodent excreta aerosol ?		*Rattus norvegicus*
	Puumala NE	rodent excreta aerosol ?		*Clethrionomys glareolus*
	Sin Nombre HPS	rodent excreta aerosol?		*Permoyscus maniculatus*
	New York HPS	rodent excreta aerosol ?		*Permoyscus leucopus*
	Black Creek Canal HPS	rodent excreta aerosol ?		*Sigmodon hispidus*
	Bayou HPS	rodent excreta aerosol ?		*Oryzomys palustris*
	Andes HPS	rodent excreta aerosol ?		*Oligoryzomys longicaudatus*
Arenaviridae *Arenavirus*	Junin (Argentine HF)	rodent excreta aerosol ?		*Calomys musculinus*; other *Calomys* spp.
	Machupo (Bolivian HF)	rodent excreta aerosol ?		*Calomys callosus*
	Lassa fever	rodent excreta		*Mastomys natalensis*
Marburg-Ebola gp. *Filovirus*	Marburg virus	infected blood via aerosol; man-man ?; infected syringes etc		? *Cercopithecus aethiops*
	Ebola virus	as above		unknown but ? monkeys

[1] The majority of haemorrhagic fevers in man are zoonotic.

[2] Adapted from Braude *et al.* (1981), Cook (1996) and Armstrong and Cohen (1999).

[3] *See also* **Table 2**.

[4] Vertical transmission occurs in vector.

[5] Hantaviruses are responsible for Haemorrhagic fever with renal syndrome (HFRS), Nephropathia epidemica (NE) and Hantavirus pulmonary syndrome (HPS). HF = haemorrhagic fever. HPS is associated with peridomestic rodent species in Argentina and probably other New World countries.

ZOONOTIC VIRAL INFECTIONS

(See **Table 25**.)

CONGO–CRIMEA HAEMORRHAGIC FEVER

1008 The cycle of infection with the virus of Congo–Crimea haemorrhagic fever
Several species of ixodid ticks transmit this arbovirus, as well as other viruses causing haemorrhagic fevers (**Table 25**). This figure shows how larvae of ticks of the genus *Hyalomma* (1) acquire the virus from birds, rodents or leporids, transmit it in the nymphal stage (2) to leporids, rodents, birds and, occasionally, humans, then via the adults (3) to humans and domestic animals. The virus can then pass to the next gen-

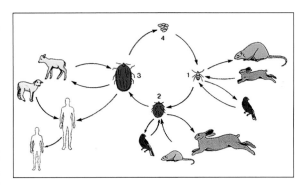

eration of larvae through transovarial transmission (4). The ticks thus serve as a reservoir for the virus. The relative sizes of the hosts in the diagram reflect their relative importance as reservoirs at the different stages of the cycle.

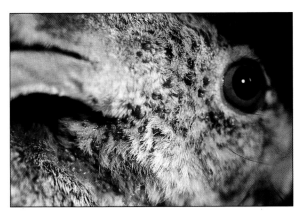

1009 *Hyalomma truncatum* nymphs and adults feeding on a West African hare, *Lepus whytei*
This African lepurid is a common vertebrate reservoir of Congo–Crimea haemorrhagic fever virus. *H. marginatum rufipes* which often lives on birds, is another host of this virus. The bird tick is widely distributed from Africa to Russia and Asia.

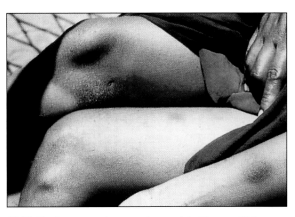

1010 Ecchymoses in a patient with Congo–Crimea haemorrhagic fever
This condition occurs in Europe, the Middle East, Asia and Africa, where it is usually acquired from tick bites by people in close contact with cattle, particularly in drier or semi-desert areas where tick infestation levels are high. A number of human to human outbreaks have also been reported among hospital staff and patients.

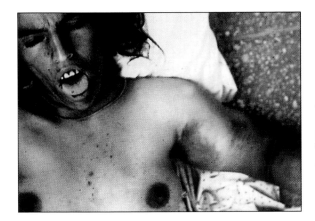

1011 Severe bleeding in Congo–Crimea haemorrhagic fever
This woman has large petechial haemorrhages on her upper chest and massive ecchymoses in the left arm and axilla. Mucosal bleeding also occurs, and death is commonly due to uncontrollable haemorrhage and shock. The fatality rate ranges between 15 and 70%.

LASSA FEVER

1012 Virus of Lassa fever

The virus of Lassa fever belongs to the genus *Arenavirus* in the family Arenaviridae. Several genetically distinct strains of this virus have been characterised from different parts of Sub-Saharan Africa. Their mode of transmission to humans is not fully understood, but human to human infections seem common. Virus particles are seen in the perisinusoidal space in this biopsy sample of liver from a fatal human case. The virions can be spherical or pleomorphic ranging from about 110 to 130 nm and contain several electron-dense ribosomes with a diameter of 20 to 25 nm ($\times 18\ 300$). (From Winn, WC Jr, Monath TP, Murphy FA, Whitfield SG. Lassa virus hepatitis: observations on a fatal case from the

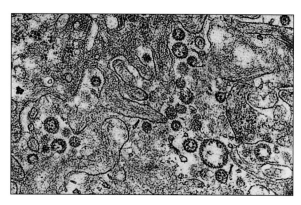

1972 epidemic in Sierra Leone. *Archives of Pathology* (1975) **99**, 599–604.)

1013 Rodent reservoir, *Mastomys natalensis*

Lassa fever occurs as an acute infectious disease in rural areas of several West African countries. During the second week of infection, toxic or vascular symptoms appear. These include pharyngitis, serous effusions, facial oedema, haemorrhagic diathesis, disorders of the central nervous system and a state of shock. The case fatality rate is high among severe cases, but benign, febrile cases of the disease also occur, as well as asymptomatic carriers. A rodent reservoir has been implicated in the epidemiology of Lassa fever.

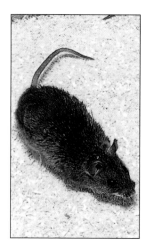

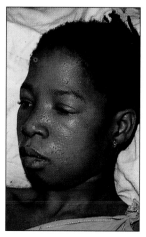

1014 Facial oedema in Lassa fever

Facial oedema is seen here in a 23-year-old Sierra Leonean woman on the 10th day of her illness; she also developed shock. These are common features of severe cases and carry a poor prognosis. The risk of human to human transmission of the virus is now considered to be less of a hazard than was originally believed. (© D.A. Warrell.)

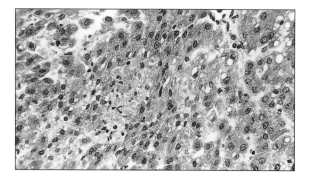

1015 Liver in Lassa fever

Liver necrosis with minimal cellular infiltrate is a marked feature of the hepatic lesion. (*H&E* × 250.)

MARBURG AND EBOLA HAEMORRHAGIC FEVERS

The precise classification of the long, filamentous viruses that are responsible for these haemorrhagic fevers is still disputed. Some authorities place them in a new family of negative-stranded, RNA viruses, the Filoviridae, genus *Filovirus*. These pathogens were first recorded in 1967 in Marburg, Germany, and in Yugoslavia, where laboratory workers were infected from the tissues of African monkeys. The Marburg virus has since been identified sporadically in patients with haemorrhagic fever in Zimbabwe, South Africa and Kenya. The Ebola virus was isolated from patients with haemorrhagic fever in Zaïre (now the Democratic Republic of Congo) and The Sudan in 1976. In those countries nearly 600 cases occurred, 88% of those in Zaïre and 53% of those in The Sudan proving fatal. Another *Filovirus* related to the Ebola group (named Ebola–Reston) was identified in cynomolgus monkeys (*Macaca fascicularis*) imported from the Philippines to the USA and to Italy in 1989 and 1990. This proved to be infective to humans but did not produce serious infection. In 1995 a further epidemic of Ebola fever infected at least 315 cases of whom 77% died. Other, iso-lated cases were identified in Côte d'Ivoire and Gabon between 1994 and 1996. In August 2000 a new epidemic began in Uganda. By the end of the first two months, 367 cases were confirmed with 149 fatalities in two districts. Although intensive containment measures limited the further geographic extension of the epidemic, 423 cases with 169 deaths (40% mortality) were recorded by mid-January 2001. The mode of primary infection in nature of the Marburg–Ebola group of viruses remains unknown. Secondary infection is by nosocomial infection, especially from blood and tissue fluids. Reston virus is probably spread also by aerosol infection. The incubation period is short, 4 to 16 days, the onset sudden and severe haemorrhagic mani-festations usually develop during the fifth to seventh days. Liver, spleen and kidneys become necrotic, and diffuse bleed-ing may occur from all orifices. In the absence of immunisa-tion or chemotherapy, the control of infection is dependent on rigidly enforced, classic containment measures, including quarantine, but these may be difficult to achieve in the unso-phisticated type of rural environment where most outbreaks are likely to occur. Intensive care, with special attention to fluid and electrolyte replacement, can reduce the mortality significantly.

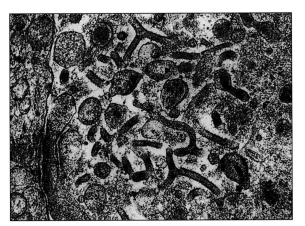

1016 Virus of Ebola haemorrhagic fever
This, and the Marburg virus (which is morphologically almost identical) in the genus *Filovirus*, are the only branched viruses so far known. The virus shown here is from human liver. (× *30 000*.)

1017 Ebola haemorrhagic fever
Haemorrhagic manifestations in the skin and internal organs are common. However, mild cases, as well as asymptomatic carriers, do also occur. In these a papular rash is seen, usually around the fifth day of the illness. The natural reservoir of the Ebola group of viruses in Africa has not yet been identi-fied, although it is suspected that certain bats in the rain forest may play a part in maintaining transmission.

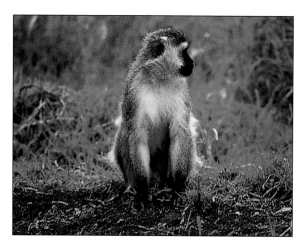

1018 *Cercopithecus aethiops,* **reservoir of Marburg virus**

The African green monkey or Vervet was the source of lethal infections contracted by laboratory workers in Europe. This species of monkey is also the host for SIV, the simian immunodeficiency virus (also known as STLV-III; simian T lymphotropic virus type III) (*see* **777, 778**). Although sporadic human infections have also occurred in Africa, the Marburg virus, unlike Ebola, has not so far been identified as the cause of epidemic, haemorrhagic fever. The causative *Filovirus* closely resembles that of Ebola fever (*see* **1016**).

HAEMORRHAGIC FEVER WITH RENAL SYNDROME

1019 Ultrastructure of Hantaan virus

This RNA hantavirus of the family Bunyaviridae (*see* **Table 25**) has been identified as the cause of a widely distributed, haemorrhagic fever with renal syndrome (HFRS), which is sometimes associated with acute nephropathy and renal failure. Hantaan virus infects nearly 150 000 Asians yearly, producing 5% mortality. Korean haemorrhagic fever (Seoul virus), Scandinavian 'nephropathia epidemica' (Puumala virus) and Balkan HFRS (Porogia virus) are related viruses, the last of these killing 15–30% of those infected. Various rodents, such as species of *Apodemus* and *Clethrionomys*, act as natural reservoirs, with the virus residing in their lungs; laboratory rats have even been found infected in several countries. Transmission may be direct or airborne via contaminated rodent urine, saliva or faeces or, possibly, through tick bite during epidemics. The hantaviruses include Prospect Hill virus (which gives rise to asymptomatic infection in humans in the USA), as well as Muerto Canyon (or 'four corners') virus—which is enzootic in deer mice (*Peromyscus maniculatus*), causing a severe, acute hantavirus pulmonary syndrome (HPS), with over 50% mortality in parts of the USA west of the Mississippi River. Several hantaviruses are also enzootic in Latin America. In the south of Argentina, for example, high infection rates have been recorded in up to 5.4% of peridomestic *Oligoryzomys longi-*

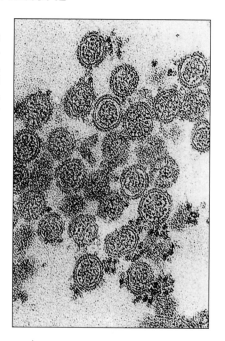

caudatus in association with HPS in rural habitats. The Hantaan virus particles seen here in section were grown in Vero E6 cells. (× *62 000.*)

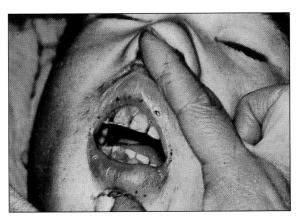

1020 Haemorrhagic fever with renal syndrome (HFRS) in a Chinese patient
Three days after the onset of his illness, severe haemorrhages occurred in the mouth of this 20-year-old man.

PARENTERALLY ACQUIRED ACUTE VIRAL HEPATITIS

(see **Table 15**.)

Four viruses associated with acute viral hepatitis are acquired by the parenteral route. Hepatitis B virus (HBV; a DNA hepadnavirus with affinities to the retroviruses), which can be transmitted from mother to infant at birth, causes the most serious infections and results in a chronic carrier state in over 40% of adults. Over one million children die from the acute infection each year. In China, Southeast Asia and Africa, 10–20% of the population are HBV carriers; there are probably over 300 million carriers worldwide. Chronic active infection with this oncogenic virus may lead to hepatic cirrhosis and is responsible for up to 80% of all cases of hepatocellular carcinoma, one of the 10 commonest tumours. HDV ('Delta virus') is a 'defective,' so-called 'piggy-back' RNA virus that develops only in the presence of HBV antigen. The combined infection can give rise to a fulminating form of hepatitis. HCV (a togavirus) and HFV (a virus which is still incompletely characterised) were formerly confused under the name of HNANB(P) (non-A, non-B virus). HCV, like HBV, can give rise to a chronic carrier state and is common in Japan. A very effective vaccine now available against HBV, which should reduce the incidence of new infections in the future, is particularly indicated for the protection of neonates.

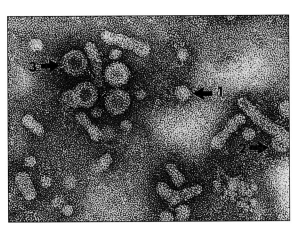

1021 Hepatitis B antigen-containing serum
Three distinct morphological entities are seen: Australia antigen surface coat in the form of (1) small, pleomorphic spherical particles measuring 20–22 nm in diameter; (2) tubular forms of varying length with a constant diameter of 20 nm (often with a terminal bulbous swelling); (3) double-shelled spheroidal Dane particles of hepatitis B virus, approximately 42 nm in diameter, with a core measuring 27 nm in diameter surrounded by surface coat. (× *167 000*.)

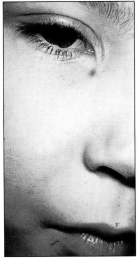

1022 Jaundiced child with hepatitis
Fever, anorexia and, later, jaundice are characteristic clinical features. The disease is particularly severe in pregnancy. Note deep jaundice and spider naevus on the cheek.

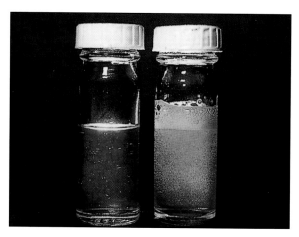

1023 Urine from child with hepatitis
The dark-coloured urine contains bilirubin and urobilinogen, which derive from conjugated bilirubin discharged into the blood from damaged hepatocytes.

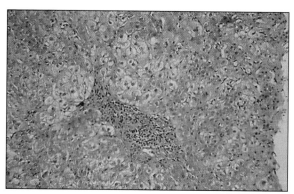

1025 Biopsy of liver in hepatitis
Histologically, the characteristic features are ballooning and a feathery degeneration of the liver parenchymal cells (×150). (See also **561–563**.)

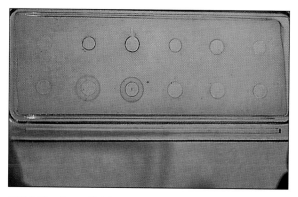

1024 Single radial immunodiffusion test
Hepatitis B virus antigen-positive serum is readily detected by this simple serological procedure.

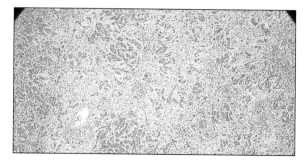

1026 Massive hepatic necrosis
Gross appearance of a liver with massive necrosis caused by hepatitis B infection. Note the wrinkled capsular surface and the 'nutmeg' appearance of the cut surface, which is due to loss of cells and congestion in the central lobular zones.

1027 Hepatic parenchyma in massive liver necrosis
Only a few isolated islands of hepatocytes remain in the liver parenchyma (H&E × 100). (AFIP No. 65–3784.)

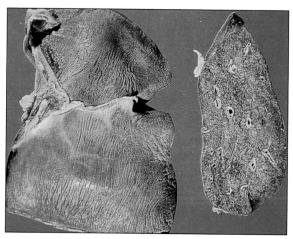

NEOPLASTIC CONDITIONS

BURKITT'S LYMPHOMA

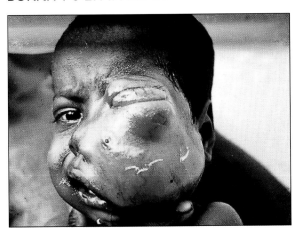

1028 African child with Burkitt's lymphoma of the maxilla

The geographical distribution of Burkitt's lymphoma in high incidence is mainly controlled by two climatic parameters: temperature and humidity. In Sub-Saharan Africa, the distribution of Burkitt's tumour is roughly the same as that of malaria. This highly malignant tumour is believed to be caused by the immunosuppression associated with chronic malaria in individuals who are carriers of the Epstein–Barr virus and characteristically show a chromosomal translocation, which leads to uncontrolled B cell proliferation. One of the most common forms of clinical presentation is that of facial swelling. The jaws are most often affected, with one or more quadrants being involved.

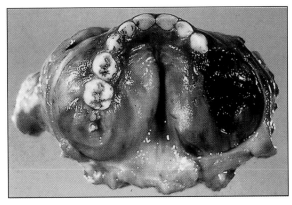

1030 Maxillary tumour at post mortem examination

The extensive infiltration of both maxillae by Burkitt's lymphoma tissue is evident in this specimen. This neoplasm, which accounts for at least half of all childhood tumours in tropical Africa, is also found in highly endemic, malarious areas of the New Guinea lowlands.

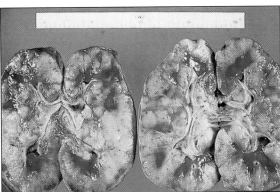

1031 Kidneys with Burkitt's lymphoma

Massive replacement of both kidneys with tumour cells is apparent in this figure. Any organ can be affected.

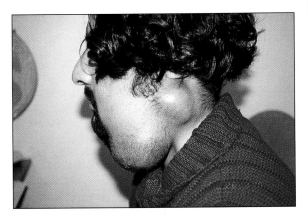

1029 Burkitt's lymphoma in an Asian adult

The figure shows enormous cervical lymphadenopathy, which was initially suggestive of tuberculous lymphadenitis but which was shown to be due to Burkitt's lymphoma by biopsy.

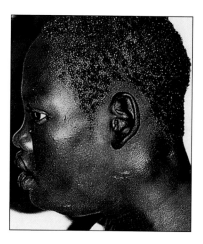

1032 Nasopharyngeal carcinoma
This condition, which is also associated with Epstein–Barr virus, has a high incidence rate in southern China. It also occurs in neighbouring countries such as Malaysia and Singapore, where it is 20 times as common in those of Chinese origin than in other races. The tumour is found also in several African countries. Massive cervical lymphadenopathy is seen in this Sudanese patient. The presenting symptoms are very variable, and depend on the precise location of the tumour. Cranial nerve involvement develops in nearly half of the cases.

HEPATOCELLULAR CARCINOMA

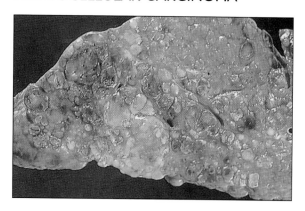

1033 Macroscopic appearance of liver
Primary, hepatocellular carcinoma of the liver (of which more than 250 000 arise yearly) is one of the 10 commonest tumours in the world and is especially common in the tropics. Coarse, nodular changes can be seen in this figure. A clear relationship has been established between hepatitis B (HBV—see **Table 15**), HCV and hepatocellular carcinoma, 85% occurring in individuals who have chronic hepatic cirrhosis. Vaccination against HBV should afford protection against hepatoma, and large-scale trials are currently in progress. Aflatoxins in certain diets seem to be an important contributory factor.

ENDEMIC KAPOSI'S SARCOMA IN AFRICA

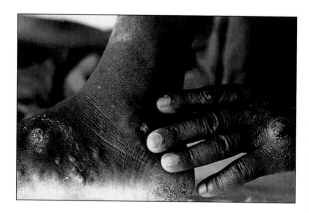

1034 Endemic (non-AIDS) Kaposi's sarcoma of the hand and foot
This malignant tumour was originally described in Austria, with its highest incidence in special ethnic communities such as southern European Jews. Later, it was recognised to be endemic in parts of Sub-Saharan Africa, particularly in Nigeria, eastern Zaïre and western Uganda. It affects mainly males, with the lesions usually starting as tumour nodules on the extremities. The lesions run a long-term course, but sometimes become more aggressive and infiltrative, causing gross lesions. Typical nodular lesions are seen on the hand and foot of this African male from Lesotho. It is now suspected that human herpesvirus 8 (in association with chronic immunodepression, especially HIV) may cause this tumour. (*See also* **803–805**.)

NEOPLASIA DUE TO CHRONIC SOLAR EXPOSURE

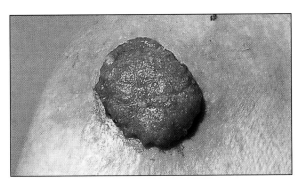

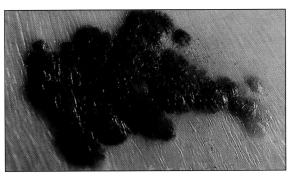

1035 Squamous cell carcinoma

Chronic exposure to solar radiation, particularly in people with light skin pigmentation, can result in various degenerative or neoplastic changes in exposed parts of the body. Increasing reduction of the ozone layer is predicted to result in an increased frequency of such conditions as squamous cell carcinoma, seen here on the shoulder of an albino patient.

1036 Malignant melanoma

A sudden increase in pigmentation and enlargement of freckles following prolonged exposure to sunlight may be precursors to the development of a malignant melanoma in a fair-skinned individual. The large melanoma seen in this 54-year-old Caucasian woman shows marked local infiltration and carries a very poor prognosis. Her skin also shows some generalised elastotic degeneration.

GENETIC BLOOD DYSCRASIAS

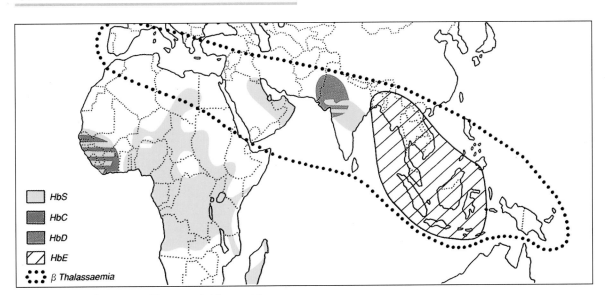

HbS
HbC
HbD
HbE
β Thalassaemia

1037 Distribution map of haemoglobinopathies

The most important abnormal haemoglobins in the tropics are Hb S, C and E. Thalassaemia, which is the result of decreased synthesis of one of the chains of haemoglobin (α or β), is also widespread. Hb D has a limited distribution and is clinically mild. The abnormal haemoglobins also occur in people in Central and South America because of migration and among blacks in the USA. The haemoglobin AS phenotype favours the survival of the gene in tropical Africa where falciparum malaria is holoendemic, but the SS phenotype increases host mortality. This is known as 'balanced polymorphism.' Alpha and β thalassaemia, Hb E and glucose-6-phosphate dehydrogenase deficiency are also believed to afford relative protection against severe *Plasmodium falciparum* infection in heterozygotes (see **97**). Alpha thalassaemia is widespread throughout all tropical areas

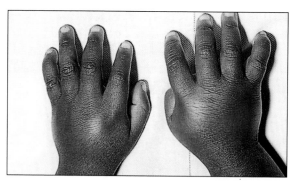

1038 Dactylitis due to sickle-cell disease
Severe bilateral dactylitis is a common presentation of sickle-cell disease in children.

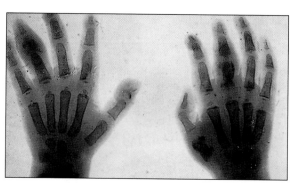

1039 Radiograph of hands in sickle-cell disease
Note the destructive changes in small bones—the result of multiple infarction complicated by infection (in this case by a *Salmonella* species).

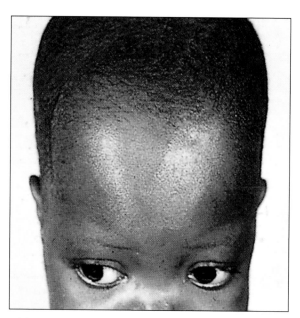

1040 Bossing of skull
Bossing of the skull due to hyperplasia of the marrow is another feature of sickle-cell disease. Similar appearances may be seen in thalassaemia and other severe, congenital haemolytic anaemias.

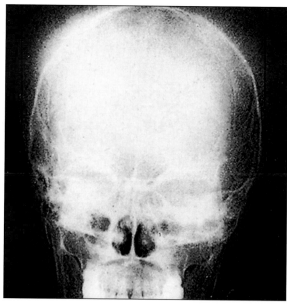

1041 Radiograph of skull in thalassaemia
Thalassaemia disease produces this typical 'hair-on-end' appearance of the skull in radiographs.

VENOMOUS BITES AND STINGS

Venomous invertebrate and vertebrate animals are to be found anywhere in the world, but are especially common in the tropics and subtropics. The following figures illustrate a few examples from various orders, including marine invertebrates and fish, scorpions, spiders, lepidoptera and snakes.

INVERTEBRATE MARINE ANIMALS

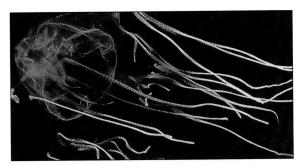

1042 The 'box jellyfish,' *Chironex fleckeri*
This venomous jellyfish, which occurs along the north Queensland coast in Australia, has caused many deaths from circulatory and respiratory failure. The tentacles, which may hang for a metre from the bell (itself about 11 cm in height), are covered with stinging nematocysts that penetrate the skin where the venom is released. The tentacles of other venomous species of jellyfish may trail for as far as 30 m.

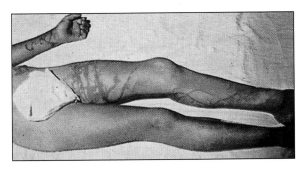

1043 Effects of contact with a 'sea wasp'
The stings of 'sea waps' are associated with intense pain. Severe stings, such as those seen here, have led to death within minutes. *Chironex fleckeri* is one of the most dangerous marine animals.

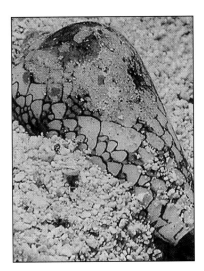

1044 A poisonous cone shell, *Conus textile*
Cone shells are common along coasts of the Indo-Pacific area. Many species have a venom apparatus that discharges through the barbed radular tooth that passes through the proboscis. This species, which has caused several fatalities, is widely distributed from the Red Sea to Polynesia.

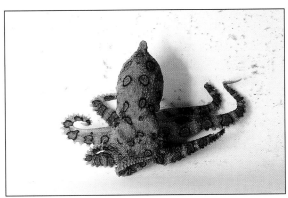

1045 Australian blue-ringed octopus, *Octopus lunulatus*
Despite the superstitions surrounding them, most octopuses are retiring, harmless animals. Exceptions are the two, small (10 cm in diameter) Indo-Pacific species, (*O. lunulatus* and *O. maculosus*), the bite of which contains tetrodoxin that can be fatal. This specimen was seen in Madang on the north coast of Papua New Guinea. (© D.A. Warrell.)

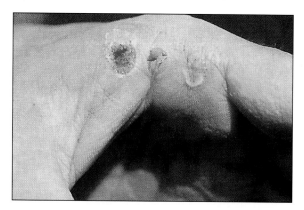

1046 Bite of an octopus
The octopus mouth has a parrot-like beak that can cause severe wounds, with even non-venomous species sometimes being very aggressive. Any octopus should be handled with care, or not at all.

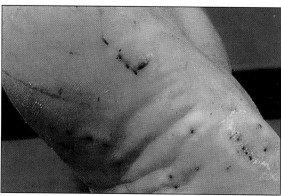

1047 Sea urchin spines in foot
Coral fishing is a popular pastime in tropical waters, but sea urchins are prevalent in such an environment. People who accidently tread on these animals with bare feet are likely to receive multiple spines deeply embedded in the skin as the brittle, sharp tips penetrate and break off easily. Some species also have venomous organs called pedicellaria between the spines.

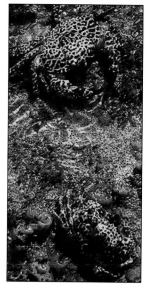

1048 *Zosimus aeneus*, a poisonous crab
This xanthid crab is common among coral in the Pacific area where it is often eaten. Its toxicity varies from region to region and it has been responsible for serious poisoning. Many contain a paralysing poison, saxitoxin, which can be lethal to humans. These crabs, as well as several other poisonous tropical shellfish ('ciguatera poisoning') and fish, may acquire the venoms from dinoflagellates in the food chain.

FISH

1049 Venomous spines of the stone fish, *Synanceja horrida*
Many species of fish, including weever fishes and stone fishes, have venomous spines. The stone fish lies well concealed in the sand of marine shores. Venom produced in glands that emerge at the tips of the dorsal spines causes intense pain if they enter the skin, and severe stings can be fatal. This species, one of the most dangerous, occurs around Indo-Pacific coasts as far south as southern Australia. Stone fishes belong to the family *Scorpionidae*, which also includes scorpion fishes and zebra fishes. Many of the species are found in the eastern Pacific and Atlantic coastal waters, as well as the Indo-Pacific region.

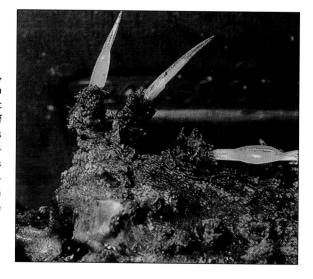

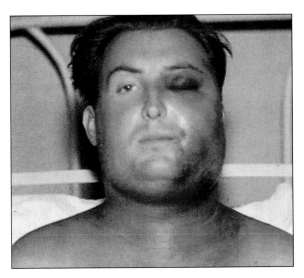

1050 Man stung by a weever fish
Weever fish, which are distributed along northeast Atlantic and Mediterranean coasts, have venomous spines over the gill covers and dorsum. The venom is both neurotoxic and haemotoxic. This man shows the haemorrhagic effects of weever fish venom.

TERRESTRIAL INVERTEBRATES

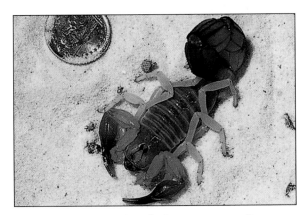

1051 A buthid scorpion, *Androctonus australis*
Most scorpions are of little danger to humans but, of the 20 or so species that are, several cause many deaths each year. This 'fat-tailed scorpion,' which occurs throughout the Mediterranean littoral, north and northwest Africa, is one of the most dangerous species. It was responsible, for example, for nearly 400 deaths among 20 000 people stung in Algeria between 1942 and 1958. The venom, which stimulates first the parasympathetic nervous system and then the sympathetic, can cause respiratory paralysis and death. Antivenoms are available against some species.

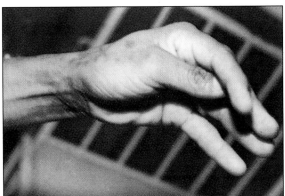

1052 Muscle spasm following a sting by *Androctonus crassicauda* on the wrist
This scorpion is also very widely distributed and has been responsible for many serious stings, especially in Turkey. The adult is slightly smaller than *A. australis* but may reach over 7 cm in length. This Iranian man made a full recovery with minimal systemic effects. Specific antivenoms against *A. australis* and *A. crassicauda* are available in some countries.

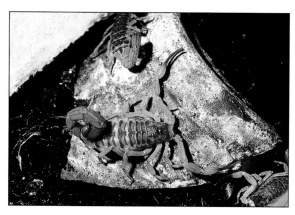

1053 *Tityus serrulatus*
This is probably the most dangerous species of this New World, largely South American genus. Like *Centruroides*, this species commonly frequents houses and is responsible for a large number of serious cases of scorpionism in Brazil, where an antivenom has been produced. Spraying houses with residual insecticides such as DDT has been beneficial in reducing its numbers. *T. serrulatus* is believed to be the only parthenogenetic species of scorpion. Adults are about 7 cm long.

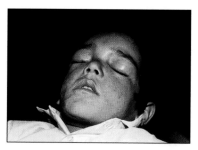

1055 Facial oedema due to cardiac dysfunction following a sting by *Hemiscorpius lepturus*
If a sufficiently high concentration of the venom of this scorpion reaches the circulation, it can exert serious changes in the central nervous and cardiovascular systems, as well as causing acute haemolysis, which may necessitate blood transfusion, and depression of the circulating lymphocytes in the blood. This Iranian boy is one of 54 who showed systemic effects among 2534 patients stung by *H. lepturus*.

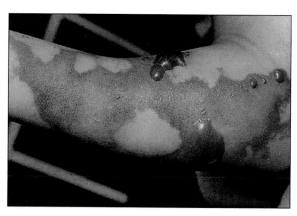

1056 Lesions following a sting by *Hemiscorpius lepturus*
The venom of chactid scorpions is mainly haemolytic and proteolytic. This child's arm shows the early stages of skin necrosis following a sting by *H. lepturus*, a species that occurs in Iran and Iraq. Sloughing of the affected skin later required extensive skin grafting.

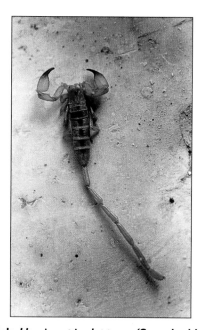

1054 Male *Hemiscorpius lepturus* (Scorpionidae)
This Middle Eastern species has exceptionally long, thin, postabdominal segments and a very small spine on the sting. Despite this it is very dangerous and accounts for 10 to 15% of all stings in Iran in the summer and most stings in the winter months. Adult males are 8.5 cm long, females 4.5 to 5 cm.

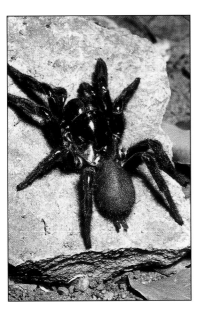

1057 Female *Atrax robustus*

This large Australian arthropod (the 'Sydney funnel web spider,' female body length up to 4 cm), one of several species of *Atrax* on that continent, is a large, nocturnal spider that often enters houses in New South Wales. Its bite is extremely painful and it has caused several deaths through the injection, by means of its large fangs, of atratoxin to which humans are peculiarly susceptible. This neurotoxin induces spontaneous action potentials in nerves supplying skeletal muscle as well as the autonomic nervous system. The clinical picture in severe envenomation is a mixture of signs starting with severe muscular twitching, profuse salivation and lachrymation, nausea and vomiting, abdominal pain and diarrhoea, followed by acute hypertension, extreme restlessness, dyspnoea possibly leading to asphyxia, confusion and finally coma and death. The initial treatment should be to apply a strong pressure bandage and immobilise the affected limb to slow the absorption of the venom, followed by the administration of specific antivenom.

1058 Female *Loxosceles laeta* (Scytodidae)

This genus, which is widely distributed throughout much of the world, contains well over 60 species of which four are especially poisonous to humans: *L. laeta*, *L. reclusa*, *L. gaucho* and *L. rufescens*, although envenomation has also been recorded from bites of other species. These spiders are also called 'violin spiders' because of the characteristic violin-like marking on the dorsal surface of the cephalothorax in many species, or 'brown spiders' because of their dull brown colouration. *Loxosceles* spin an irregular web and feed mainly on small arthropods that they ensnare. However, they are mainly nocturnal and, because they seek dark places to shelter, they are commonly attracted to human habitations. If accidentally handled, they bite with their inwardly pointing fangs, at the same time actively ejecting venom. This is essentially cytolytic as it is normally used to partially digest the bodies of prey, which can then be ingested through the mouth. However, in mammals it can also be haemolytic. This

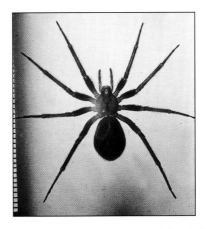

species is found over much of South America except the extreme northern parts and is responsible for hundreds of severe injuries, with up to about 10% of fatalities. (× 2.3.)

1059 Girl bitten by *Loxosceles laeta*

Loxoscelism presents in two forms, the first limited to the skin and subcutaneous tissues and the second systemic due to the haemolytic effects of the venom when absorbed. This Chilean child who was bitten on the right cheek shows the effects of severe intravascular haemolysis, as well as the beginning of blistering and necrosis of the skin. The massive facial oedema is evident, and she is comatose. This type of response to envenomation occurs in about 13% of the victims of *L. laeta* bites. Up to one third of such cases die with haematuria, anuria and other evidence of haemolysis unless treated urgently with antivenom and general supportive therapy.

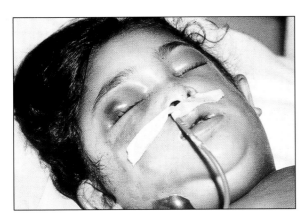

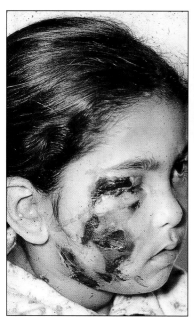

1060 Sloughing of skin following spider bite
This Chilean child was bitten by *Loxosceles laeta*. Necrosis and sloughing followed severe blistering at the site of the bite and generalised facial oedema.

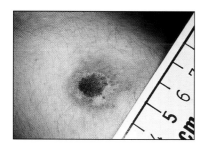

1061 Bite by *Loxosceles gaucho* on the thigh after 48 hours
Initially the site of the bite, which is very painful, shows an area of oedema with a central violaceous plaque. After a while the centre becomes necrotic and is surrounded by an area of ischaemia, beyond which is an erythematous halo. (© D.A.Warrell.)

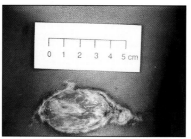

1062 Lesion caused by *Loxosceles gaucho* 25 days after the bite
The affected skin was removed surgically as the area surrounding the bite is now known to have a high content of venom. Debridement can assist by removing this material, although skin grafting is often required later to promote healing. Antibiotics to control secondary bacterial infection are indicated, and sometimes cortico-steroids. (© D.A.Warrell.)

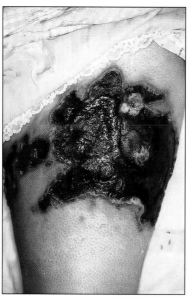

1063 Severe necrosis following a bite by *Loxosceles reclusa* in the western USA

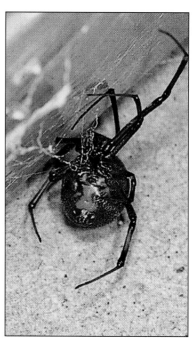

1064 'Black widow' spider
Among the best known poisonous spiders is the 'black widow,' *Latrodectus mactans*. Humans are bitten only by the females, which produce α-latrotoxin, a venom that causes the rapid release of acetylcholine at neuromuscular junctions. Noradrenaline is also released, causing signs of overstimulation of the sympathetic nervous system. A transient acute psychosis may follow, but most victims make a full recovery. (× 1.)

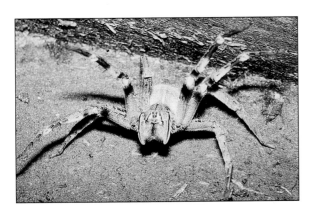

1065 Female *Phoneutria* in fighting stance

The chelicerae and fangs are very clear in this picture of a specimen seen in Cayenne. These species inhabit the Amazonian part of Brazil and neighbouring countries. The banana spiders are aggressive creatures and will attack their attacker, moving very rapidly and climbing anything available to reach them. (× *0.75.*)

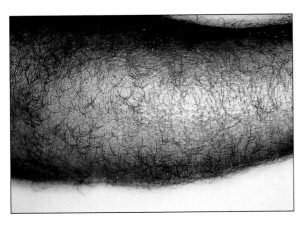

1066 Bite by *Phoneutria nigriventer*

One of the bite marks is visible. The venom is neurotoxic and functions in a similar manner to atratoxin by causing the release of acetylcholine and catecholamines that stimulate the parasympathetic and sympathetic nervous systems. About two hours after the bite there is marked local swelling, sweating and piloerection due to the release of cat-echolamines. The associated signs are similar to those described for poisoning by atratoxin but, in addition, pri-apism often occurs in boys. Death caused by *Phoneutria* occurs rarely. In Brazil a polyvalent antivenom is available against *Phoneutria, Lycosa* and *Loxosceles*. (© D.A. Warrell.)

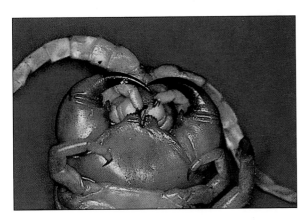

1067 Head of a venomous centipede

A few of the large species of tropical centipedes are capable of inflicting an intensely painful but probably non-lethal sting. The venom is passed through the piercing forcipules seen on the ventral surface of the head of this large *Scolopendra* species from Singapore. (× 2.)

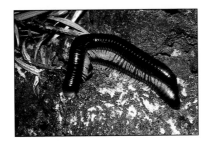

1068 *Epibolus pulchripes* (Spirobolida)

These giant millipedes from East Africa are harmless unless provoked, preferring to hide in moist earth or humus where they feed on vegetable matter. The glossy male is readily dis-tinguished from the female, which has a comparatively matt surface. The pairs of orange legs on each segment and the bright orange, jointed antennae of the male are well illustrated here. Some tropical species such as the African *Graphidostreptus gigas* can exceed 28 cm in length.

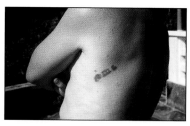

1069 'Burn' caused by contact with *Epibolus pulchripes*
The victim unwittingly slept on the millipede which had
entered his bed. Within an hour he noted itching and discomfort, and the following morning the site was erythematous. It
subsequently turned purple. Five days later the hardened skin
cracked and peeled leaving a raw patch, which eventually
healed, leaving no residual pigmentation.

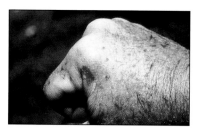

**1070 'Burn' caused by fluid droplets squirted by
*Polyconoceras alokistus***
This giant streptobolid is endemic in Papua New Guinea, the
child whose fist is shown here being attacked at Lae on the
north coast. Like that of *Epibolus pulchripes*, the liquid that
this species can eject for some 25 cm causes immediate pain
and brown staining on contact with the skin, followed by
erythema and oedema, which may remain visible for a week
or more. If the fluid reaches the conjunctiva or cornea it can
cause serious and very painful conjunctivitis, with subsequent ulceration of the conjunctiva and cornea.

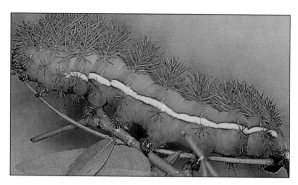

1071 Poisonous spines on a caterpillar
The larvae of many species of moths are protected with
venomous spines. The toxin of many species (including the
Saturniid species, *Automeris liberia*, from Cayenne, seen here)
contains histamine. (× 0.7.)

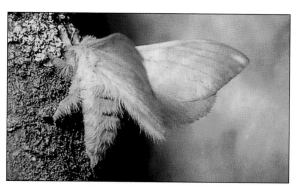

1072 Female *Hylesia metabus* (Saturniidae)
The abdomens of adult moths of this genus are covered with
strongly barbed, urticating hairs (fléchettes), which are
readily shed if the insects are damaged. The presence of
large numbers of these moths has caused epidemics of
'lepidopterism' or 'erucism' of sufficient gravity that several
tropical tourist centres have had to be temporarily abandoned. (× 1.1.)

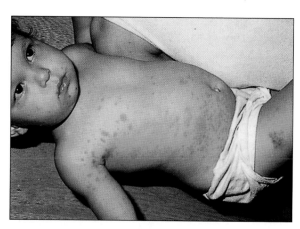

1073 Rash caused by contact with *Hylesia*
This child in São Paulo State, Brazil, was probably affected by
H. paulex, which is common in that area. The venom of
another Brazilian moth, *Lonomia achelous*, contains a fibri-
nolysin. Stings from the caterpillar spines can cause severe
ecchymoses and profuse bleeding from the body orifices.
(© D.A. Warrell.)

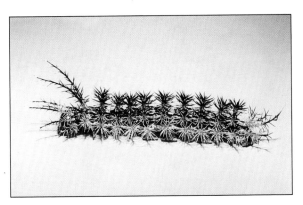

1074 Caterpillar of *Lonomia achelous* (Saturniidae)

This Hemileucine species, which occurs in the Amazon region of Brazil, has poison spines that deliver a potent fibrinolytic toxin. Similar toxic responses to Saturniid caterpillars have been reported from Venezuela.

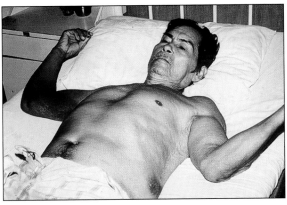

1075 Brazilian adult with severe haemorrhagic syndrome after being stung by a larva of *Lonomia achelous*

Following contact with the insect there is a localised burning sensation, then headache and generalised discomfort. Extensive ecchymoses appear from eight to 72 hours in the affected area and then over other parts of the body. There may be profuse bleeding from the orifices.

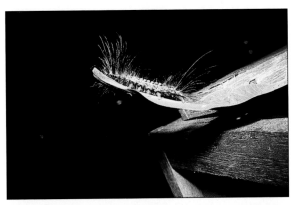

1076 Larva of *Premolis semirufa* (Arctiidae)

Stinging by this Brazilian caterpillar causes a condition known as 'pararama.' The long barbed hairs at both ends of the insect are prominent in this picture as are the brown dorsal tufts. The latter carry short, venomous hairs that cause a severe inflammatory reaction at the sites of the skin that are penetrated. (× 0.5)

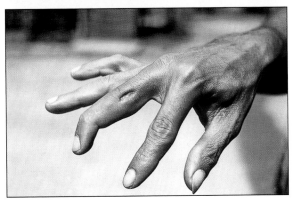

1077 Deformation of the hand in a Brazilian rubber tapper

Premolis semirufa feeds on the leaves of the rubber tree, *Hevea brasiliensis*, and is commonly encountered by plantation workers. The stings cause deep inflammation around the joints that may leave the victim permanently disabled.

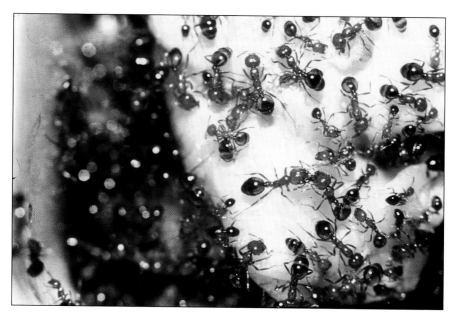

1078 Workers of *Solenopsis* (Myrmicinae)
Two sizes of workers of this unidentified species of 'fire ant' from Cayenne are seen feeding on a piece of meat. *Solenopsis* species have gained their name because of the extremely painful stings they inflict. The venom is composed largely of various 2,6-dialkylpiperidines, the exact compounds being species dependent. They are haemolytic and cytolytic. Some proteinaceous material and a small quantity of phospholipase A and hyaluronidase are also present. Like all Myrmicinae, they also possess mandibular gland venoms that are rich in ethyl ketones. ($\times$ 2.4.)

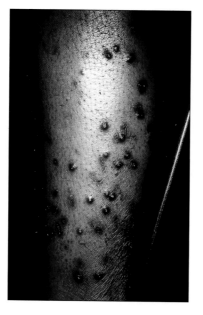

1079 Healing bites of *Solenopsis* in a dark-skinned individual
The pustules rupture leaving a crust that heals in three to 10 days. As with other hymenopterous stings, some individuals become sensitised, and repeated stings by *Solenopsis* can lead to severe anaphylactic responses. In the southern USA it has been estimated that one million people are stung every year by *S. geminata*.

1080 Acute renal failure following multiple stings by *Vespa affinis*

Hornets in this genus occur worldwide and are generally large, very aggressive insects. They often attack in large numbers and are responsible for many deaths. *V. orientalis* occurs from North and East Africa, through the Middle East and Central Asia to Southeast Asia. This Thai soldier who was stung by over 100 hornets, developed intravascular haemolysis associated with frank haemoglobinuria and acute renal tubular necrosis leading to renal failure. He eventually recovered after dialysis. Such serious consequences of multiple hornet stings are not uncommon. Another effect of hornet venom is rhabdomyolysis associated with myoglobinuria and renal failure. Recovery can be achieved with prompt dialysis and other supportive measures. Phospholipase A associated with kinins in the venom is believed to trigger the red cell lysis and may also have a direct toxic effect on the renal tubular epithelium. Wasp venom also contains a mast-cell degranulating peptide called mastoparan. This is also a potent stimulator of endogenous phospholipase activity

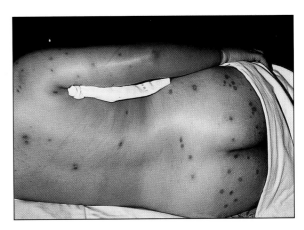

(comparable to the mellitin in bee venom). Such severe responses can be distinguished from hypersensitivity reactions as the latter are almost immediate and may follow even a single sting. Purely toxic effects may take 24 hours or more to become evident.

1081 Fatal, multiple bee stings by *Apis mellifera scutellata*, the African 'killer bee'

This highly aggressive bee was introduced into Brazil in 1956 because of its good honey productivity. It has competed with the local subspecies of *Apis mellifera* and is now colonising other countries of both South and North America where the aggressive behaviour of its swarms has caused many casualties and deaths. The colony seen here were in Cayenne. As distinct from the stings of wasps, those of bees are barbed and cannot be removed from the site of the attack in skin. Unlike the venom of wasps, that of the Apidae is constituted by mellitin (about 50%), phospholipase A (12%), histamine (0.1 to 1.5%), hyaluronidase (1 to 3%), apamin (2%) and a mast-cell discharging peptide (MCD) (1 to 2%). Histamine produces the acute pain following bee stings. Mellitin is a stimulator of endogenous phospholipase A (like the mastoparan of wasps, which also combines the action of MCD). Apamin has a neurotoxic action. Mellitin is actually a mixture of several peptides that seem to be antigenic but not anaphylactogenic. Apamin, which may also contain several small peptides, acts on polysynaptic reflexes at the level of the spinal cord. The figure shows a Brazilian boy aged 13 years, 48 hours after he was attacked by a swarm of *A. mellifera scutellata* in São Paulo State, Brazil. He received more than 1500 stings. At first he developed extensive oedema and bruising, his consciousness was impaired and he became oliguric. The remains of many bee stings can

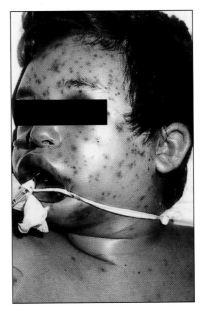

still be seen in the skin and hair. Later the boy developed bronchospasm, hypotension and intravascular haemolysis with haemoglobinuria and myoglobinuria. He also had spontaneous bleeding from the mouth and other sites. Soon he became anuric and hypertensive, dying on the third day after being stung. (© D.A. Warrell.)

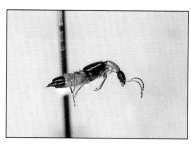

1082 *Paederus fusca*
(Staphylinidae)
These small, colourful staphylinids
produce vesicating lesions if crushed
on the skin due to the release from
their bodies of pederin, an extremely
toxic alkaloid. *P. fusca* is common in rice
fields in Thailand and other countries
of Southeast Asia and causes blisters in
rice pickers during the harvest season.
(× 4.5.)

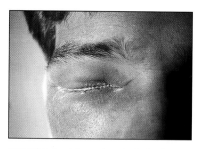

**1083 'Nairobi eye,' ophthalmia
caused by** *Paederus sabaeus*
Severe periorbital swelling is seen,
associated with a linear vesication of
the upper eyelid and adjacent bridge of
the nose, as well as a purulent conjunctivitis. The patient was affected by a
beetle that flew into his eye 39 hours
before this photograph was taken.

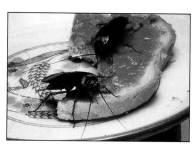

1084 Adult *Periplaneta americana*
feeding
Cockroaches such as these and *Blatella
germanica*, which frequent houses and
feed on rotting organic matter, food,
excrement and other debris, can carry
pathogens mechanically on their feet,
legs and mouthparts. There is increasing evidence that antigens derived from
cockroaches such as these are responsible for asthma, especially among
people living in highly infested, poor
quality housing. (× 0.5.)

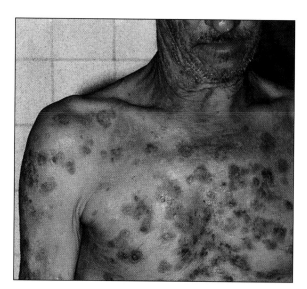

1085 Brazilian man with 'fogo selvagem'
This chronic form of pemphigus is endemic in a number of
localities in central and western Brazil, northern Argentina,
Peru, Bolivia and Venezuela. It is commonest in young women
in hot, humid rural areas, but about 15% of those affected
are children. The burning sensation in the skin gives rise to
the name. It is now believed to be caused by massive and
repeated bites by the tiny blackfly, *Simulium oyapockense* s.l.
in the Amazon lowlands. Another, more acute condition
known as haemorrhagic syndrome of Altamira is probably
caused by the bites of large numbers of *S. minusculum* in
northern Brazil.

SNAKE BITE

(See **Table 26**.)

Venomous snakes include members of four families: sea snakes (*Hydrophiidae*); cobras, mambas, kraits and taipans (*Elapidae*); vipers and rattlesnakes (*Viperidae*); and the boomslang (*Colubridae*). Travellers to remote areas where venomous snakes are prevalent should be informed of the steps to be taken in the event of a bite and of antivenins available locally against the main species. Snake bites account for an estimated 50 000–100 000 deaths every year. Some 25 000–35 000 of these occur in Asia where the Russell's viper, *Daboia russelii*, and the 'saw-scaled' or 'carpet viper,' *Echis carinatus*, are the main culprits.

Table 26 Principal venomous snakes responsible for morbidity and mortality

Family	Subfamily	Genus and species	English name	Distribution
ATRACTASPIDIDAE		*Atractaspis* spp.	burrowing asps, stiletto snakes	Africa, Middle East
ELAPIDAE		*Naja nigricollis*	black-necked spitting cobra	Africa
		N. haje	Egyptian cobra	Africa
		N. naja	Indian cobra	Southeast Asia, Far East
		N. kaouthia	Asian cobra	Southeast Asia
		Dendroaspis spp.	mambas	Africa
		Bungarus caeruleus	Indian krait	Southeast Asia
		Acanthophis spp.	death adders	Australasia
		Oxyuranus scutellatus	common taipan	Australasia
		Pseudechis australis	mulga, king brown snake	Australasia
		Pseudonaja textilis	eastern brown snake	Australasia
		Notechis scutatus	eastern tiger snake	Australasia
HYDROPHIIDAE		*Enhydrina schistosa*	beaked sea snake	Southeast Asia
VIPERIDAE	CROTALINAE	*Crotalus adamanteus*	eastern diamondback rattlesnake	North America
		C. atrox	western diamondback rattlesnake	North America
		C. viridis subspp.	western rattlesnakes	North America
		C. durissus durissus	Central American rattlesnake	Central America
		C. durissus terrificus	South American rattlesnake	South America
		Bothrops atrox asper	terciopelo, caissaca	Central America
		B. jararaca	jararaca	South America
		Calloselasma (Agkistrodon) rhodostoma	Malayan pit viper	Southeast Asia
		Trimeresurus spp.	green pit vipers	Southeast Asia
		T. flavoviridis	habu	Far East
		T. mucrosquamatus	Chinese habu	Far East
	VIPERINAE	*Vipera berus*	viper, adder	Europe
		V. ammodytes	long-nosed viper	Europe
		V. palaestinae	Palestine viper	Asia, Middle East
		Macrovipera lebetina	levantine viper	Asia, Middle East, North Africa
		Daboia russelii	Russell's viper	Indian sub continent, Southeast Asia
		Echis spp.	'saw-scaled' or 'carpet' viper	Africa, Middle East, Southeast Asia Indian subcontinent
		Bitis arietans	puff adder	Africa
COLUBRIDAE		*Dispholidus typus*	boomslang	Africa

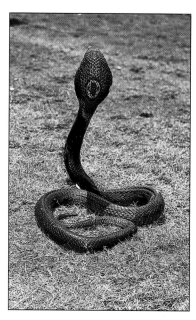

1086 Elapidae: monocellate cobra from Southeast Asia

The venom of Asian cobras (genus *Naja*), such as the *Naja kaouthia* shown here, contains both post-synaptic neurotoxins that cause paralysis and cytotoxic components that produce local tissue necrosis at the site of the bite. (© D.A. Warrell.)

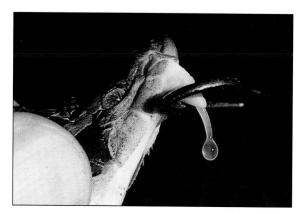

1087 Viperidae: venom being squeezed from the tip of the fang of a Malayan pit viper (*Calloselasma rhodostoma*) by gentle pressure over the venom glands

Venoms of *Viperinae* and *Crotalinae* (pit vipers) contain toxins mainly affecting blood coagulation, damaging vascular endothelium and lowering blood pressure. (© D.A. Warrell.)

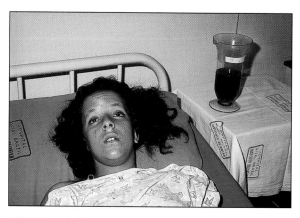

1088 Myoglobinuria following a rattlesnake bite

This patient was bitten by a tropical rattlesnake (*Crotalus durissus terrificus*) in Brazil. Eighteen hours after the bite she had 'myasthenic facies' resulting from paralysis of muscles innervated by the cranial nerves and was passing myoglobin in the urine. Both features are the result of venom phospholipases A_2, which damage nerve endings and skeletal muscle. (© D.A. Warrell.)

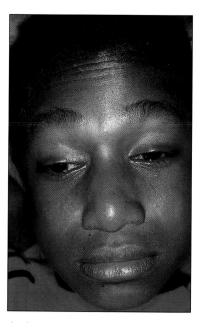

1089 Ptosis due to elapid bite

This boy was bitten by a Papuan taipan (*Oxyuranus scutellatus canni*) 4½ hours earlier. Elapid venom results in neuromuscular block, initially of muscles innervated by the cranial nerves, progressing to bulbar respiratory and, finally, generalised paralysis. This patient shows bilateral ptosis (inability to open the eyes despite contraction of the temporalis muscle puckering the brow), external ophthalmoplegia (divergent squint), paralysis of facial muscles and inability to open the mouth and protrude the tongue. (© D.A. Warrell.)

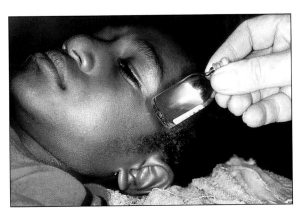

1090 Twenty minute, whole blood clotting test
This is an invaluable bedside test to detect incoagulable blood, resulting from consumption coagulopathy caused by the venom of Viperidae and some species of Colubridae and Australasian Elapidae. Blood taken by venepuncture from the patient shown in **1089** was left undisturbed in a new, clean, dry, glass vessel for 20 minutes. It remained liquid, indicating systemic envenoming. (© D.A. Warrell.)

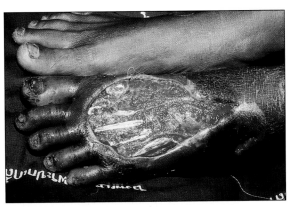

1092 Cobra bite on the foot
This is the same patient as seen in **1091**, 10 days later, after spontaneous sloughing of the necrotic skin and subcutaneous tissue exposing the tendons (© D.A. Warrell.)

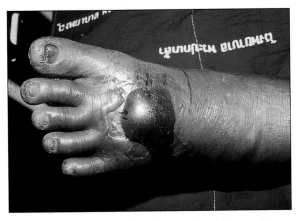

1091 Local necrosis following a cobra bite on the foot
This patient was bitten four days earlier by a monocellate cobra (*Naja kaouthia*) in Thailand (*see also* **1086**). There is a darkened, anaesthetic area surrounded by blisters, smelling of putrefaction (rotting flesh), an early sign of tissue necrosis.

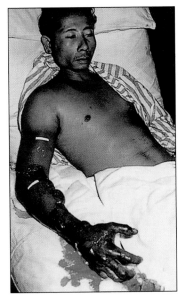

1093 Severe tissue damage caused by a viper bite
This Malaysian, who was bitten on the hand by a Malayan pit viper (*Calloselasma rhodostoma*), developed massive oedema, spreading onto the trunk, extensive bruising, blistering and bleeding.

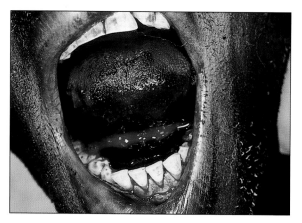

1094 Spontaneous systemic bleeding after viper bite
This man had been bitten by a saw-scaled viper (*Echis ocellatus*) 2½ hours previously in Nigeria. Bleeding from the gums and into the floor of the mouth indicates the effects of circulating venom haemorrhagins (metalloproteinases that damage vascular endothelium) that were also responsible for an intracranial haemorrhage from which he died three hours later. He had a high blood venom antigen level, but the decisive factor in this fatal outcome was probably the dose of procoagulants (prothrombin and factor X activators), as well as the haemorrhagin. (© D.A. Warrell.)

DISEASES OF UNUSUAL OR UNCERTAIN AETIOLOGY

ENDOMYOCARDIAL FIBROSIS

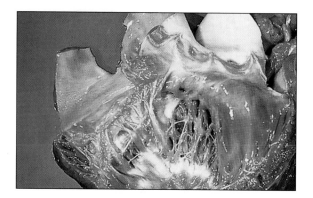

1095 Fibrotic changes in the heart of an African
Endomyocardial fibrosis is a common cause of heart disease in the tropics. It presents in three clinical forms: mainly left sided, as mitral incompetence; right sided, with features suggestive of constrictive pericarditis; a form involving both sides of the heart, presenting as congestive cardiac failure.

AINHUM

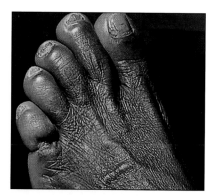

1096 Ainhum of small toe
This condition of unknown aetiology is a progressive encircling fibrosis of a toe, usually the fifth. In this patient, the lesion was bilateral, affecting also the fifth toe of the right foot.

SPRUE

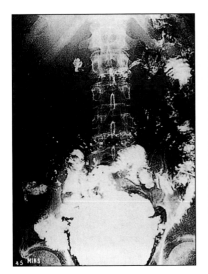 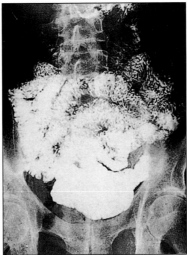 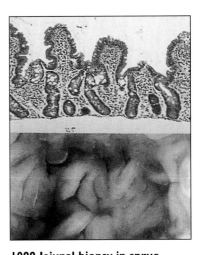

1097 & 1098 Radiographs of patient with tropical sprue
Sprue is characterised by chronic steatorrhoea of unknown aetiology, with associated abdominal symptoms, glossitis and anaemia. Fat, bulky faeces are characteristic of this condition. The figures show loss of normal intestinal pattern before treatment (**1097**, left) and then recovery after three months of treatment (**1098**, right).

1099 Jejunal biopsy in sprue
Partial villous atrophy with squat villi are seen in this biopsy sample from a patient with tropical sprue. The lower figure shows a section of the biopsy seen before fixation. Upper figure shows that the ratio between the villus height and the crypt depth is about 1:0. (*H&E × 40.*)

ENDEMIC BLADDER STONE DISEASE

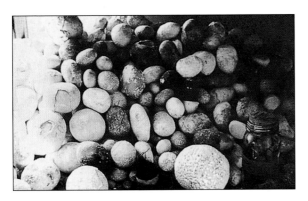

1100 Collection of bladder stones
Bladder stones are very common in children in Thailand, Indonesia and the Middle East. The aetiological factors involved include a low milk–high cereal diet, low urinary volume, high ambient temperature, ingestion of certain local vegetables and ingestion of leaves of forest plants that have a high oxalate content.

PODOCONIOSIS

1101 Advanced podoconiosis in an Ethiopian

Podoconiosis ('non-filarial elephantiasis') is a debilitating condition caused by the passage of microparticles of silica and alumino-silicates through the skin of bare footed people who walk in terrain with a high content of red laterite of volcanic origin. It is especially prevalent in certain highland areas of Ethiopia and other African countries, but has also been recorded in other continents where such soils occur (such as the high plateau of central Brazil). The cytotoxic microparticles pass into the lymphatics of the foot and lower leg where they become deposited in macrophages. The destruction of the phagocytes serves as a stimulus for excessive collagen formation, which culminates in local oedema and fibrosis of the dermis and other tissues. In late cases, such as that shown here, a thickened, leathery, verrucose change develops, while obstruction of the regional lymph nodes gives rise to more generalised lymphoedema in the affected limbs. The disease can be prevented and early changes reversed through the use of appropriate footwear.

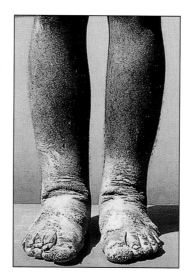

Treatment of later cases may include compression to reduce the lymphoedema and surgical removal of excessive tissue where indicated.

Bibliography

We have found the following references invaluable in preparing this edition. Some of the older textbooks that appeared in earlier editions have been omitted as they are either out of date or difficult to obtain. Although the list is by no means exhaustive, further references will be found in each of these works.

General works

Armstrong D and Cohen J (eds) *Infectious Diseases. 2 Vols.* Mosby: London, Philadelphia, St Louis, Sydney, Tokyo.

Ash LR and Orihel TC (1997) *Atlas of Human Parasitology. 4th edn.* American Society for Clinical Pathology Press, Chicago.

Binford CH and Connor DH (1976) *Pathology of Tropical and Extraordinary Diseases. 2 Vols.* Armed Forces Institute of Pathology, Washington, DC.

Caramello P (ed) (2000) *Atlas of Medical Parasitology – a Project for the Year 2000.* Infectious Diseases Clinic: University of Torino and Carlo Denegri Foundation Torino. Available electronically from www.cdfound.to.it.

Centers for Disease Control (1994 onwards) *Emerging Infectious Diseases.* Bimonthly journal available from CDC/NCID/MS, Atlanta and electronically from www.cdc.gov/eid.

Cheesbrough M (1987) *Medical Laboratory Manual for Tropical Countries, 2nd edn.* Tropical Health Technology and Butterworths: London, Boston, Durban, Singapore, Sydney, Toronto, Wellington.

Cook GC (ed) (1996) *Manson's Tropical Diseases, 20th edn.* Saunders: London, Philadelphia, Toronto, Sydney, Tokyo.

Cox FEG (ed) (1996) *The Wellcome Trust Illustrated History of Tropical Diseases.* Wellcome Trust: London.

Cox FEG, Kreier JP and Wakelin D (eds) (1998) *Topley and Wilson's Microbiology and Microbial Infections, 9th edn. Vol. 5. Parasitology.* Arnold: London, Sydney, Auckland.

Farrar WE, Wood MJ, Innes JA and Tubbs H (1992) *Infectious Diseases: Text and Color Atlas, 2nd edn.* Gower Medical: London, New York.

Forbes CD and Jackson WF (1993) *A Colour Atlas and Text of Clinical Medicine.* Wolfe: London.

Gilles HM (ed) (1999) *Protozoal Diseases.* Arnold: London, Sydney, Auckland.

Guerrant RL, Walker DH and Weller PF (eds) (1999) *Tropical Infectious Diseases. Principles, Pathogens and Practice.* Churchill Livingstone: Philadelphia, London, Toronto, Montreal, Sydney, Tokyo, Edinburgh.

Gutierrez Y (1990) *Diagnostic Pathology of Parasitic Infections with Clinical Correlations.* Lea and Febiger: Philadelphia, London.

Hendrickse RG, Barr DGD and Matthews TS (eds) (1991) *Paediatrics in the Tropics.* Blackwell: London, Edinburgh, Boston, Melbourne, Paris, Berlin, Vienna.

Hutt MSR and Burkitt DP (1986) *The Geography of Non-Infectious Disease.* Oxford University Press: Oxford, New York, Tokyo.

Kean BH, Sun T and Ellsworth RM (1991) *Color Atlas/Text of Ophthalmic Parasitology.* Igaku-Shoin Medical: New York.

Lang W (ed) (1993) *Tropenmedizin in Klinik und Praxis.* Georg Thieme Verlag: Stuttgart, New York.

Mandell GL, Douglas RG and Bennett JE (eds) (2000) *Principles and Practice of Infectious Diseases, 5th edn.* Churchill Livingstone: New York, Edinburgh, London, Melbourne.

Marcial-Rojas RA (1971) *Pathology of Protozoal and Helminthic Diseases with Clinical Correlations.* Williams and Wilkins: Baltimore.

Mims CA (1998) *Medical Microbiology, 2nd edn.* Mosby-Wolfe: London.

Muller R (1975) *Worms and Disease. A Manual of Medical Helminthology.* William Heinemann Medical: London.

Spicer WJ (2000) *An Illustrated Colour Text of Clinical Bacteriology, Mycology and Parasitology*. Churchill Livingstone: Edinburgh, London, New York, Philadelphia, St Louis, Sydney, Toronto.

Stanfield P, Brueton M, Chan M, Parkin M and Waterston T (eds) (1991) *Diseases of Children in the Subtropics and Tropics 4th edn.* Arnold: London, Melbourne, Auckland.

Strickland GT (ed) (2000) *Hunter's Tropical Medicine and Emerging Infectious Diseases, 8th edn.* Saunders: Philadelphia, London, Toronto, Montreal, Sydney, Tokyo.

UNAIDS (2000) *Report on the Global HIV/AIDS Epidemic June 2000.* UNAIDS: Geneva.

Warren KS (ed) (1993) *Immunology and Molecular Biology of Parasitic Infections, 3rd edn.* Blackwell: Oxford, London, Edinburgh, Melbourne, Paris, Berlin, Vienna.

Chapter 1

Birtles RJ, Harrison TG and Taylor AG (1993) Cat scratch disease and bacillary angiomatosis: aetiological agents and the link with AIDS. *Communicable Disease Report* **3**, review 8, R108–110.

Curtis CF (ed) (1991) *Control of Disease Vectors in the Community.* Wolfe: London.

Danis M and Mouchet J (eds) (1992) *Paludisme.* Ellipses: Paris.

Dumler JS, Dawson JE and Walker DH (1993) Human ehrlichiosis: hematopathology and immunohistologic detection of *Ehrlichia chaffeensis*. *Human Pathology* **24**, 391–396.

Gilles HM and Warrell DA (eds) (1993) *Bruce-Chwatt's Essential Malariology, 3rd edn.* Arnold: London, Boston, Melbourne, Auckland.

Gubler DJ (1998) Dengue and dengue haemorrhagic fever. *Clinical Microbiology Reviews* **11**, 480–496.

Lane RP and Crosskey RW (eds) (1993) *Medical Insects and Arachnids.* Chapman and Hall: London.

Mulligan HW (ed) (1970) *The African Trypanosomiases.* Allen and Unwin: London.

Peters W (1987) *Chemotherapy and Drug Resistance in Malaria, 2nd edn. 2 Vols.* Academic Press: London.

Peters W (1992) *A Colour Atlas of Arthropods in Clinical Medicine.* Wolfe: London.

Peters W and Killick-Kendrick R (eds) (1987) *The Leishmaniases in Biology and Medicine. 2 vols.* Academic Press: London.

Vainio J and Cutts F (1998) *Yellow Fever.* WHO, Geneva (available from WHO Internet website).

Wernsdorfer WH and McGregor I (1988) *Principles and Practice of Malariology. 2 Vols.* Churchill Livingstone: Edinburgh, London, Melbourne, New York.

World Health Organization (1984) The leishmaniases. *Technical Report Series No. 701.* WHO: Geneva.

World Health Organization (1985) Arthropod-borne and rodent-borne viral diseases. *Technical Report Series No. 719.* WHO: Geneva.

World Health Organization (1985) Viral haemorrhagic fevers. *Technical Report Series No. 721.* WHO: Geneva.

World Health Organization (1989) *Geographical Distribution of Arthropod-Borne Diseases and their Principal Vectors.* WHO Vector Biology and Control Division: Geneva.

World Health Organization (1990) Control of the leishmaniases. *Technical Report Series No. 793.* WHO: Geneva.

World Health Organization (1992) Lymphatic filariasis: the disease and its control. *Technical Report Series No. 821.* WHO: Geneva.

World Health Organization (1995) Onchocerciasis and its control. *Technical Report Series No. 852.* WHO: Geneva.

World Health Organization (1995) Vector control for malaria and other mosquito-borne diseases. *Technical Report Series No. 857.* WHO: Geneva.

World Health Organization (1998) Control and surveillance of African trypanosomiasis. *Technical Report Series No. 881.* WHO: Geneva.

World Health Organization (2000) *Yellow fever.* In: *WHO Report on Global Surveillance of Epidemic-Prone Infectious Diseases WHO/CDS/CSR/ISR/2000.1* WHO: Geneva (available from WHO Internet website).

World Health Organization (2000) *Management of Severe Malaria, 2nd edn.* WHO: Geneva.

World Health Organization (2000) Severe falciparum malaria. *Transactions of the Royal Society of Tropical Medicine and Hygiene*, **94**, supplement 1.

World Health Organization (2000) WHO expert committee on malaria. 20th report. *Technical Report Series No. 892.* WHO: Geneva.

World Health Organization (2000) *Malaria Diagnosis. New Perspectives. Report of a Joint WHO/USAID Informal Consultation 25–27 October 1999.* WHO:

Geneva (document WHO/MAL/2000.1091 available from WHO Internet website).

World Health Organization (2000) *Bench Aids for the Diagnosis of Malaria Infections, 2nd Edn.* WHO: Geneva.

Chapter 2

Crompton DWT, Nesheim MC and Pawlowski ZS (eds) (1985) *Ascaris and its Public Health Significance.* Taylor and Francis: London, Philadelphia.

Prociv P and Croese J (1990) Human eosinophilic enteritis caused by dog hookworm *Ancylostoma caninum. Lancet* **335**, 1299–1302.

Chapter 3

Doumange JP, Mott KE, Cheung C, Villenave D, Chapuis O, Perrin MF and Reaud-Thomas G (1987) *Atlas of the Global Distribution of Schistosomiasis.* CEGET-CNRS, Talence. WHO: Geneva.

Jordan P, Webbe G and Sturrock RF (eds) (1993) *Human Schistosomiasis.* CAB International, Wallingford.

Miyazaki I (1991) *Helminthic Zoonoses.* International Medical Foundation of Japan: Tokyo.

Sen-Hai Y and Mott KE (1994) Epidemiology and morbidity of food-borne intestinal trematode infections. *Tropical Diseases Bulletin* **91**, R126–R150.

World Health Organization (1993) The control of schistosomiasis. *Technical Report Series No. 830.* WHO: Geneva.

World Health Organization (1995) Control of foodborne trematode infections. *Technical Report Series No 849.* WHO: Geneva.

Chapter 4

Canning EU and Hollister WS (1992) Human infections with microsporidia. *Reviews in Medical Microbiology* **3**, 35–42.

Dance DAB (2000) Melioidosis as an emerging global problem. *Acta Tropica* **74**, 115–119.

Evangelopoulos A, Spanakos G, Patsoula E, Vakalis N and Legakis N (2000) A nested, multiplex, PCR assay for the simultaneous detection and differentiation of *Entamoeba histolytica* and *Entamoeba dispar. Annals of Tropical Medicine and Parasitology* **94**, 233–240.

Hopkins DR, Ruiz-Tiben E, Kaiser RL, Agle AN and Withers PC Jr (1993) Dracunculiasis eradication: beginning of the end. *American Journal of Tropical Medicine and Hygiene* **49**, 281–289.

Kammerer WS and Schantz PM (1993) Echinococcal disease. *Infectious Disease Clinics of North America* **7(3)**, 605–618.

Ortega YR, Sterling CR, Gilman RH, Cama VA and Díaz F (1993) *Cyclospora* species—a new protozoan pathogen of humans. *New England Journal of Medicine* **328**, 1308–1312.

Polderman AM and Blotkamp J (1995) *Oesophagostomum* infections in humans. *Parasitology Today* **11**, 441–481.

Wachsmuth IK, Blake PA and Olsvik O (eds) (1994) *Vibrio cholerae and Cholera.* American Society of Microbiologists: Washington.

Xiao L, Morgan UM, Fayer R, Thompson RCA and Lal AA (2000) *Cryptosporidium* systematics and implications for public health. *Parasitology Today* **16**, 287–292.

Zuckerman AJ and Thomas HC (eds) (1998) *Viral Hepatitis. Scientific Basis and Clinical Management, 2nd edn.* Churchill Livingstone: Edinburgh, London, Madrid, Melbourne, New York, Tokyo.

Chapter 5

Ansary MA, Hira SK, Bayley AC, Chintu C and Nyaywa SL (1989) *A Colour Atlas of AIDS in the Tropics.* Wolfe: London.

Arya OP and Hart CA (1998) *Sexually Transmitted Infections and AIDS in the Tropics.* CAB International: Wallingford.

De Cock KM, Soro B, Coulibaly IM and Lucas SB (1992) Tuberculosis and HIV infection in sub-Saharan Africa. *Journal of the American Medical Association* **268**, 1581–1587.

Farthing CF, Brown SE and Staughton RCD (1988) *A Colour Atlas of AIDS and HIV Disease, 2nd edn.* Wolfe: London.

Ioachim HL (1989) *Pathology of AIDS.* Lippincott, Philadelphia and Gower, New York, London.

Lucas SB, Hounnou A, Peacock C, Beaumel A, Djomond G, N'Gbichi JM, Yebove K, Honde M, Dismonde M, Giordano C *et al.* (1993) The mortality and pathology of HIV infection in a West African city. *AIDS* **7**, 1569–1579.

Morse SA, Moreland AA and Thompson SE (1990) *Atlas of Sexually Transmitted Diseases.* Lippincott, Philadelphia and Gower, New York, London.

Schaller KF (ed) (1993) *Colour Atlas of Tropical Dermatology and Venerology.* Springer: Heidelberg.

UNAIDS (2000) *Report on the Global HIV/AIDS Epidemic June 2000*. UNAIDS: Geneva.

Wakefield AE, Peters SE, Banerji S, Bridge PD, Hall GS, Hawksworth DL, Guiver LA, Allen AG and Hopkin JM (1992) *Pneumocystis carinii* shows homology with the ustomycetous red yeast fungi. *Molecular Microbiology* **6**, 1903–1911.

World Health Organization (2000) Leishmania/HIV co-infection. South-western Europe 1990–1998. WHO/LEISH/2000.42. WHO: Geneva.

Chapter 6

Alexander JO'D (1984) *Arthropods and Human Skin*. Springer–Verlag: Berlin, Heidelberg, New York, Tokyo.

Breman JG, Kalisa-Ruti Steniowski MV, Zanotto E, Gromyko AI and Arita I (1980) Monkeypox in man, 1970–79. *Bulletin of the World Health Organization* **58**, 165–182.

Du Vivier A (1991) *Atlas of Infections of the Skin*. Gower: London, New York.

Bücherl W and Buckley EE (1971) *Venomous animals and their venoms. Vol 3. Venomous Invertebrates*. Academic: New York, London, Toronto, Sydney, San Francisco.

Keegan HL (1980) *Scorpions of Medical Importance*. University Press of Mississippi: Jackson.

Lane RP and Crosskey RW (eds) (1993) *Medical Insects and Arachnids*. Chapman and Hall: London.

Peters W (1992) *A Colour Atlas of Arthropods in Clinical Medicine*. Wolfe: London.

Schaller KF (ed) (1993) *Colour Atlas of Tropical Dermatology and Venerology*. Springer: Heidelberg.

Schlossberg D (1999) *Tuberculosis and Non-Tuberculosis Mycobacterial Infections, 4th edn*. W.B. Saunders: Philadelphia.

Visvesvara GS, Schuster FL and Martinez AJ (1993) *Balamuthia mandrillaris*, n.g., n.sp., agent of amebic meningoencephalitis in humans and other animals. *Journal of Eukaryotic Microbiology* **40**, 504–514.

World Health Organization (1994) Chemotherapy of leprosy. *Technical Report Series No. 847*. WHO: Geneva.

World Health Organization (2000) Leprosy—global situation. *Weekly Epidemiological Record* **75**, 226–231.

Zumpt F (1965) *Myiasis in Man and Animals in the Old World*. Butterworths: London.

Chapter 7

Braude AI, Davis CE and Fierer J (eds) (1985) *Infectious Diseases and Medical Microbiology, 2nd edn*. Saunders: Philadelphia.

Gorbach SL, Bartlett JG and Blacklow NR (eds) (1992) *Infectious Diseases*. Saunders: Philadelphia, London, Montreal, Sydney, Tokyo.

Mandell GL, Douglas RG and Bennett JE (eds) (2000) *Principles and Practice of Infectious Diseases, 5th edn*. Churchill Livingstone: New York, Edinburgh, London, Melbourne.

Schlossberg D (1999) *Tuberculosis and Non-Tuberculosis Mycobacterial Infections, 4th edn*. W.B. Saunders: Philadelphia.

Chapter 8

McClaren D (1992) *A Colour Atlas and Text of Diet Related Disorders, 2nd edn*. Wolfe: London.

McClaren DS and Meguid MM (1988) *Nutrition and its Disorders*. Churchill Livingstone: Edinburgh.

Stephenson L (1993) The impact of schistosomiasis on human nutrition. *Parasitology* **107**, S107–123.

Stephenson LS, Latham MC, Adams EJ, Kinoti SN and Pertet A (1993) Weight gain of Kenyan school children infected with hookworm, *Trichuris trichiura* and *Ascaris lumbricoides* is improved following once- or twice-yearly treatment with albendazole. *Journal of Nutrition* **123**, 656–665.

Chapter 9

Bettini S (ed) (1978) *Arthropod Venoms. Handbook of Experimental Pharmacology, Vol. 48*. Springer-Verlag: Berlin, Heidelberg, New York.

Birtles RJ, Harrison TG and Taylor AG (1993) Cat scratch disease and bacillary angiomatosis: aetiological agents and the link with AIDS. *CDR Review*, **3**, review 8, R107–110.

Bösner S (1993) *Das Burkitt-Lymphom. Erforschungsgeschichte und Epidemiologie*. Basilisken-Presse: Marburg.

Habermehl GG (1981) *Venomous Animals and their Toxins*. Springer-Verlag: Berlin, Heidelberg, New York.

Halstead BW, Auerbach PS and Campbell D (1990) *A Colour Atlas of Dangerous Marine Animals*. Wolfe: London.

Lane RP and Crosskey RW (eds) (1993) *Medical Insects and Arachnids*. Chapman and Hall: London.

McKee KT Jr, LeDuc JW and Peters CJ (1991) Hantaviruses. In: *Textbook of Human Virology. Ed. R.B. Belshe*, pp. 615–632. Mosby: St Louis.

Peters CJ (1991) Arenaviruses. In: *Textbook of Human Virology, Ed. R.B. Belshe*, pp. 541–570. Mosby: St Louis.

Price EE (1990) *Podoconiosis. Non-Filarial Elephantiasis*. Oxford University Press: Oxford, New York, Tokyo, Nairobi, Dar es Salaam, Cape Town.

Serjeant GR (1992) *Sickle-Cell Disease, 2nd edn.* Oxford University Press: Oxford.

World Health Organization (1985) Arthropod-borne and rodent-borne viral diseases. *Technical Report Series No. 719*. WHO: Geneva.

World Health Organization (1985) Viral haemorrhagic fevers. *Technical Report Series No. 721*, WHO: Geneva.

Zuckerman AJ and Thomas HC (eds) (1998) *Viral Hepatitis. Scientific Basis and Clinical Management, 2nd edn.* Churchill Livingstone: Edinburgh, London, Madrid, Melbourne, New York, Tokyo.

Index

References in **bold** are to figure and table numbers, those in light type to page numbers of text material. (*See* page xi for List of Tables).